Red Cell Transfusion

CONTEMPORARY HEMATOLOGY

1. Red Cell Transfusion: *A Practical Guide*

edited by *Marion E. Reid* and *Sandra J. Nance,* 1998

Red Cell Transfusion

A Practical Guide

Edited by

Marion E. Reid, PhD

New York Blood Center, NY

and

Sandra J. Nance, MS, MT(ASCP)SBB

American Red Cross Blood Services, Philadelphia, PA

Humana Press **Totowa, New Jersey**

© 1998 Humana Press Inc.
999 Riverview Drive, Suite 208
Totowa, New Jersey 07512

This publication is printed on acid-free paper. ∞
ANSI Z39.48-1984 (American Standards Institute) Permanence of Paper for Printed Library Materials.

Cover design by Patricia F. Cleary.

For additional copies, pricing for bulk purchases, and/or information about other Humana titles, contact Humana at the above address or at any of the following numbers: Tel.: 973-256-1699; Fax: 973-256-8341; E-mail: humana@mindspring.com; Website: http://humanapress.com

Printed in the United States of America. 10 9 8 7 6 5 4 3 2 1

Library of Congress Cataloging in Publication Data

Red cell transfusion: a practical guide / edited by Marion E. Reid and Sandra J. Nance.
       p. cm. -- (Contemporary hematology)
     Includes index.
     ISBN 0-89603-412-7 (alk. paper)
     1. Erythrocytes--Transfusion.   I. Reid, Marion E. II. Nance, Sandra J.   II. Series.
        [DNLM: Erythrocyte Transfusion. WB 356 R311   1998]
    RM171.4.R43   1998
    615'.39--dc21
    DNLM/DLC   97-39691
    for Library of Congress   CIP

Preface

Red Cell Transfusion: A Practical Guide is designed to describe the procedures involved in obtaining, selecting, and transfusing red cells to patients. The chapters are organized to detail the usual circumstances surrounding blood transfusion in a hospital transfusion setting. These chapters are written by transfusion medical experts renowned for their experience and expertise. The tables and flow charts provide a useful and readily available source of information. Throughout the book, the importance of effective communication is emphasized.

As a background review and introduction, Chapter 1 surveys the steps taken to procure donor blood and describes all aspects of its testing, including discussion of restricted blood orders. Chapter 2 gives an overview of immunology with concentration on the immunologic aspects of transfusion medicine. Parts of the chapter deal with the role of antigen-presenting cells, idiotypes, cytokine release, and irradiation effects. Chapter 3 focuses on approaches to and limitation of compatibility testing for red cell products. A discussion of different crossmatch protocols and the identification of alloantibodies is presented.

The ensuing six chapters (4–9) discuss transfusion in a variety of patient groups. Transfusion difficulties in patients with autoantibodies is covered in Chapter 4, with differentiation between benign and clinically significant autoantibodies. Red cell transfusion of immunocompromised and other anemic patients is the topic of Chapter 5. Concentration is given to immunocompromised patients with regard to special products needed, e.g., leukoreduced red cells. Chapter 6 describes protocols for the transfusion of infants with hemolytic disease of the newborn and approaches to the minimization of donor exposures in children. Chapter 7 delves into protocols for transfusion and transplantation of solid organs. Specific examples of transfusion situations are given with clear recommendations from the literature and the author. Stem cell transfusions are the focus of Chapter 8, where a discussion of autogeneic and allogeneic transplantation is given. Other areas of interest treated are the types of cells used for transfusion, i.e., peripheral blood and bone marrow. The particular challenges of massive transfusions are discussed in Chapter 9, where the configurations of blood products, including ABO and D types in massively transfused patients, are covered.

In preparation for the transfusion of red cells, autogeneic cells are often collected, stored, and used. Chapter 10 describes indications for their use, limitations, and alternatives. Chapter 11 discusses the laboratory and clinical criteria that should be considered before ordering a transfusion of red cells.

Chronic transfusion support for patients requiring red cells is a concern for most transfusion services. Chapter 12 describes processes for patient diagnostic groups that frequently require long-term red cell transfusion. Some of the groups discussed include patients with leukemia, thalassemia, sickle cell disease, aplastic anemia, and cancer.

Chapter 13 focuses on the adverse effects of red cell transfusions and their management. The types of transfusion reaction and their treatment are discussed, as well as the products currently recommended for transfusion.

The final chapter reviews topics that are sometimes most thought-provoking to transfusion medicine specialists: blood group antigens, their association with disease, and their differential diagnosis.

Red Cell Transfusion: A Practical Guide, with its expert authors, is intended to become the standard review and reference source in transfusion medicine. Neophytes will find it an important tool in their learning of the many facets of red cell transfusion, while those already adept in the field will find fresh insights and information designed to maximize and extend their current capabilities.

We thank Paul Dolgert for his help and patience during the production of this book. We also acknowledge the medical editing of Jeffrey McCullough, MD, whose in-depth review of the chapters involving medical practice was insightful, thorough, and much appreciated.

Marion E. Reid
Sandra J. Nance

Contents

Contributors

ELLEN M. AREMAN, MS, SBB(ASCP) • *Laboratory Medicine Department, Georgetown University Medical Center, Washington, DC*

BEAT M. FREY, MD • *Immunochemistry Laboratory, New York Blood Center, New York, NY*

DENNIS GOLDFINGER, MD • *Division of Transfusion Medicine, Department of Pathology and Laboratory Medicine, Cedars-Sinai Medical Center, Los Angeles, CA*

NANCY M. HEDDLE, MSC, ART • *Department of Hematology, Coagulation, and Transfusion Medicine, McMaster University Medical Center, Hamilton, Ontario, Canada*

ELAINE K. JETER, MD • *Department of Pathology and Laboratory Medicine, Medical University of South Carolina, Charleston, SC*

KAREN E. KING, MD • *Department of Transfusion Medicine, Johns Hopkins Hospital Blood Bank, Baltimore, MD*

PATRICIA M. KOPKO, MD • *Division of Transfusion Medicine, Department of Pathology and Laboratory Medicine, Cedars-Sinai Medical Center, Los Angeles, CA*

PATRICIA L. KOTULA, MT(ASCP) • *Laboratory Medicine Department, Georgetown University Medical Center, Washington, DC*

SANDRA J. NANCE, MS, MT(ASCP)SBB • *Musser Blood Center, American Red Cross Blood Services, Philadelphia, PA*

PAUL M. NESS, MD • *Department of Transfusion Medicine, Johns Hopkins Hospital Blood Bank, Baltimore, MD*

MARION E. REID, PHD • *Immunochemistry Laboratory, New York Blood Center, New York, NY*

RONALD A. SACHER, MD, FRCP(C) • *Laboratory Medicine Department, Georgetown University Medical Center, Washington, DC*

KATHLEEN SAZAMA, MD, JD • *Department of Pathology and Laboratory Medicine, Allegheny University of the Health Sciences, Philadelphia, PA*

WILLIAM C. SHERWOOD, MD • *Musser Blood Center, American Red Cross Blood Services, Philadelphia, PA*

LESLIE E. SILBERSTEIN, MD • *Blood Bank, Hospital of University of Pennsylvania, Philadelphia, PA*

STEVEN R. SLOAN, MD • *Blood Bank, Hospital of University of Pennsylvania, Philadelphia, PA*

MARY ANN SPIVEY, MHS, MT(ASCP)SBB • *Department of Pathology and Laboratory Medicine, Medical University of South Carolina, Charleston, SC*

RICHARD K. SPENCE, MD • *Department of Surgery, Staten Island University Hospital, Staten Island, NY*

CHRISTOPHER P. STOWELL, MD, PHD • *Blood Transfusion Service, Massachusetts General Hospital, Boston, MA*

DARRELL J. TRIULZI, MD • *Institute for Transfusion Medicine, Pittsburgh, PA*

PEARL T. C. Y. TOY, MD • *Department of Laboratory Medicine, University of California Medical Center, San Francisco, CA*

1

From Donor to Patient

Sandra J. Nance

1. INTRODUCTION

This chapter gives the reader an overview of the relationship between the blood donor and the blood transfusion recipient. The text includes a review of the recruitment, collection, and testing of the donors and their blood. There is a discussion of the red cell components that can be made from the whole blood, including the routinely manufactured products and the boutique products that are becoming the norm. The cycle involved in the transfusion of red cells is discussed, as are patients' needs, testing required for transfusion, patients with problem crossmatches, and the importance of the order of issue of products especially for surgical use. There is a discussion of transfusion alternatives for difficult immunohematologic problems and the use of rare blood. Finally, there is a section that details the importance of communication. Pertinent references and a flow chart (Figs. 1 and 2) are given. The reader is also referred to larger discussions elaborating on the regulations and standards of practice (1–5).

2. RECRUITMENT OF WHOLE BLOOD DONORS

This section is not meant to be a primer on the recruitment of blood donors, but rather a brief discussion of some recruitment issues. It should give the reader an idea of the considerations involved in the procurement of blood for use in transfusion.

2.1. Routine Donor Recruitment

In the normal course of blood distribution, there is sufficient time between the collection and use of the whole blood to allow for the manufacture of products, testing of donor samples, labeling steps, and distribution to the transfusing facility. These steps must be performed with strict adherence to current good manufacturing practices (cGMPs) (6). At the transfusing facility, further testing ensures compatibility of the donor blood with the recipient. An important part of recruitment is tapping into the motivation of blood donors. An interesting report reviewed findings of a survey instrument designed to explore the motivation of longtime donors (7,8). External recognition did not serve as a motive for the committed donor, rather self-image and community service were important to these donors.

From: *Red Cell Transfusion: A Practical Guide*
Edited by: M. E. Reid and S. J. Nance Humana Press Inc., Totowa, NJ

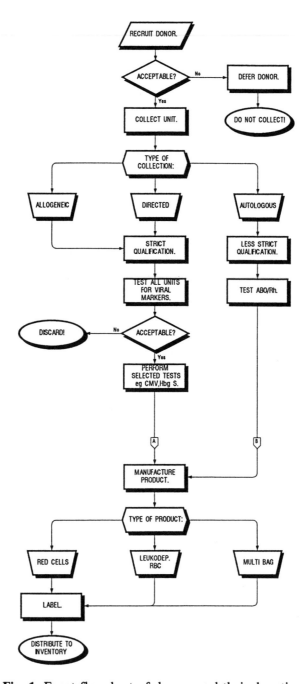

Fig. 1. Event flowchart of donors and their donation.

One of the key elements of any donor recruitment effort is the ability to consistently recruit repeat donors. Although it is optimal in terms of financial outlay of recruitment dollars, it also offers other tangible benefits. One of the biggest benefits is that with control of the recruitment, only donors with previously negative viral marker tests will be recruited and drawn. Another potential benefit of repeat donors is the use of previous antigen typing results to allow inventory management of

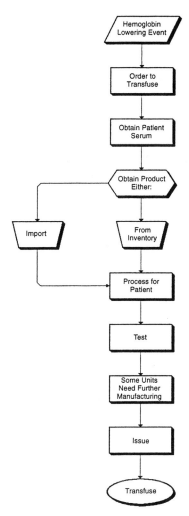

Fig. 2. Event flowchart of transfusion recipients (split from Fig. 1).

phenotyped blood for use in patients with problems obtaining compatible red cell products. A controversial study has reported that paid apheresis donors were no more likely to have positive infectious disease markers than volunteer whole blood donors *(9)*. One drawback to this article, pointed out in the accompanying editorial, was that the paid apheresis donors had previously been whole blood donors, and therefore, may have had a longer previous donor history *(10)*. There are studies that indicate that an incentive as small as a T-shirt can result in increased rates of positive infectious disease markers *(11)*. This report shows that a T-shirt giveaway also resulted in increased rates of medical deferrals, self-deferrals, and donations from previously deferred donors.

2.2. Rare Blood Donor Recruitment

Recruitment of rare blood donors is usually handled in a similar way as routine donor recruitment. Often, there is a need to selectively recruit donors of a certain red-cell antigen phenotype for a specific patient need. Although not a wholesale recruitment, this selected recruitment often yields a better percent return of recruitment efforts. This may be because the recruiter is informed of the details surrounding why the blood is needed, and can use this knowledge in conversations with the donor. The timing of this type of recruitment is critical, for frequently there is a patient need for transfusion of blood from this phenotype only. Another important adjunct to this process is a system in the collecting facility (usually computer-based) that can recognize and hold blood from this rare donor, independent of human intervention, if possible. By using the donor recruitment personnel to recruit rare donors, a consistency in recruitment is maintained, and the donor recruiter and the donor are rewarded for their efforts.

If the blood is not needed immediately, the red cells may be kept in the frozen state for up to 10 yr after collection. This allows the collecting or transfusing facility to store blood for later use. It also facilitates inventory management from a national perspective.

2.3. Restricted Donor Exposure

There are circumstances in which restricted donor exposure is desired. This may be driven by the patient's family or by special programs designed to designate certain donors to a patient. Long-term support of a patient with a restricted number of donors can be performed with the commitment of the donor and adequate advance scheduling of the transfusion. Section 3.4. discusses designated donor processes.

3. COLLECTION

The collection of blood from eligible volunteer donors is a highly regulated procedure. Most often, special needs must be accommodated within the mold of the regulations. Some special collection needs include use of multibag collection devices, leukoreduction filters, directed donations, designated donations, and autogenic donations. These areas are more fully discussed in other chapters (*see* Chapters 5, 6, 10, and 12) of the book. Blood donation is not without some adverse reactions. A 1995 report showed that there is a small but measurable risk of blood donation *(12,13)*.

3.1. Routine Donor Collection

Most of the country's transfusion needs are met by routine whole blood collection. In the past few years, blood collections have not increased greatly. A 1994 report showed that the total supply of blood grew more slowly from 1988 through 1992 than in the years before 1988 *(14)*. The collection of allogeneic blood decreased 0.2% annually and autogeneic collections increased by 23.2% annually. Autogeneic blood accounted for 5.7% of the total 1992 collections.

When a donor has been recruited and presents at the collection site, a medical history and vital signs are taken. Local, state, and federal regulations govern the requirements at the collection site. Many collection facilities can perform a computer check of the donor to ascertain the last collection date and deferral information from the facility's files. Once accepted for donation, appropriate paperwork and labeling is completed and the donor is drawn. A single phlebotomy is usually performed; however, collection by apheresis technology has also been described *(15)*. The activities that follow the collection are important in the preparation of components. It is necessary to know the intended disposition of the whole blood so that appropriate temperature storage requirements are met. Certain time and temperature requirements must be met for blood to be optimally used. In addition to the unit, samples for testing are obtained at the time of the draw. Integral tubing is used to prepare segments that will be used at the transfusing facility for type confirmations and crossmatching.

3.2. Collection into Multibag Containers

The decision to collect into multibag (e.g., quad or quint) containers occurs at the time the donor presents to the collection site. An optimal number of group O collections are desired to be collected into multibag containers to support the transfusion needs of neonates. This requires that the donor be of known ABO type and present a donor card with this information. The containers are more costly, so it is desirable to have minimal wastage owing to positive tests for infectious disease markers. Sterile connection devices can also be used to attach additional bags after donation, but this also comes as an additional cost. However, these devices are very useful to select units for neonatal transfusion if other needs are present (e.g., leukoreduced, antigen negative, and so on). For utilization reasons, group O units are widely used for transfusion to neonates, blood-group-specific units are used less often. Therefore, the optimal multibag donor is one who has been a frequent donor previously, is group O (D positive or, even better, D negative), and has the collection facility's donor card to provide this information at the collection site.

3.3. Directed Donor Collection

Collection of blood in this category requires extreme coordination by the patient, his or her doctor, the selected donors, the collection facility, and the transfusing facility. Optimally, information about the availability of directed donors is provided to the patient by the responsible physician the first time the possibility of transfusion is discussed with the patient *(16,17)*. There are many ways facilities manage directed donors. In the simplest of models, patients are advised of the need for transfusion by their physician. Alternatives to allogeneic transfusion are discussed, and appropriate permission paperwork for the directed donors is obtained. This paperwork contains the patient's name, and the time and location of the prospective transfusion. The prospective directed donors are given the permission paperwork, preferably by the patient. These donors present to the collection site at the appropriate time with the paperwork. Once the unit is collected, it is tested and made available to the transfusing facility. As most readers know, coordinating collection and distribution of directed donations is much more an art than a science. The quagmires that exist are many, including positive viral marker testing, incompatible ABO/Rh types, Cytomegalovirus (CMV) test results, inappropriate collection dates, and the regulation that donors not be collected more frequently than every 56 d. A 1991 study of 1990 data from the American Association of Blood Bank's (AABB) institutional members showed that 3.1% of total donations were directed and 51% of units could be used in allogeneic transfusion *(18)*.

3.3.1. Routine Directed Donors

In the routine setting, sufficient time is given to allow collection, testing, and issue. Generally 3 d are used for these activities, 1 d to collect, 1 d to test, and 1 d to make the blood available to the patient. The most convenient circumstance is that of elective surgery or scheduled transfusion. In these cases, the time and estimated usage is known. The most difficult scheduling is for urgent or fresh blood transfusion.

3.3.2. Urgent Need/Fresh Blood Transfusion

The most extreme case of rapid processing occurs when a "walking donor" is used for collection. There are risk/benefit arguments to this circumstance, but it is a quick way to obtain blood, albeit not tested for infectious disease markers at the time of collection. Alternatively, a rapid processing mechanism for donor units is in place at some testing facilities. In the rapid processing scenario, the blood is collected, tested as soon as it returns to the testing facility, and made available for transfusion within 8 h after collection. The rapid processing scenario has a primary client, the thoracic surgeon convinced of the need for fresh whole blood. These surgeons frequently require a segment of the inventory of predetermined ABO/Rh types to be processed rapidly and made available for transfusion for the operating room. This model has been routinely used in Philadelphia *(19)*. Often though, the rapidly processed bloods used for this scenario are not from directed donors.

3.3.3. Collection Within 56 D of Last Donation

Requests for repeated phlebotomy after an interval < 56 d may be requested by the patient's family to meet the transfusion needs of the patient. These cases should be referred for medical judgment for the donor's protection. If an exception is granted, this must be documented and become part of the donor's record.

3.4. Designated Donor Units

There are two frequent ways that red-cell units are designated to be transfused to patients. Some programs exist to link the chronic transfusion recipient with several donors of known phenotype. Often these protocols are established for patients with sickle-cell anemia, in the hope that alloimmunization to red-cell antigen can be prevented or limited. Several donors willing to participate in the program are selected based on their red-cell phenotype matching the patient's types.

Another way a donor unit becomes designated is in the selection of donor units for neonates to reduce donor exposure. A donor unit, usually containing multiple bags, is assigned to a baby. This unit is commonly used until expiration date or until the contents are used. A report of this process has been published *(20)*.

3.5. Autogeneic Units

The logistics of collecting autogeneic units can be challenging given the characteristics of many autogeneic donors. Blood donated for autogeneic use costs more to prepare than allogeneic units *(21)*. Also, since most facilities do not allow autogeneic units to be used for other patients, the procurement costs are borne by the facility *(22)*. A 1993 study showed that basic costs were $24/unit higher for autogeneic procurement *(23)*. In October 1992, a National Heart, Lung and Blood Institute of the National Institutes of Health conference discussed trends and controversial aspects of autogeneic transfusion *(24)*. The chair of the conference, P. Toy, is the author of Chapter 10.

There is a different set of donor requirements for donation of autogeneic units that are less restrictive than for allogeneic donations *(5)*. If the donor unit tests positive for an infectious disease marker, then special notification and documentation steps are required. Often a positive Hepatitis B or HIV test precludes shipment to the transfusing facility based on their acceptance requirements. There are facilities that do accept such units to maximize the use of the autogeneic program, so procedures must be in place to facilitate the shipment.

Autogeneic donation is highly encouraged for donor/patients who have a rare blood type and who are sensitized to the antigen(s) they lack. Often these donations are stored and frozen for up to 10 yr for use by the donor or other patients with the same alloimmunization problem. Frequently, patients in this situation are asked to contact eligible siblings for donation. In a given nuclear family, there is a one in four chance that a sibling will inherit the same genetic material coding for the absence of a high-frequency antigen matching the patient's type.

Although not truly an autogeneic donation, there are circumstances when maternal blood is used for intrauterine transfusion. Often this is performed in a case of maternal sensitization to a paternal antigen. The procedure is dependent on the mother being an acceptable donor and her health permitting the collection. These collections are often frozen in aliquots (frequently three) to allow multiple intrauterine transfusion events.

4. TESTING

A series of tests on the blood from donors is mandated and/or recommended by various agencies. For the purposes of this section, the text is divided into two categories or tests performed on all donor blood (nonviral and viral) and one for tests done on selected donor bloods. The nonviral tests are discussed first.

4.1. Nonviral Tests

4.1.1. ABO/Rh

ABO/Rh testing is performed on all donor samples. The vast majority of donors are clearly typed by automated or manual methods. Infrequently, weakened expressions of antigens, or weakened or unexpected antibodies interfere with the determination of type. In these cases, further testing is required to resolve the type. The outcome is usually a subgroup of A or a weakly reactive anti-A or anti-B. Most often these typing discrepancies can be easily resolved by serologic methods designed to determine type. The cost is relatively low if the facility has the means to use the blood, once typed, for transfusion. If the typing cannot be easily reconfirmed by the transfusing facility (if different than the collecting facility), then the transfusing facility cannot make use of these units. The best outcome so as not to waste these otherwise acceptable units, is when the transfusing facility is the collecting facility and can rely on facility records to use the unit. Donor centers are also frequently able to use such units in cases in which they provide crossmatched units for transfusion.

The use of monoclonal antibody-derived products for routine typing has shown variant results in testing the blood of some donors, when compared to results obtained using human source reagents. As long as human source reagent is available, it can be used to resolve discrepancies between current type determined by monoclonal source reagents and historic type determined by human source reagent. Decisions to change the ABO/Rh record of a donor based solely on the typing obtained with monoclonal reagents should not be hastily made.

4.1.2. Antibody Screen

Antibody screening tests performed on the blood of donors have fewer restrictions than antibody screens performed on the blood of patients. Donor samples may be tested using pooled reagent red cells or using pooled sera. Often, units are tested using a technique that includes a 37 °C incubation read only at the antihuman globulin phase of testing. For these reasons, samples from autogeneic donors may yield different results when tested as a donor than when tested as a patient. This can present difficulties and delays at the transfusing facility unless the antibody screen test parameters of the donor testing are quickly realized. This is one of the challenges that faces manufacturers of automated instruments for antibody screen tests.

There are some conversions of antibody screening results that may occur throughout the life cycle of the donor. There should be little concern about changes from historic positive to current negative and vice versa unless erroneous testing is suspected. The only result that should be considered pertinent for the donor unit is the current result.

4.2. Viral Markers

There are a litany of viral tests and donor medical history questions for viral markers required for donor. A chronology table of the steps taken since 1983 to protect the blood supply appeared in a 1992 publication *(25)*. An editorial discussing the newest infectious disease test was discussed in a 1995 editorial *(26)*.

An important repository of donor serum has been established by the Retrovirus Epidemiology Donor Study (REDS) supported by The National Heart, Lung and Blood Institute *(27)*. This repository has the potential to enhance our current knowledge as samples are available for the evaluation of new infectious disease agents or new testing strategies for existing infectious diseases.

Meanwhile, infectious disease tests should be performed as mandated by regulating agencies. As new tests are licensed and recommended for use in donor screening, new challenges face inventory management personnel. The implementation plan established for new testing should include the logistics of inventory switchout if required and testing of stored samples for inventory retrieval (or for rare frozen units of blood). Special consideration should be given to the chronology of testing stored samples and the notification to the transfusing facility and transfusing physicians for the transfusion of these units.

4.3. Selected Testing

Selected numbers of donations are subjected to other tests (e.g., anti-CMV, hemoglobin S, red cell antigen typing, and platelet antigen typing) according to inventory requirements. The reasons for this testing are covered in other chapters of this book according to patient need (Chapters 5–7, 14). Often, these tests are required to retain an inventory of products or for a specific known need. The impetus for use of anti-CMV negative, or hemoglobin S negative blood is generally driven by the ordering practices of the physician or hospital, but may be enhanced in certain patient diagnostic categories, e.g., transplant cases or patients with sickle cell disease *(28–31)*.

The reason for ordering red cell products negative for specific antigens (red cell or platelet) is usually a decision made after consultation with the blood bank. It is important that the inventory management staff have the ability to obtain these products with little delay to allow for optimal patient care. More often than ever before, a delay in product transfusion may result in a longer hospital stay. In these fiscally restrictive times, the shortest time between order and transfusion of product is essential.

There are situations involving extremely rare units that lack high incidence antigens that may require use of alternate blood suppliers. If the inventory management staff cannot obtain a specific unit required for transfusion, consultation with the Rare Donor Registry of the American Red Cross (soon to be the American Rare Donor Program) is necessary. This registry contains a list of donors listed by collecting facility with rare blood types. Prior to a request for a search, the patient's antibody should be confirmed by an accredited reference laboratory. In a time of urgent need, the serologic confirmation can follow the request.

5. COMPONENTS

Red cell products come in a variety of "flavors" according to physician request and patient need. The patient populations requiring various red cell products are quite diverse. Often, products are requested to be leuko-reduced; in some hospitals reduced products are covered in other chapters (*see* Chapters 5–7, 12, and 14) of this book.

Some other varieties of red cells include those listed. With a little imagination, it is easy to see how complex an order could be, dependent on the number of product types needed. Varieties of red cells include:

1. Leuko-reduced.
2. Anti-CMV negative.
3. Hemoglobin S negative.
4. Antigen negative.
5. Less than 5-d old.
6. Multibag.
7. Washed.
8. Frozen-deglycerolized.

6. REQUESTS FOR TRANSFUSION

Transfusion requests differ in the urgency required for treatment of the patient. The routine inpatient use and preadmission testing allow for batching of tests. The stat request for a trauma case, operating room case, or medical emergency case must be filled immediately.

6.1. Routine Inpatient Use

Frequently, the orders for routine inpatient transfusion follow the results of routine morning or evening blood draws. The urgency of the transfusion may lie in the discharge time of the patient. In general, these requests can be batched in large institutions. Batching of tests decreases the cost of performing the test and leads to more productive technologist time. Therefore, for a cost-efficient transfusing facility, test batching is a desired outcome.

6.2. Preadmission Testing

Elective surgery patients are often candidates for preadmission testing. Preadmission testing in some facilities means day of or the eve of the surgical day, whereas in others it can be up to 6 wk before surgery. In the latter facilities, the type and screen is performed, then the serum/plasma is frozen for crossmatching later. Preadmission surgical cases are often easily batched, especially in the hospitals with a long lead time before surgery. The only danger in batching tests received the eve of surgery is the potential of delaying the discovery of a patient with an antibody problem.

6.3. Surgical Use

Use of blood in the surgical suite has a few important rules in identification of recipient and unit. If there is a refrigerator for storage of red cells in the operating room, these rules are also the responsibility of the operating room staff. The standard operating procedures (SOPs) for use of the refrigerator are often jointly written by the blood bank and operating room directors.

If autogeneic, directed, and allogeneic units are available for the patient, the order of issue is of paramount importance. Some blood bank computer systems police the order of issue, but when the blood is stored offsite, these rules are more difficult to enforce.

Off-site storage becomes a daily cooperative endeavor between the blood bank and the operating room staff. The SOPs should address the critical control points for use of this tool, e.g., release of blood to the operating room refrigerator, labeling requirements, access to the refrigerator, order of issue, length of time out of the refrigerator, monitoring of the refrigerator, use in the recovery room, and return of unused units to the blood bank.

6.4. Emergency Red Cell Transfusion

In emergency situations, e.g., trauma or medical emergency, SOPs should clearly dictate the course of action. The recommendations for patient specimen labeling are covered in Chapter 3. In some institutions, coolers packed with multiple units of group O blood for emergency transfusion are ready to be released. This blood has already been tagged with the necessary paperwork, segments have been removed, and it has been packed and stored in the refrigerator. Other institutions may stock group O blood in an offsite trauma refrigerator. The needs for such policies are best addressed jointly by the transfusing department and the blood bank. In a few years, perhaps, emergent needs may be met by a pharmaceutical oxygen carrier, and red cell transfusion with group O blood in the trauma situation may be history.

6.5. Rare Blood

Order for transfusion of rare antigen-negative blood can usually be met if the need is not urgent. If the need is critical (<8 h), then it is essential that dialog among the transfusing facility, patient's physician, and the sending institution be well understood. In some cases, this means mass screening random units, but it can mean retrieving units from frozen inventory, shipping blood from other locations, and in extreme circumstances, shipping blood from other countries. There may be the need to transfuse antigen-positive or antigen-untested units until the rare blood can be obtained at the transfusing facility.

7. COMMUNICATION

At the base of all well-run facilities and blood banks is good communication. In the area of red-cell transfusion, this is particularly important. In small institutions, the blood-bank technologist may have knowledge of a patient with a low red-cell count even before the physician, because he or she performed the test. In larger facilities, the first knowledge may come from a request to draw specimens for type and crossmatch, or by phone, or pneumatic carrier. Whatever the means, it is important to be able to rely on the accuracy of the information. Problem patients, time, and availability issues can cause delays in transfusion. It is necessary to minimize delays as much as possible by effective communication. Some facilities have dedicated telephones, ''hot lines,'' to emergency transfusion departments like the operating room, trauma, or emergency room. Perhaps the most difficult times to ensure effective communications are the off-hours when the usual management team is not on location. Often this is handled by individuals empowered to make decisions that can be located by a pager. Use of a communication network, e-mail, voicemail, logbooks, and bulletin boards have all been used to maintain good communication and to ensure messages are given and received. It is imperative that two-way communication be efficient between the blood bank and the transfusion location as well as blood supplier.

8. SUMMARY

This introductory chapter is intended to be an overview of activities that occur in the course of the provision of blood for transfusion. The reader is referred to the reference list of recent publications for a larger discussion of the subtopic areas.

REFERENCES

1. U.S. Department of Health and Human Services, Food and Drug Administration. *The Code of Federal Regulations,* 21 CFR 600 series, current editor, Washington, DC: U.S. Government Printing Office, 1997.
2. *Standards for Blood Banks and Transfusion Services* (16th ed.). Bethesda, MD: American Association of Blood Banks, 1994.
3. Walker RH, ed. *Technical Manual,* 10th ed. Arlington, VA: American Association of Blood Banks, 1990.
4. Nance ST, ed. *Transfusion Medicine in the 1990s.* Arlington, VA: American Association of Blood Banks, 1990.
5. Nance ST, ed. *Blood Supply: Risks, Perceptions and Prospects for the Future.* Bethesda, MD: American Association of Blood Banks, 1994.
6. Miller WV. Controversies in transfusion medicine, blood banks should use good manufacturing practices and the pharmaceutical manufacturing approach. *Transfusion* 1993;33:435–438.
7. Royse D, Doochin KE. Multi-gallon blood donors: who are they? *Transfusion* 1995; 35:826–831.
8. Gardner WL, Cacioppo JT. Multi-gallon blood donors: why do they give? (Editorial) *Transfusion* 1995;35:79–798.

9. Strauss RG, Ludwig GA, Smith MV, et al. Concurrent comparison of the safety of paid cytapheresis and volunteer whole blood donors. *Transfusion* 1994;34:116–121.

10. Huestis DW, Taswell HF. Donors and dollars (Editorial). *Transfusion* 1994;34:96–97.

11. Read EJ, Herron RM, Hughes DM. Effect of nonmonetary incentives on safety of blood donations. *Transfusion* 1993;33(Suppl.):45S.

12. Popovsky MA, Whitaker B, Arnold NL. Severe outcomes of allogeneic and autologous blood donation: frequency and characterization. *Transfusion* 1995;35:734–737.

13. Scott EP. The safety of blood donation—is it what it should be? (Editorial). *Transfusion* 1995;35:717,718.

14. Forbes JM, Laurie ML. Blood collections by community blood centers, 1988 through 1992. *Transfusion* 1994;34:392–395.

15. Meyer D, Bolgiano DC, Sayers M, Price T, Benson D, Slichter SJ. Red cell collection by apheresis technology. *Transfusion* 1993;33:819–824.

16. Oberman HA. The patient's decision to receive a blood transfusion (Editorial). *Transfusion* 1993;33:540–541.

17. Eisenstaedt RS, Glanz K, Smith DG, Derstine T. Informed consent for blood transfusion: a regional hospital survey. *Transfusion* 1993;33:558–561.

18. Devine P, Linden JV, Hoffstadter LK, Postoway N, Hines D. Blood donor-apheresis-, and transfusion-related activities: results of the 1991 American Association of Blood Banks Institutional membership questionnaire. *Transfusion* 1993;33:779–782.

19. Manno CS, Hedberg KW, Kim HC, et al. Comparison of the hemostatic effects of fresh whole blood, stored whole blood and components after open heart surgery in children. *Blood* 1991;77:930–936.

20. Wang-Rodriquez J, Mannino FL, Liu E, Lane TA. A novel strategy to limit blood donor exposure and blood waste in multiply transfused premature infants. *Transfusion* 1996;36:64–70.

21. Forbes JM, Anderson MD, Anderson GF, Bleecker GC, Ross EC, Moss GS. Blood transfusion costs: a multicenter study. *Transfusion* 1991;31:318–323.

22. Renner SW, Howanitz PJ, Bachner P. Preoperative autologous blood donation in 612 hospitals. A College of American Pathologists' Q-Probes study of quality issues in transfusion practice. *Arch Pathol Lab Med* 1992; 116:613–619.

23. Birkmeyer JD, Goodnough LT, Aubuchon JP, Noordsij PG, Littenberg B. The cost effectiveness of pre-operative autologous blood donation for total hip and knee replacement. *Transfusion* 1993;33:544–551.

24. Conference Report, National Heart, Lung and Blood Institute Autologous Transfusion Symposium Working Group. Autologous transfusion; current trends and research issues. *Transfusion* 1995;35:525–531.

25. Zuck TF. The case of Arthur Ashe: that was then, this is now. *J Natl Inst Health Res* 1992;4:94–101.

26. Busch MP, Alter HJ. Will human immunodeficiency virus P24 antigen screening increase the safety of the blood supply and, if so, at what cost? (Editorial) *Transfusion* 1995;35:536–539.

27. Zuck TF, Thomson RA, Schreiber GB, et al. The Retrovirus Epidemiology Donor Study (REDS): rationale and methods. *Transfusion* 1995;35:944–951.

28. Vichinsky EP, Earles A, Johnson RA, et al. Alloimmunization in sickle cell anemia and transfusion of racially unmatched blood. *N Engl J Med* 1990;3221:1617–1621.

29. Tahhan HR, Holbrook CT, Braddy LR, Brewer LD, Christie JD. Antigen matched donor blood in the transfusion management of patients with sickle cell disease. *Transfusion* 1994;34:562–569.

30. Ness PM. To match or not to match: the question for chronically transfused patients with sickle cell anemia (Editorial). *Transfusion* 1994;34:558–560.

31. Rosse WF, Gallagher D, Kinney TR, et al. Transfusion and alloimmunization in sickle cell disease. The Cooperative Study of Sickle Cell Disease. *Blood* 1990;76:1431–1437.

2

Overview of Immunology

Nancy M. Heddle

1. INTRODUCTION

The immune response is a highly evolved system that can recognize foreign material or pathogens that invade the body, and can initiate a sequence of events to eliminate these invaders. Fortunately, this process usually occurs with minimal or no long-lasting morbidity to the host.

There are many components to the immune system that work in a delicate balance to ensure that foreign bacteria, viruses, and abnormal (malignant) cells produced within the body are destroyed, thereby maintaining a state of health. Sometimes, this delicate balance is disrupted. Overactivity of the immune system can result in allergies, or autoimmune diseases in which the body attacks its own tissue. Under-activity, which can be caused by viruses, drugs, or malnutrition, leave the host susceptible to a wide range of infectious agents. The components of the immune system are extremely complex; however, in this chapter an attempt has been made to provide a simplistic overview of both the cellular and soluble components of the immune system, including their structure and how they interact and function to maintain a state of health. Specific examples of some issues encountered in the practice of transfusion have also been discussed.

2. TERMINOLOGY

It is important to understand some of the terminology that will be used to describe the cellular and soluble components of the immune system. For this reason, the cluster of differentiation (CD) nomenclature, the immunoglobulin supergene family, and the major histocompatibility complex (MHC) are briefly described at the beginning of this chapter.

2.1. CD Nomenclature

The CD nomenclature is used to describe specific markers found on the surface of various components of the immune system. The nomenclature originated when human leukocytes were injected into mice, resulting in the formation of antibodies specific for cell surface markers on the leukocyte surface. This finding resulted in the production of many different antibodies that were specific for these markers

From: *Red Cell Transfusion: A Practical Guide*
Edited by: M. E. Reid and S. J. Nance Humana Press Inc., Totowa, NJ

using monoclonal technology. Certain groups, or "clusters" of monoclonal antibodies (MAbs) appear to recognize the same surface molecule, and have been given the same CD number. There are over 120 different CD markers that have been described on hemopoietic cells using these antibodies. Many of these CD markers are important receptors that facilitate the intercell communication required to maintain a functional immune system *(1)*.

2.2. The Immunoglobulin Supergene Family

Foreign antigen recognition is critical to the effective functioning of the immune system and is accomplished through "receptors" that are expressed on lymphoid cells, and are found in a soluble form. Many of these receptors have been characterized at both the structural and molecular levels and it is obvious that they share similar structural and genetic features. The similarities are so striking that it has been postulated that the receptors arose from a common ancestral gene. Because the basic structure of these receptors is modeled on the immunoglobulin domains, the receptors (and their genes) are classified as members of the immunoglobulin supergene family. Some of the antigen receptors included in this family are: antibody/immunoglobulin; MHC class I and class II molecules; and the T-cell receptor (TCR). There are many other family members, including: receptors that bind to the constant domains of the immunoglobulin molecule; receptors for growth factors, cytokines, viruses, and tumor cell antigens; neural receptors; and molecules that regulate lymphocyte function. In total, there are several hundred members of the supergene family that are involved with recognition and interaction events between cells *(2)*.

2.3. The Major Histocompatibility Complex

The MHC consists of the genetic loci involved in the rejection of foreign tissue. The MHC in humans is also known as the human leukocyte antigen (HLA) system *(3)*. There are three classes of MHC molecules known as class I, II, and III. The genes that code for these molecules are located on the short arm of chromosome 6.

2.3.1. MHC Class I Molecules

There are three major class I loci (A,B,C). Within each loci there are many different alleles: at least 26 alleles for the A locus, 35 for the B locus, and 14 for the C locus. As each individual inherits two A, B, and C loci genes, a maximum of six different MHC class I genes can be inherited. This, in turn, results in a maximum of six different versions of the MHC class I molecules that can be expressed on an individual's cells. Recently, several other class I genes have been identified (E, F, G); however, their exact function is not well understood *(4)*.

MHC class I molecules are present on almost all body cells. They are comprised of a glycosylated heavy chain (45 kDa) and a smaller polypeptide (12 kDa) called β_2-microglobulin (Fig. 1). The heavy chain has three extra cellular domains called α_1, α_2, and α_3, a transmembrane region, and a cytoplasmic tail. The α_1 and α_2 domains form the antigen binding groove within the molecule. Their structure consists of eight parallel β strands forming a platform that supports two α helices *(5)*. The long groove that exists between the two α helices is the binding site for antigen peptides that have been processed by the cell. This groove can accommodate peptides that are approx 10–12 amino acids long. The shape of the binding site varies depending

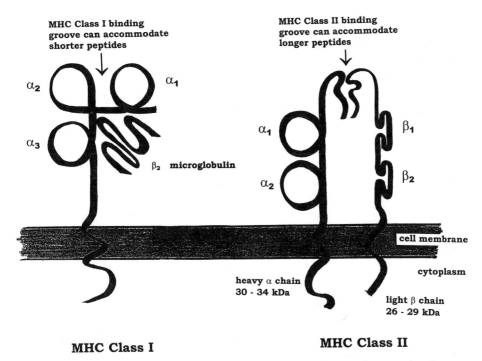

MHC Class I binding groove can accommodate shorter peptides

MHC Class II binding groove can accommodate longer peptides

α_2

α_1

α_3

α_1

β_1

β_2 **microglobulin**

α_2

β_2

cell membrane

cytoplasm

heavy α chain 30 - 34 kDa

light β chain 26 - 29 kDa

MHC Class I

MHC Class II

Fig. 1. Illustration of the MHC class I and class II antigens. These molecules present foreign and self peptides to T-cells. T-helper cells (CD4 +) recognize class II MHC structures; whereas T-cytotoxic cells (CD8 +) recognize class I MHC molecules.

on the different amino acid sequences encoded by the various alleles at the A, B, and C loci. The α_3 domain is homologous to the constant (C) domain on the immunoglobulin molecule, which is discussed in Section 3.1. *(4)*. The structure of β_2-microglobulin is identical in all individuals and is similar to the C domain on the immunoglobulin molecule. β_2-microglobulin is required for class I MHC molecules to be expressed on the cell surface.

2.3.2. MHC Class II Molecules

There are three major class II gene loci termed DR, DQ, and DP. Like the class I genes, there are numerous alleles for each of the three loci: 43 different alleles at the DR locus, 31 for DQ, and 23 for DP. These genes code for a heterodimic glycoprotein structure consisting of an α heavy chain (30–34 kDa) and a β light chain (26–29 kDa). The structures of the two chains are similar, each having an extracellular portion with two domains (α_1 and α_2, β_1 and β_2), a short transmembrane region and a cytoplasmic tail (Fig. 1) *(4)*.

Like the immunoglobulin molecule (Section 3.1.), the α_2 and β_2 domains are constant, whereas the α_1 and β_1 domains have a diverse structure. Class II molecules appear only on certain types of cells involved in the immune response such as macrophages, B-lymphocytes, and some activated T-cells. The antigen-binding groove created by the diversity of the α_1, and β_1 domains is similar in structure to the class I molecules. However, the groove is more open; thus allowing for longer peptides (15–20 amino acids long) to be bound *(4)*.

2.3.3. *Formation of Class I and II MHC Molecules*

The class I and class II MHC molecules are synthesized in the endoplasmic reticulum of the cell. Once produced, the binding groove on the molecule attaches to small peptides that have been degraded inside the cell. When a cell is healthy, all of the degraded peptides will be "self." When a cell is infected with a foreign agent or is a phagocytic cell that has engulfed foreign particles, some of the peptides that bind to the MHC molecules will be foreign. The peptides that are bound by class I and class II molecules originate in different places within the cell. The peptides that bind to class I molecules originate from proteins in the cytosolic compartment of the cell. Proteins in the cytosolic compartment can be self proteins which are digested as part of the natural process of cell renewal, or may be foreign proteins from viruses, or microbes that have invaded and replicated in the cell. As the class I molecules are formed, they fold around one of these peptide fragments and the entire complex is transported to the cell surface where it can interact with T-cells *(6)*.

The peptides that are bound by class II molecules are found in vesicles that are sealed off from the cytoplasm by a membrane. These peptides are from proteins on bacteria or other foreign matter that has been internalized into the cell. In the macrophage, internalization occurs through phagocytosis. The internalized material is sealed into vesicles where the foreign matter can be safely degraded without causing harm to the cell. With B-lymphocytes, the entire immunoglobulin receptor that binds to foreign antigen proteins is internalized through a process called endocytosis. When class II molecules are synthesized in the endoplasmic reticulum, their peptide binding groove is held in check by a special chain of amino acids termed the invariant chain. As the class II molecules move to the vesicles, the invariant chain is removed, allowing the MHC class II molecules to bind peptides and hold them within their goove. The peptide-class II complex is transported to the cell surface where it can be recognized by T-cells (Section 4.1.2.) *(6)*.

2.3.4. *MHC Class III Molecules*

There is a diverse collection of approx 20 genes in the class III region of the MHC. Some of these genes code for proteins in the complement system and others are involved in antigen processing *(4)*.

3. SOLUBLE COMPONENTS OF THE IMMUNE SYSTEM

3.1. *Immunoglobulins*

Immunoglobulins are proteins that are expressed on the surface of B-cells. These proteins can also be secreted by B-cells following cell stimulation. These soluble forms of the immunoglobulin molecule are termed antibodies. The development and function of immunoglobulins is discussed in the section on B-lymphocytes (Section 4.1.1.); however, the structure of the immunoglobulin molecule is presented now, as the basic elements of its structure are shared by all members of the immunoglobulin supergene family.

All immunoglobulin molecules are similar, consisting of two identical light chains and two identical heavy chains. The light chains, consisting of approx 212 amino acids, have a molecular weight of 25 kDa, and exist as two distinct types—kappa (ϰ) and lambda (λ). Within one immunoglobulin molecule, the two light chains are always the same type. The heavy chain, comprised of 450 amino acids, has a molecular weight of 50–77 kDa and can be categorized into five different classes (isotypes): mu (μ), gamma (γ), alpha (α), delta (δ), and epsilon (ϵ). The two heavy chains of an immunoglobulin molecule are always identical. The heavy and light chains are held together by disulphide bonds. On each light and heavy chain, there are regions where the polypeptide chains are looped, forming globular structures called domains. Each light chain has two domains. The amino acid sequence in the constant light-chain domain (C_L) is similar in all $\varkappa$ or λ chains; whereas the structure of the variable light-chain domain (V_L) is extremely diverse. The heavy chains have four domains: a variable region (V_H) which has a diverse structure; and three constant domains termed C_H1, C_H2, and C_H3, which have minimal variability between immunoglobulin molecules (Fig. 2). The constant domains of a specific isotype of Ig may show slight amino acid variability from one individual to another. The epitopes expressed as a result of these amino acid substitutions result in allotypic variation. The amino acid variations in the variable regions of Ig are much more diverse and determine the binding specificity of the Ig. The epitopes expressed in this region are termed "idiotypes" *(4)*.

The variable region (V_H and V_L) of the heavy and light chains allow the immunoglobulin to function as an antigen-binding receptor. The hinge area between the C_H1 and C_H2 domains ensures that the molecule has flexibility, allowing the two antigen-binding receptors to operate independently. A number of different biological functions are associated with the constant heavy-chain domains: macrophage binding; placental transfer, and complement activation.

The immunoglobulin molecule can be cleaved into fragments using proteolytic enzymes. The enzyme papain generates two antigen binding fragments (Fab) and one fragment that is crystalizable (Fc) from each immunoglobulin molecule. Other enzymes such as pepsin, produce a larger fragment containing both antigen binding sites [F(ab')$_2$]. This property of proteolytic cleavage has both experimental and therapeutic applications *(4)*.

3.1.1. Immunoglobulin Isotypes

The heavy-chain composition of the constant region of the molecule will determine the immunoglobulin class: IgG (γ chains), IgM (μ chains), IgA (α chains), IgD (δ chains), or IgE (ϵ chains) *(4)*.

3.1.1.1. IgG

IgG is the most abundant immunoglobulin, accounting for approx 75% of the total immunoglobulin concentration in human serum. There are four subclasses of IgG (IgG1, IgG2, IgG3, and IgG4), each having slight structural differences in the γ heavy chain. Individuals have all four subclasses. IgG is distributed equally in the intravascular and extravascular compartments and is the major class of Ig produced during a secondary immune response *(4)*.

3.1.1.2. IgM

IgM makes up approx 10% of the immunoglobulin pool. It has a pentameric structure consisting of five immunoglobulin subunits held together by a joining chain (J chain) and disulphide bonds. IgM is produced primarily during the initial immune response and is found in the intravascular compartment *(4)*.

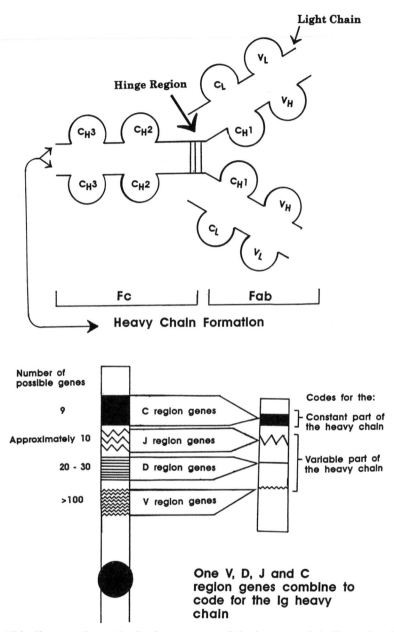

Fig. 2. This diagram shows the basic structure of the immunoglobulin molecule and the heavy-chain gene recombination that takes place in the B-cell during development. Similar light-chain gene recombination also occurs; however, only three gene segments are involved (V, J, and C). This shuffling process creates over a million different possible combinations.

3.1.1.3. IgA

IgA, representing 15–20% of the total Ig pool, can exist as a monomer, but usually occurs as a dimer (two Ig subunits). IgA is found in secretions such as colostrum, milk, and saliva, and is also found in tracheobronchial and genitourinary secretions. There are two IgA subclasses: IgA1, which predominates in serum; and IgA2, located primarily in secretions. The two Ig subunits of IgA are also connected by a J chain. Another protein termed a secretory component binds to the molecule to facilitate its transport across epithelial cell layers into secretions *(4)*.

3.1.1.4. IgD

IgD makes up < 1% of the serum Ig, but is abundant on the surface of naive B-lymphocytes as an antigen receptor. Its monomeric structure is susceptible to proteolysis as there is only one disulphide bond connecting the heavy (δ) chains. The function of IgD is unknown, but it may be important in lymphocyte differentiation, which is triggered by antigen binding *(4)*.

3.1.1.5. IgE

The monomeric structure of IgE is found predominantly on the surface of basophils and mast cells. IgE may be an important defense mechanism for helminthic parasites, but is more commonly recognized for its role in allergic reactions *(4)*.

3.2. Cytokines

Cytokines are low molecular weight proteins that are produced by a variety of cells. Their functions include important biological processes such as cell growth, cell activation, immunity, tissue repair, inflammation, fibrosis, and morphogenesis. Some cytokines also have chemotactic ability and are called chemokines. Over 80 different cytokines have been described. Each cytokine can have several different functions, depending on the type of cell to which it binds. Binding occurs when a cell expresses a specific receptor for a cytokine. This cytokine–receptor interaction sends a signal into the cell, which will activate specific genes and change the cell's activity. Some of the cytokines involved in immune functions are summarized in Table 1 *(2,4)*.

3.3. Complement

The complement system consists of at least 20 proteins that act in sequence to bring about or facilitate the destruction of foreign or malignant cells. There are two main pathways by which complement can be activated: the classical pathway and the alternative pathway. They differ in the initiation of complement activation but merge as a common pathway.

3.3.1. The Classical Pathway

Complement activation by the classical pathway is initiated by immune complexes, or cellbound IgG and/or IgM (Fig. 3). The initial step in the pathway occurs when two or more of the globular domains of the C1q molecule binds to the C_H2 domain on IgG molecules or the C_H3 domains of a single IgM. This binding leads to conformational changes in the C1 complex, causing activation of the two $\overline{C1r}$ molecules, which then cleave the two C1s molecules resulting in activated $\overline{C1s}$ (a strong serine esterase). This complex ($\overline{C1s}$) cleaves C4 into two fragments: C4a, which has weak anaphylatoxic activity, and a larger fragment C4b. Most of the C4b generated is inactivated; however, the C4 that binds to the cell membrane acts as a binding site for C2. The bound C2 is also cleaved by $\overline{C1s}$, releasing a fragment called C2b. The remaining C2a segment is bound to C4b forming $\overline{C4b2a}$ which is also known as C3 convertase. The C3 convertase cleaves C3, releasing the small C3a fragment that has

Table 1
Summary of Major Cytokines Involved in the Immune System,
Their Site of Production, and Function[a]

Cytokine	Site or Product	Primary functions
Interleukins		
IL-1	Many cells (e.g., APC, endothelial cells, B-cells, fibroblasts)	T-cell activation, neutrophil activation, stimulates bone marrow, pyrogenic, acute phase protein synthesis.
IL-2	Activated T_H cells	T-cell growth, chemotaxis, macrophage activation.
IL-4	Activated T_H cells	B-cell activation, B-cell differentiation, T-cell growth, T_H2 differentiation.
IL-6	Many cells (e.g., T-cells, APC, B-cells, fibroblasts, and endothelial cells)	B-cell differentiation, pyrogenic, acute phase protein synthesis.
IL-8	Many cells (e.g., macrophages and endothelial cells)	Inflammation, cell migration/chemotaxis.
IL-10	Activated T_H cells	Suppression of T_H1 cells, inhibits antigen presentation, inhibits cytokine production, (IL-1, IL-6, TNFα, and IFN).
Others		
TNF	Macrophages and lymphocytes	Neutrophil activation, pyrogenic, acute phase protein synthesis.
Interferon γ (IFN-γ)	T-cells	Phagocyte activation.
Transforming growth factor-β (TGF-β)	Various cells	Stimulate connective tissue growth and collagen formation, inhibitory function.
Colony-stimulating factors (GM-CSF, M-CSF, G-CSF)	Various cells	Growth and activation of phagocytic cells.

[a]Abbreviations: APC, antigen-presenting cell; GM-CSF, granulocyte macrophage-colony-stimulating factor; G-CSF, granulocyte-colony-stimulating factor; M-CSF, macrophage-colony-stimulating factor; TNF, tumor necrosis factor.

anaphylatoxic activity, and exposing a binding site on the C3b fragment, which attaches to proteins and sugars on the surface of adjacent cells *(2,4)*.

3.3.2. *The Alternative Pathway*

The alternative pathway of complement activation occurs spontaneously in the plasma at a slow but steady rate. This has been referred to as tickover activation

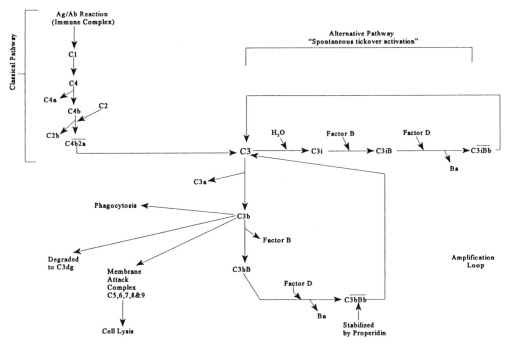

Fig. 3. Diagram illustrating the activation of complement by the classical and alternative pathways.

(Fig. 3). Soluble C3 undergoes spontaneous hydrolysis by water resulting in C3i. The C3i generated acts as a binding site for Factor B, producing C3iB. The Factor B can be cleaved by Factor D, releasing a fragment called Ba. The fluid phase component that remains (C3iBb) is the C3 convertase of the alternative pathway, cleaving the C3 molecule into C3a and C3b. Most of the C3b generated in this fluid phase is inactivated; however, if the C3b binds to a foreign surface such as a bacterial cell wall, an amplification process takes place, accelerating the activation of the complement cascade.

When C3b binds to a cell surface, Factor B is bound to give C3bB. Factor D can also react with this cell-bound substrate, releasing the small Ba fragment leaving cell-bound C3bBb. This complex will dissociate rapidly unless it is stabilized by properdin resulting in the complex C3bBbP. Like the C4b2a complex of the classical pathway, C3bBbP is capable of converting more C3 into C3b. In summary, both the classical and alternative pathways result in C3b generation. The C3 convertase of the classical pathway is C4b2a; whereas, the C3 convertases of the alternative pathway are C3iBb in the fluid phase and C3bBbP when cell bound. The C3 convertases formed create a positive feedback loop that amplifies complement activation *(4)*.

3.3.3. The Common Pathway—Membrane Attack Complex

Once C3b has been cleaved by the convertase of either the classical or alternative pathway, the final phase of activation involving the membrane attack complex can occur. The C5 molecule is bound and cleaved by C3 convertase into two fragments: a small peptide, C5a, which is a potent anaphylatoxin; and a larger fragment, C5b. This C5b fragment binds C6, C7, C8, and up to 14 monomers of C9, resulting in a lytic hole in the membrane. Small amounts of lysis can occur when C8 is bound, but the binding of C9 rapidly facilitates the lytic process and cell death *(4,7)*.

The binding of C3b to a cell membrane is the pivital stage of the pathway. The cell-bound C3b can proceed to activate the membrane attack complex (C5–C9) and cause cell lysis; however, in some situations the inhibitors of the cascade may stop the activation sequence, leaving the cell coated with C3b. The cell-bound C3b is cleaved by Factor I, leaving iC3b on the membrane, which is further cleaved, leaving only C3dg. These three subcomponents of C3 (C3b, iC3b, and C3dg) are opsonins, facilitating the phagocytosis or clearance of the cell. A variety of phagocytic cells have receptors that can bind to C3 subcomponents on the cell. Four different receptors have been identified: CR1, CR2, CR3, and CR4 *(4,7)*.

3.3.4. Complement Receptors

3.3.4.1. CR1 Receptor

The CR1 receptor is found on a variety of cells. On red cells and platelets, the CR1 receptor plays an important role in clearing immune complexes. On phagocytic cells and B-lymphocytes, it is an opsonic receptor that is involved in lymphocyte activation. CR1 also has a regulatory role in protecting self cells from damage to further complement activation by assisting Factor I in cleaving C3b into iC3b and C3dg *(4,7)*.

3.3.4.2. CR2 Receptor

The CR2 receptor is found on B-cells, some epithelial cells, and follicular dendritic cells. It plays an important role in mediating B-cell activation. It is also the receptor for interferon α and the Epstein Barr virus *(4,7)*.

3.3.4.3. CR3 Receptor

CR3 receptors are found on cells of the myeloid lineage. CR3 mediates phagocytosis of particles coated with iC3b and is also an important adhesion molecule capable of binding to certain types of bacteria and yeast *(4,7)*.

3.3.4.4. CR4 Receptor

The CR4 receptor is found on both lymphoid and myeloid cells. Its function is not well characterized but it appears to have opsonic activity for iC3b, and it plays a role in adhesion.

3.3.5. Complement Regulation

The potential for complement to cause cell death through lysis or phagocytosis is tremendous; therefore, it is critical to have a mechanism that ensures that complement-mediated cell destruction is focused on foreign and malignant cells and not the body's self cells and healthy tissue. To accomplish this task, there are several regulatory and inhibitory mechanisms specifically designed to prevent complement from binding to self-cell surfaces or to inhibit complement if this binding occurs (Table 2). The surface of foreign organisms lack some of these regulatory proteins. In addition, the surface of many self cells are coated with acidic sugars such as sialic acid which resist C3b deposition *(4,8)*.

Table 2
Summary of the Inhibitors of Complement Activation

Complement control proteins	Function
C1 inhibitor	A serine proteinase inhibitor that binds and activates C1r and C1s.
Factor I plus C4 binding protein (C4-bp)	Catabolize C4 in the fluid phase.
C4-bp	Causes dissociation of C2a from C4b2a.
Decay accelerating factor	Inhibits the binding of C2 to C4b.
(DAF, CD55)	Causes dissociation of C2 from C4b.
Complement receptor 1 (CR1, CD35)	Accelerates the dissociation of C3bBb.
Membrane cofactor protein	Prompts catabolism of C4b by Factor I and is a cofactor with Factor I to cleave C3b
Factor H	Causes dissociation of Bb from C3i and C3b and is a cofactor to Factor I for catabolism of C3i and C3b.
Factor I	Cleaves and degrades C3b using one of three cofactors: Factor H (plasma), CR1, or MCP (membrane-bound)
S protein (Vitronectin)	Binds to the C5b67 complex preventing insertion into the lipid bilayer.
C8 binding protein (CD59)	This cell-bound protein binds to C8 preventing C9 from inserting into the membrane.
Homologous restriction factor (HRF)	Inhibitor of C9

4. CELLULAR COMPONENTS OF THE IMMUNE SYSTEM

The primary cellular components of the immune system are B-lymphocytes, T-lymphocytes, natural killer (NK) cells, and phagocytotoxic cells. Each of these cells is derived from a single progenitor called a hemopoietic stem cell. Stem cells first appear in the human embryo in the yolk sac, migrate to the liver as the fetus develops, and then move to the bone marrow. Stem cells are found only in the bone marrow after birth. Hemopoietic stem cells are able to repeatedly reproduce themselves; however, some stem cells have limited ability to differentiate (totipotent stem cells). Stem cells that can differentiate into several lineages are termed pluripotent stem cells. An antigen called CD34 is expressed on pluripotent stem cells, thus the CD34 marker is a useful indicator to estimate the number of stem cells that have been collected from a donor when stem cell transplantation is being performed *(9)*.

From the stem cell, all types of blood cells are generated. As illustrated in Fig. 4, the hemopoietic stem cell can give rise to two main lineages: myeloid cells and lymphoid cells. From the myeloid progenitor arises platelets, granulocytes (eosinophils, neutrophils, basophils), mast cells, and macrophages. T- and B-lymphocytes are formed from the lymphoid progenitors. Dendritic cells and NK cells also arise from the hemopoietic stem cell; however, their precise origin is unknown. The rate at which hemopoietic cell replication and differentiation occurs is astounding with

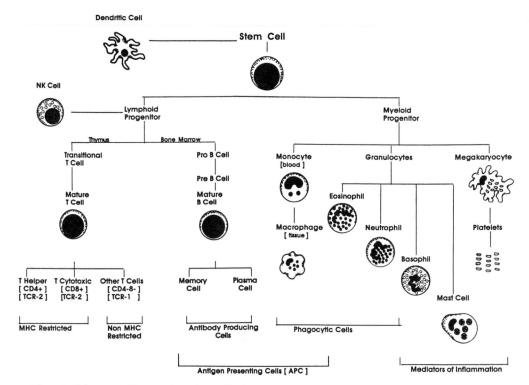

Fig. 4. Diagram illustrating the cells involved in the immune response that originate from the pluripotent stem cells.

3–10 billion red cells, platelets, neutrophils, and lymphocytes produced each hour. The rate of production can increase 10-fold if needed *(9)*.

4.1. Lymphocytes

The stem cell can differentiate into two lineages of lymphocytes: B-cells, which are derived from the bone marrow; and T-cells, which arise in the thymus. The T- and B-cells have distinct differences in structure and function. As a result of this individuality, T- and B-cells have different approaches for responding to foreign invaders. B-cells can recognize a specific epitope on intact antigen. This recognition occurs through the specific antibody receptor on the surface of the B-cell. In contrast, T-cells can recognize only small fragments of antigen proteins (peptides 10–20 amino acids long) that have been processed by antigen-presenting cells and are presented in association with the MHC. These two mechanisms to recognize foreign material complement each other, making the T- and B-lymphocytes perfect partners to fight off foreign invaders *(10)*.

4.1.1. B-Lymphocytes

The lymphoid stem cell in the bone marrow progresses through a number of stages of differentiation before it reaches a mature B-cell. These stages include: the progenitor B-cell (pro-B-cell); pre-B-cell; an immature B-cell; and finally a mature B-cell. Each B-cell in the body is able to recognize one or a limited set of related antigenic epitopes via a receptor on its surface. These receptors are immunoglobulin

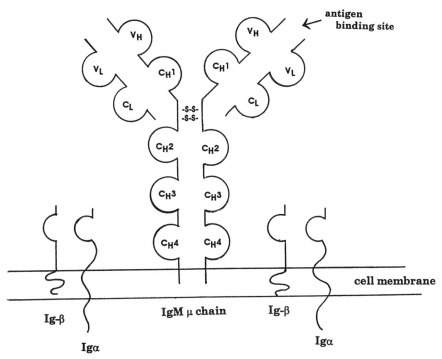

Fig. 5. Illustration of the immunoglobulin receptor found on the surface of B-cells. This receptor has one additional heavy-chain domain compared to secreted antibody, which is required to anchor the molecule to the cell membrane. Several accessory molecules (Ig-α and Ig-β) are closely associated with the receptor and play a role in signal transduction, which results in IL-2 production and cell differentiation.

molecules that have been produced in the B-cell and inserted into the cell by a transmembrane domain. Once the antibody receptor on the B-cell binds to an antigen, the B-cell (with the help of T-cells) can be stimulated to divide and differentiate into a plasma cell that is able to secrete a soluble form of the cell-bound immunoglobulin receptor (antibody) *(4)*.

If each B-cell has receptors with limited specificity, and the body's immune system may be called on to recognize thousands of different foreign antigens over a lifetime, how does our immune system know which specific antigen receptors will be needed? The answer to this question is now understood. It is known that the human genome contains approx 100,000 genes. It is also estimated that 10 trillion B-cells in the body make more than 100 million different antibody proteins. It is obvious from this model that one individual does not inherit enough genes to code for the millions of different foreign proteins that the immune system must be capable of recognizing. Such diversity is achieved through a process called gene rearrangement *(11,12)*.

As discussed in Section 3.1., each immunoglobulin receptor is comprised of two identical heavy chains and two identical light chains. The genes that code for segments of these chains combine to form the entire gene complement necessary for immunoglobulin synthesis by the B-cell. The three genes that contribute to the diversity of the immunoglobulin receptor are termed V (variable), D (diversity), and J (joining). The final C (constant) gene affects the function of the molecule, but not its antigen-binding affinity (Fig. 5) *(11,12)*.

There are four different gene segments coding for the Ig heavy chain: V_H; D_H; J_H; and C_H. The V_H gene codes for a major portion of the variable part of the heavy-chain protein. Several hundred different V_H genes exist, with one being randomly selected for the heavy chain produced by an individual B-cell. The D_H gene provides further diversity to the heavy chain with 20–30 different D_H genes available for random selection. The joining part of the heavy-chain gene (J_H) can be selected from approx six different J genes, and the constant part of the heavy chain (C_H) can be selected from one of nine different possibilities. These nine types include μ, δ, γ_1, γ_2, γ_3, γ_4, ϵ, α_1, and α_2. The selection of one of these C_H segments will determine the isotype of the antibody (e.g., IgM, IgG, IgA, IgE, or IgD). At the pre-B-cell stage, the heavy-chain genes are shuffled and one member from each set of genes (V_H, D_H, J_H, and C_H) are randomly selected. Because of the large number of genes available for selection, the number of possible combinations is greater than 10^4 *(6,11,12)*.

The light-chain gene is comprised of three gene segments V_L (variable), J_L (joining) and C_L (constant), which are selected through a shuffling process similar to the heavy-chain gene. Over a thousand different combinations of light chains could be formed. When the diversity of the heavy- and light-chain genes are combined ($10^4 \times 10^2$), over a million different combinations are possible. Further diversity also occurs through several other mechanisms. During the joining process of each fragment, enzymes add random DNA bases to the ends of the genes being joined, resulting in the formation of new or additional genetic information. Diversity also occurs during the assembly of the heavy and light protein chains that form the immunoglobulin receptor on the B-cell membrane (combinatorial shuffling), and through somatic mutations that occur when the B-cell is activated. Through these mechanisms of shuffling, random selection, and gene rearrangement, each B-cell in the body is able to create and express a different and unique immunoglobulin receptor on its surface. This is the immune system's way of ensuring that there is at least one B-cell in the body specific for any foreign invader *(6,11,12)*.

Each B-cell has approx 10^5 identical surface immunoglobulin receptors on its membrane. Most peripheral blood (naive) B-cells express two immunoglobulin isotypes on their surface IgM (monomers) and IgD. B-cells expressing the IgG, IgA, or IgE isotypes occur in larger numbers in specific locations. For example, B-cells expressing IgA on their surface are concentrated primarily in the intestinal mucosa. In addition to immunoglobulin receptors, there are also other molecules associated with the B-cell receptor that collectively are termed the B-cell antigen receptor complex. There are also a number of CD markers that have been identified on B-cells. CD5 was originally detected only on T-cells; however, it is now known that a subset of B-cells also express this marker. It is believed that this CD5-positive B-cell subset is predisposed to autoantibody production. The components of the B cell antigen receptor complex and their functions are summarized in Table 3 *(4)*.

Because of the random rearrangement of the B-cells genes, some B-cells will produce immunoglobulin receptors that react to the body's own cells. These cells must be eliminated or downregulated or the body would have uncontrolled production of autoantibodies. The mechanism of elimination occurs through a process of negative selection or the induction of anergy.

Table 3
Summary of the Surface Markers
and Receptors on Peripheral Blood B-Cells and Their Function

Receptor/marker	Function/role
IgMα	Transport and assemble IgM monomers in the cell membrane.
Igβ	Accessory molecules that interact with the transmembrane segments of IgM.
MHC class II (DP, DQ, DR)	Play a role in activation of B-cells and are important for cooperative interactions with T-cells.
Complement receptors C3b (CR1, CD35); C3d (CR2, CD21)	Play a role in cell activation and "homing" of cells.
Fe receptors (FcδRII, CD32)	Exogenous receptors for IgG and negative signaling to B-cell.
CD19, 20, and 22	Primary cell markers used to distinguish B-cells.
CD72–78	Other cell markers that identify B-cells.
CD5	Cell marker that identifies a subset of B-cells predisposed to autoantibody production.

4.1.1.1. NEGATIVE SELECTION

This process begins when a newly formed B-cell encounters large quantities of antigen in the body's environment which can bind to the immunoglobulin receptors on the cell's surface. When strong binding occurs, the immunoglobulin receptor sends a signal into the cell, causing it to commit suicide or apoptosis (programmed cell death). Apoptosis occurs because the signals transmitted by the antibody receptors activate enzymes that cleave nuclear DNA. It is estimated that 75% of the B-cells that mature in the bone marrow do not reach the circulation, but undergo apopotosis. B-cells whose receptors do not react strongly to self-antigens are able to survive and mature, creating the B-cell repetroire that can respond to foreign invaders *(13)*.

4.1.1.2. B-CELL ACTIVATION

Mature B-cells migrate from the bone marrow into the peripheral blood where they act as sentries looking for foreign antigen that is specific for their Ig receptor. When the immunoglobulin receptor recognizes and binds to an antigen, a signal occurs, causing the receptor-antigen complex to be internalized. Once in the cell, the antigen is degraded into small peptides that bind to MHC class II molecules. This MHC-peptide complex is transported to the cell membrane where it can interact with a receptor on T-cells (*see* Section 4.1.2.). This interaction stimulates cytokine production that signals the B-cell to proliferate. Proliferation is rapid, with approx 10^4 cells produced within 3–4 d. The newly formed B-cells leave the germinal center of the lymph node either as a memory cells or as plasma cell precursors that eventually differentiate into plasma cells. Antibodies produced by a single plasma cell always have the same specificity and are of the same immunoglobulin class; however, each time proliferation occurs and daughter cells are formed, somatic mutations occur, resulting in slight differences in the binding affinity of the immunoglobulin receptor. Because the Ig receptors with the highest binding affinity will be most likely to interact with antigen and cause more cell proliferation, the cycle will continue with preferential proliferation of cells with the highest affinity for the foreign antigen. This is referred to as a focused immune response *(4,10,14)*.

4.1.1.3. CLASS SWITCHING

Following activation, most B-cells secrete IgM antibodies, the Ig that is characteristic of the primary immune response. At some point, many of these B-cells will switch, making antibodies of a different class. When this switch occurs, the antibody has the same specificity (as it uses the same VDJ genes), but selects a different constant region gene that determines the Ig class isotype. The ability to select a different gene for the constant part of the protein results from a variety of interactions, including repeated antigen stimulation and cytokines produced by helper T-cells *(4)*.

4.1.2. *T-Lymphocytes*

Stem cells in the thymus divide and differentiate into two major types of T-cells: T-helper cells and cytotoxic T-cells. A third type of large granular lymphocytes called natural killer (NK) cells are also produced (*see* Section 4.2.). As the T-cell matures in the thymus, several different events take place. The T-cell's first challenge is to determine if it recognizes self MHC antigens presented by antigen-presenting cells. If the T-cell is able to recognize self MHC antigens as it scans the thymic environment, the T-cell survives. If self MHC antigens are not recognized by the T-cell, it dies. The next challenge during T-cell development is to selectively destroy T-cells that react too well with self MHC antigens. The ultimate goal is to select mature "educated" T-cells with receptors that recognize self MHC molecules without reactivity to self peptides. These T-cells are then ready to react with self MHC molecules that have foreign peptides bound to their groove. This goal is not always achieved, thus a small percentage of T-cells ($< 10\%$) are able to react with nonself (foreign) MHC complexes. The receptor on the T-cell that is involved in the recognition process is called TCR *(4,10,15,16)*.

There are two types of TCR: TCR-1 and TCR-2. TCR-1 is a heterodimer consisting of a γ and α chain that are linked by disulphide bonds. T-lymphocytes that express the TCR-1 receptor comprise 5–15% of T-cells and are found predominantly in the mucosal epithelia. It is believed that T-cells expressing TCR-1 receptors play an important role in protecting the body's mucosal surfaces against foreign bacteria. These cells do not express CD4 or CD8, which are found on T-cells with TCR-2. The TCR-2 has a similar structure, but consists of two heterodimers: α and β. Each chain comprising the TCR has two domains similar to those found on immunoglobulin molecules. One domain is variable, the other is constant. The T-cells that express the TCR-2 receptors can be further subdivided into two populations—those that express the CD4 marker and are termed T-helper cells and those that express the CD8 marker and are called cytotoxic T-cells, since they can cause direct cell death. Antigen recognition by each of these T-cell subsets is different *(4)*.

Both the TCR-1 and TCR-2 receptors are associated with a complex called CD3, which consists of at least five polypeptide chains (Fig. 6). The structure of CD3 is

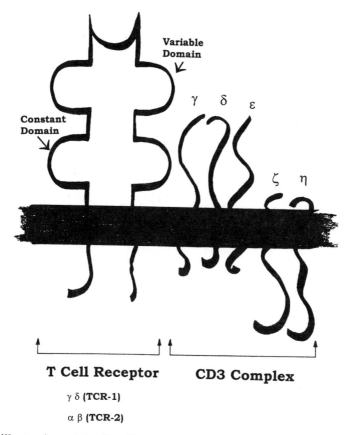

T Cell Receptor　　**CD3 Complex**

γ δ (TCR-1)

α β (TCR-2)

Fig. 6. An illustration of the T-cell receptor (TCR) that is found on T-helper cells and cytotoxic T-cells. The TCR recognizes foreign peptides bound to MHC antigens. It is associated with an accessory molecule called CD3, which is comprised of five polypeptide chains. The CD3 molecule appears to be responsible for signal transduction. The genes that code for the heavy chains that make up the TCR are formed from recombination of gene segments (a process similar to the Ig heavy-chain genes).

identical on all T-cells. Three of the five chains that make up the CD3 molecule (γ, δ, and ε), have a long extracellular domain, a transmembrane region, and a short cytoplasmic tail. The two remaining chains, ζ(zeta) and η(eta), also span the cell membrane but have a short extracellular component and a long cytoplasmic tail. When antigen is recognized by the TCR, the CD3 complex is responsible for signal transduction *(17)*.

4.2.1.1. Recognition by T-Helper Cells

T-helper cells (CD4+) recognize foreign peptides in association with MHC class II structures. As mentioned previously, the peptides bound to MHC class II proteins may come from self or foreign extracellular antigens that have been ingested by a phagocytic cell. The process of recognition requires two signals. The first signal involves an interaction between the TCR-2 and the class II MHC/peptide complex. The CD4 protein also acts as a coreceptor binding to the MHC class II complex. The second signal involves interaction between other surface markers. An example of costimulatory surface markers that can provide this second signal is the interaction of the B7 protein that can be expressed on the surface of B-cells and macrophages binding to CD28 on the cytotoxic T-cell *(14,18)*. When the double signal occurs, the T-cell releases a number of different cytokines such as interleukin (IL)-2 and IL-4 that causes B-cell proliferation and antibody production. Interferon-γ (IFN-γ) is also produced and signals the macrophage to produce tumor necrosis factor (TNFα) and other chemicals that can destroy foreign microbes ingested by the cell *(4)*.

4.2.1.2 RECOGNITION BY CYTOTOXIC T-CELLS

Cytotoxic T-cells (CD8+), recognize foreign peptides in association with MHC class I structures. As discussed previously, the foreign peptides bound to MHC class I complexes come from proteins in the cytosolic compartment of the cell. These may be self proteins, or foreign proteins derived from viruses or microbes that have invaded the cell. The TCR-2 interacts with foreign peptide bound to MHC class I structures. The CD8 protein on the T-cell acts as a coreceptor and also binds to the MHC class I molecule. These interactions send a signal to the cell resulting in the production of perforin and other proteins that disrupt the integrity of the target cell membrane causing cell death. Cytokines, such as interferon-γ and TNFα, that are capable of limiting viral replication are also produced. This mechanism prevents replication of intracellular virus that may be shed during cell death; thereby stopping the infective process. Although this is an effective mechanism of killing virally infected cells, it has the potential to cause extensive harm to the host. This is the case with hepatitis B infections. The hepatitis B virus is quite harmless; however, cytotoxic T-cells attempting to kill liver cells that harbor the hepatitis B virus cause extensive damage to the host's cells, resulting in progressive liver disease *(4,6,10,14)*.

4.2. NK Cells

NK cells represent approx 15% of the lymphocyte population, but do not express T- or B-cell receptors; however, they do express some CD surface markers that are also found on granulocytes, some macrophages, monocytes and T-cells. The NK cell's function is to recognize and kill some cells infected with virus and some tumor cells. The mechanism by which recognition and death occurs is not completely understood; however, the role of certain membrane receptors has been suggested. For example, HLA-C antigens probably play a role in viral/tumor recognition; CD16, which is the FcγRIII receptor for IgG, may destroy target cells coated with IgG through a process termed antibody-dependent cellular cytotoxicity; and the production and release of cytokines such as IL1, granulocyte macrophage-colony stimulating factor (GM-CSF), and IFN-γ from NK cells appears to play a regulatory role in immune function *(4)*.

4.3. Mononuclear Phagocytes

This group of phagocytic cells includes blood-borne cells such as monocytes and polymorphonuclear granulocytes (neutrophils, eosinophils, and basophils), and macrophages that are located in a variety of body tissues such as the liver (Kupffer cells), kidney, lungs, spleen, lymph nodes, and brain. These cells have two primary functions: phagocytosis of particulate matter; and, processing and presentation of

Table 4
Receptors/Markers Present on Macrophages and Monocytes

Marker	Function
Manosyl–fucosal receptors (MFR)	Binds to sugars on microorganisms.
Complement receptors	
CR1 (C3b receptor, CD35)	Binds to cells coated with C3b.
CR3 (C3bi receptor, CD11b)	Adhesion and activation.
Leukocyte function antigen	Adhesion and activation.
(LFA1 or CD11a)	
P150,95 (CD11c)	Adhesion and activation.
MHC class II antigen	Presents antigen to T-cells.
Fc receptors	
FcγRI (CD64)	High affinity for IgG.
FcγRII (CD32)	Medium affinity for IgG.
FcγRIII (CD16)	Low affinity for IgG.
Cytokine receptors (IL-1, IL-4, IFNγ)	Receptors that bind cytokines signaling
and migration-inhibition factor	activation and other cells functions.
FcεRII (CD23)	Low-affinity receptor for the Fc of IgE.

antigen to T-cells. This phagocytic network has been termed the reticuloendothelial system.

4.3.1. Macrophages/Monocytes

Blood-borne monocytes differentiate from the myeloid progenitor stem cells in the bone marrow. Some of these cells migrate through blood vessel walls into tissues and become macrophages. The purpose of these cells is to phagocytose and proteo-lytically digest particulate matter. The particulate matter that is ingested is housed within the walled-off vesicles to protect the rest of the cell from destructive enzymes. The killing and processing of this particulate matter is accomplished by the intra-cellular lysosomes that contain various digestive enzymes such as peroxidase and various types of acid hydrolases. The ability of these cells to phagocytose is accomplished through the presence of receptors on the cell membrane. One receptor termed MFR (manosyl–fucosyl receptor) can bind to sugars present on the surface of micro-organisms. Other types of important receptors are the complement receptors and the Fc receptors for IgG which can be of three types: FcγRI which has high affinity for IgG; FcγRII having medium affinity for IgG; and FcγRIII with low binding affinity for IgG. A summary of the major membrane receptors on macrophages and monocytes is presented in Table 4 *(4)*.

4.3.2. Polymorphonuclear Granulocytes (PMNs)

These bone-marrow-derived cells are rapidly produced (80 million/min) but live for a very short time (2–3 d). The most abundant granulocyte is the neutrophil. These cells respond to chemotactic agents, such as complement fragments and cyto-kines such as IL8, that signal them to migrate to the site of inflammation. Eosinophils represent only 2–15% of the blood leukocytes. Although their primary function is one of regulating the inflammatory response through the release of an enzyme that inactivates histamine, they appear to be capable of phagocytosing and killing microorganisms. The third type of PMN cell is the basophil, which constitutes < 0.2% of the total leukocyte pool. These cells also respond to chemotactic factors. The stimulus for both eosinophils and basophils to release their intracellular granules is often an antigen which causes an allergic reaction (allergen) *(4)*.

4.4. Antigen Processing and Presentation

Antigens must be degraded and split into small peptides before they can be presented to T-cells. Antigens that are taken into the cell by phagocytosis are digested within the lysosomal compartment, then travel to the endoplasmic reticulum where they bind to the groove in the MHC class II molecules, and are then transported to the cell surface where they can be presented to CD8+ T-cells. When the cell is infected by virus or foreign pathogens, antigens from this foreign matter are digested, travel to the endoplasmic reticulum where they bind to MHC class I molecules, are transported to the cell surface and are recognized by CD4+ T-cells. Proteins that are synthesized within the cell (self or viral proteins) are degraded in the Golgi apparatus. The heavy chain of the MHC class I molecules forms around these small peptides, then carries them to the cell surface where the complex associates with β_2 microglobulin and presents the peptide to T-cells *(6)*.

B-cells are also efficient antigen-presenting cells. When an antigen binds to the Ig receptor on the B-cell, the receptor–antigen is internalized and the antigen is degraded into peptides. A peptide binds to the MHC class II molecules and the complex is then transported to the surface of the cell *(4)*.

5. IMMUNOLOGY RELATING TO TRANSFUSION MEDICINE

This basic information on the components of the immune system and their function can be applied to explain certain observations that are encountered in transfusion medicine practice. To illustrate this application, three specific examples are given: red cell alloimmunization; platelet alloimmunization, and febrile nonhemolytic transfusion reactions.

5.1. Red Cell Alloimmunization

When allogeneic red cells are transfused, a certain percentage of the red cells will be nonviable, depending on the age of the product. These old cells can be fragmented as they pass through the spleen and degraded in the plasma, resulting in many different soluble red blood cell proteins being released. B-lymphocytes are constantly surveilling this material and if they encounter foreign antigen or an antigenic epitope that is the correct specificity for their Ig receptors, binding occurs. This antigen–immunoglobulin bond sends a signal to the cell to internalize the Ig receptor through a process called endocytosis. Once internalized, the antigen bound to the Ig receptor is degraded into small peptide chains that then bind to the groove in the MHC class II molecules. This complex is transported to the cell surface where it is recognized by the TCR on CD4+ T-helper cells. In combination with the CD4 coreceptor, this MHC–TCR interaction stimulates cytokine production (IL1, IL2, and IL4), which signals the B-cell to proliferate into plasma cells and produce antibody specific for the antigen that was originally bound to the cell (Fig. 7). Initial

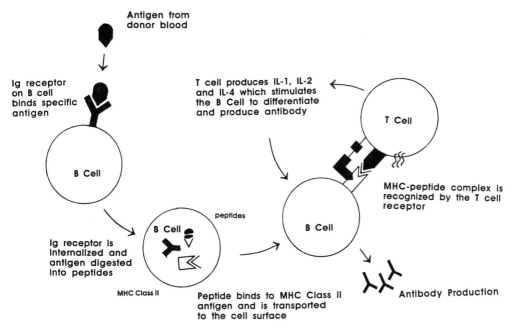

Fig. 7. Diagram illustrating the mechanism of red-cell alloantibody production following interaction of B-cells with antigen.

antibody production is predominantly IgM; however, class switching eventually occurs and IgG antibody is produced. In the transfusion laboratory, this antibody is detected by the antibody screen or crossmatch indicating that posttransfusion red cell alloimmunization has occurred.

There is also a second mechanism by which red cell alloimmunization can occur. Like the previous model, old allogeneic red cells that have been transfused can be cleared from the circulation by macrophage endocytosis in the liver and spleen. As the allogeneic red cells are phagocytosed, the proteins (some representing blood-group antigens) are broken down and degraded into small peptides. The peptides bind to MHC class II antigens and are transported to the cell membrane. The TCR in combination with the CD4 protein recognizes the foreign peptide bound to self MHC and secretes cytokines. The cytokines produced have a stimulating effect on any B-cells in the microenvironment that have the same antigen bound in their Ig receptors (Fig. 8). Thus, the classical model of antigen presentation and cell proliferation results in antibody production. If the Ig receptor on the stimulated B-cell is specific for a red cell blood-group antigen, then red cell alloantibodies are produced.

In the first mechanism that was described, the B-cell directly stimulates T-cells to produce cytokines that will promote B-cell proliferation. This is the predominate mechanism of red cell antibody production when the antigenic stimulus is small (i.e., fetal maternal bleeds). In the second mechanism, the T-cell is stimulated to produce cytokines following interaction with MHC class II antigens on macrophages. B-cells in the microenvironment that have bound antigen to their Ig receptors, benefit from this tripartite interaction as cell proliferation can occur without B-cells degrading the antigen and expressing the digested peptides on its surface. This is probably the dominant mechanism of red cell alloantibody production when the antigen stimulus is large (i.e., red cell transfusions).

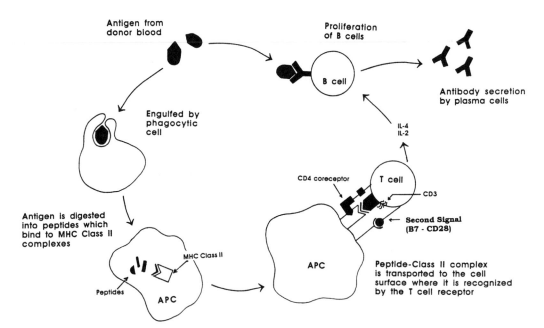

Fig. 8. Diagram illustrating the mechanism of red-cell alloantibody production when macrophages present donor antigenic peptides to T-cells.

5.2. HLA Alloimmunization to Platelets

It has been well documented that reducing the number of leukocytes in red cells and platelets to a threshold of 5×10^6/product will prevent HLA alloimmunization in many transfused individuals *(19)*. Why is this intervention effective? Donor allogeneic leukocytes express both MHC class I and class II antigens. Some of the MHC class II antigens will contain peptides that originated from the MHC class I antigens on the donor's cells. Most of the transfusion recipient's T-cells recognize self MHC, carrying foreign peptides; however, as mentioned in Section 4.1.2., a small percentage of T-cells (< 10%) are able to recognize foreign MHC-carrying peptides *(4)*. When platelets are transfused, the TCR-2 on the patient's CD4+ T-cells recognizes the foreign MHC class II complex on the donor leukocytes. If the dual signal occurs, the T-cells activate nearby B-cells that have also bound MHC class I antigen fragments to their Ig receptor, resulting in cell proliferation and MHC class I (HLA) antibody production (Fig. 9). In this scenario, the donor's leukocytes can serve as the antigen-presenting cells rather than going through the process of cell clearance and presentation of peptides by the recipient's macrophages. Because antigen is being presented primarily by donor leukocytes, the process of antibody production can often be prevented by removing most of the leukocytes from the donor blood product. However, some patients receiving leuko-reduced blood products may produce HLA antibodies through the same mechanism by which red cell alloimmunization occurs.

5.3. Febrile Nonhemolytic Transfusion Reactions

There is strong evidence to suggest that the primary pathophysiology of febrile nonhemolytic transfusion reactions (FNHTRs) to red cells and platelets is different.

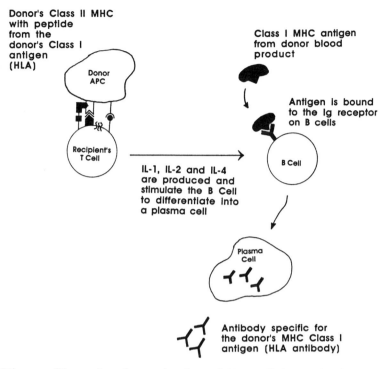

Fig. 9. Diagram illustrating the mechanism of HLA alloimmunization due to leukocytes present in platelet transfusions.

This evidence evolved from the observation that platelet reactions were strongly dependent on the age of the platelets, and the observation that poststorage leukoreduction was effective for preventing most FNHTRs to red cells, but was often ineffective in preventing platelet-associated reactions *(20,21)*.

5.3.1. Red Cell Reactions

Most FNHTRs to red cells are the result of an antigen/antibody incompatibility. Antileukocyte antibody (HLA or granulocyte) in the transfusion recipient's plasma binds to specific antigens on the surface of the donor leukocyte. The presence of IgG on the cell surface may lead to complement activation leaving both IgG and C3b present on the cell surface. The FcγR1 and CR1 receptors on macrophages bind to and phagocytose the sensitized cells. This process results in the secretion of a number of different cytokines by the recipient such as IL-1, IL-6, and TNFα that are endogenous pyrogens capable of causing the febrile response that is typical of these reactions *(21)*.

5.3.2. Platelet Reactions

Although some FNHTRs associated with platelet reactions can be mediated by antigen–antibody incompatibility, like red-cell transfusions, the majority of FNHTRs to platelets appear to be caused by biological response modifiers present in the plasma portion of the platelet product *(22)*. Platelet concentrates are contaminated with variable numbers of leukocytes depending on the method of collection and preparation. The majority of the leukocytes are lymphocytes (>90%), with the remainder being predominantly monocytes. During platelet storage, the leukocytes produce a number of cytokines such as IL-1, IL-6, TNFα, and IL-8. Production of these cytokines appears to be temperature dependent and affected by agitation; thus, storage of platelets at room temperature with gentle agitation facilitates cytokine production and release. The exact mechanism of cytokine production is not clear. When the platelets are transfused, the overall concentration of cytokines with pyrogenic activity is sufficiently high to cause a febrile response in some patients. Although cytokines have been implicated in causing FNHTRs, other biological response modifiers that accumulate during storage may also play a role *(21)*.

6. SUMMARY

These are only a few examples of how the immune system relates to situations that are encountered in transfusion medicine practice. A basic comprehension of the concepts presented in this chapter will allow individuals involved in transfusion medicine practice to have a better understanding of some of the adverse complications that occur with blood transfusion and the role that the immune system plays in these events.

ACKNOWLEDGMENTS

Special thanks to Mike Heddle for the illustrations included in this chapter, Greg Dennome for his many suggestions and comments, and Janice Butera and Barbara Lahie for their clerical assistance.

REFERENCES

1. Kaczmarski RS, Mufti GJ. The cytokine receptor superfamily. *Blood Rev* 1992;5: 193–203.
2. Staines N, Brostoff J, James K. *Introducing Immunology,* 2nd ed. St. Louis: Mosby-Yearbook Europe Ltd, 1993.
3. WHO Nomenclature Committee on Leukocyte Antigens. Nomenclature for factors of the HLA system, 1987. In: Dupont B, ed. *Immunobiology of HLA.* New York: Springer-Verlag, 1989.
4. Roitt I, Brostoff J, Male D. *Immunology,* 4th ed. St. Louis: Mosby YearBook, 1993.
5. Santos-Aguado J, Barbosa JA, Biro A, Strominger JL. Molecular characterization of serologic recognition sites in the human HLA-A2 molecule. *J Immunol* 1988;141: 2811–2818.
6. Janeway CA, Jr. How the immune system recognizes invaders. *Scientific American* 1993;269(3):73–79.
7. Roitt I. *Essential Immunology,* 8th ed. Oxford: Blackwell Scientific Publication, 1994.
8. Devine DV. The regulation of complement on cell surfaces. *Transf Med Rev* 1991;V: 123–131.
9. Golde DW. The stem cell. *Scientific American* 1991;265(3):86–93.
10. Weissman IL, Cooper MD. How the immune system develops. *Scientific American* 1993;269(3):64–71.
11. Tonegawa S. Somatic generation of antibody diversity. *Nature* 1983; 302:575–581.
12. Alt FW, Backwell TK, Yancopoulos GD. Development of the primary antibody repertoire. *Science* 1987;238:1079–1087.
13. Russell DM, Dembic Z, Morahan G, Miller JFAP, Buki K, Nemazee D. Peripheral deletion of self-reactive B cells. *Nature* 1991;354:308–311.

14. Paul WE. Infectious diseases and the immune system. When bacteria, viruses and other pathogens infect the body, they hide in different places. *Scientific American* 1993;269(3):90–97.
15. Nossal GJV, Pike BL. Cellular mechanisms of immunological tolerance. *Proc Natl Acad Sci USA* 1981;78:38–44.
16. Marrack P, Lo D, Brinster R, Palmiter R, Burkly L, Flavell RH, Kappler J. The effects of thymus environment on T cell development and tolerance. *Cell* 1988;53:627–634.
17. Clevers H, Alarcon B, Willeman T, Terhorst C. The T cell receptor/CD3 complex: a dynamic protein ensemble. *Ann Rev Immunol* 1988;6:629–662.
18. Marrack P, Kappler JW. How the immune systems recognizes the body. *Scientific American* 1993;269(3):81–89.
19. Heddle NM. The efficacy of leukodepletion to improve platelet transfusion response: a critical appraisal of clinical studies. *Transf Med Rev* 1994;VIII:15–28.
20. Heddle NM, Klama LN, Griffith L, Roberts R, Shukla G, Kelton JG. A prospective study to identify the risk factors associated with acute reactions to platelet and red cell transfusions. *Transfusion* 1993;33:794–797.
21. Heddle NM, Kelton JG. Febrile non-hemolytic transfusion reactions. In: Popovsky MA, ed. *Transfusion Reactions*. Bethesda, MD: AABB Press, 1996, pp. 45–80.
22. Heddle NM, Klama L, Singer J, Richards C, Fedak P, Walker I, Kelton JG. The role of the plasma from platelet concentrates in transfusion reactions. *N Engl J Med* 1994; 331:625–628.

3

Compatibility Testing
for Red Blood Cell Components

Approaches and Limitations

Kathleen Sazama

1. INTRODUCTION

Compatibility testing for red blood cell transfusion in U.S. health care facilities consists of a specified series of steps, defined in the American Association of Blood Banks' (AABB's) Standards for Blood Banks and Transfusion Services (Standards) *(1)* and further described in the AABB's *Technical Manual (2)*. The elements of this process include assuring that a physician order exists and that a proper request has occurred, obtaining or receiving a properly collected and labeled patient sample, testing the patient sample for ABO and Rh, performing a historical check of prior patient ABO, testing of donor unit for ABO (and D, if D-negative), screening patient serum for unexpected antibodies, identifying any unexpected antibodies, and performing a crossmatch between donor cells and patient serum (or an electronic crossmatch if specific conditions are met). At every step in this process, choices occur (Fig. 1). To ensure that all appropriate actions occur, a checklist is helpful. Table 1 is an example of a checklist based in part on the AABB's Quality Program, System I: Compatibility Testing *(3)*.

2. REQUEST FOR TRANSFUSION

2.1. Physician Order

Before any compatibility testing occurs, a physician must write an order requesting a red blood cell transfusion, specifying number of units and urgency of need.

2.2. Laboratory Request

The laboratory/blood bank must receive a completed request form (written on paper or electronically transmitted) or a properly authorized verbal request with followup documentation.

Recommendation: Your facility should have a written procedure and/or policy requiring that a written order exist for transfusion of red blood cells. A written order is required by federal regulation for every transfusion.

From: *Red Cell Transfusion: A Practical Guide*
Edited by: M. E. Reid and S. J. Nance Humana Press Inc., Totowa, NJ

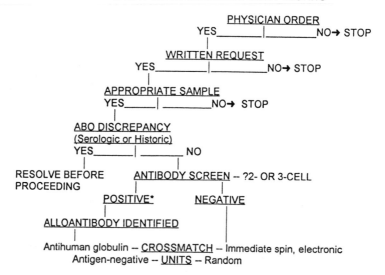

Fig. 1. Decision tree for compatibility testing. *If autoantibody found, *see* Chapter 4; if polyagglutination, further studies needed.

3. SAMPLE ACCEPTABILITY

Because fatalities can result from failure to properly identify patients at the sample collection phase, organizations should insist on developing and maintaining systems that ensure a high degree of confidence that patient identification is correct. To ensure that a proper sample is available, the process must include establishing the unique identity of the patient, obtaining a sufficient volume of properly anticoagulated (or nonanticoagulated) whole blood, and recording *on the sample label* the name and unique identifying number (as specified in the standard operating procedure), the date (and sometimes the time), and the identity of the person obtaining the sample. When the sample is time critical, such as at the onset of a massive transfusion protocol or when therapeutic interventions may alter blood constituents in a way that masks the patient's true condition, every effort should be made to obtain the maximum sample volume required before any intervention begins.

3.1. Patient Identification

3.1.1. Routine Inpatient

For inpatients, proper identification of the patient should be obtained from objective sources, particularly from an institution-issued identification band, because the patient can be confused, semiconscious, heavily medicated, or physically unable to properly respond when asked to state his or her name.

3.1.2. Emergency

In the emergency room (and during transportation when samples are obtained from massively bleeding patients), many institutions provide for a substitute identi-

Table 1
Checklist for Compatibility Testing

Order and Request for Transfusion
  Physician order
    Written
    Oral
    Oral with follow-up written
  Request form
    Patient's name (first, last)
    Unique identification number
    Type and amount of blood ordered
    Name of requesting physician
    Statement of priority
Sample
  Patient identification
    Objective system
    Alternative used
  Sample characteristics
    Acceptable collection
      Serum and/or plasma
      Nonhemolyzed
      Not diluted
      Other, specify _____
    Sample Age
      Up to 3 d old
      Older than 3 d for appropriate patients
    Label on sample
      Patient name (first, last)
      Unique identification number
      Both name and number identical with request form
      Date of phlebotomy
      Time of phlebotomy (if necessary)
      Identity of phlebotomist
      Single label
  ABO Testing
    Current sample
      Patient forward ABO and reverse agree
      Donor segment forward ABO and reverse agree
      Donor ABO test result matches donor ABO on label
    Historical records
      Patient has prior record
      Patient's prior record and current serologic results agree
      No prior record, duplicate typing agree
  Rh Testing
    Patient sample
    Donor sample, only if Rh negative

(continued)

Table 1 (*continued*)

Antibody Screening
    Two- or three- cell screen: Any or all cells reactive
        Control negative, proceed to antibody identification and use antigen-negative units
            for crossmatch
        Control positive, resolve problem with control before proceeding
    Two- or three-cell screen: All cells negative, use random units and IS crossmatch
Direct Antiglobulin Testing
    Not routinely performed
    Test positive, refer for special studies
    Test negative
Antibody Identification
    Red cell panels (commercial/in-house) reactions
        All cells: Refer for special studies
        No cells: Recheck screen and methodology, re-identify patient sample
        Some cells: identify antibod(ies); perform AHG crossmatch using antigen-negative unit
Crossmatching
    Nonemergencies
        No antibodies (current or past):
            Immediate spin crossmatch
            Electronic crossmatch
        Alloantibodies (current and/or past):
            AHG crossmatch required
    Emergency situations
        Life-threatening hemorrhage: No crossmatch, no sample (or no time to type sample)
            Group O, D-positive for all except women of childbearing years
            Group O, D-negative for women of childbearing years
            Retrospective antibody screen, if sample available
            Retrospective antibody identification, if indicated
            Retrospective crossmatch, if sample available
        Life-threatening hemorrhage: No crossmatch, time to type sample:
            Type specific or compatible blood except for Rh negative women of
                childbearing years
            Type identical blood for Rh negative women of childbearing years
            Retrospective antibody screen
            Retrospective antibody identification
            Retrospective crossmatch
        No life-threatening hemorrhage
            No alloantibodies (current or past)
                Immediate spin crossmatch
                Electronic crossmatch
            Alloantibodies (current or past)
            AHG crossmatch
                Antigen-negative units
                Random units
            Immediate spin (or electronic) crossmatch, followed by retrospective
                AHG crossmatch
                Antigen-negative units
                Random units
Massive Transfusion
    Written protocol
    Documentation
    Conversion of "unknown" to known patient

fication process (often called a "Doe" or temporary alias process) to accommodate the time exigencies attendant to such patients. Systems to ensure appropriate record keeping for converting the "Doe" or "alias" to the specific patient information must minimize risk of harm during time critical ongoing activities.

3.1.3. Outpatient and Out-of-Hospital

In the outpatient and out-of-hospital setting, patients and/or family and friends can assist in making a proper identification for sample collection. Some facilities use an additional identification process at the time of sample collection, in one or more settings.

3.2. Samples

3.2.1. Type

The patient samples required for laboratory testing usually include an ethylene-diamine tetraacetic acid (EDTA)-anticoagulated sample and a serum sample. The EDTA tube should provide an adequate volume of whole blood for laboratory testing procedures when the tube is filled appropriately. Underfilling of the EDTA tube may result in an improper anticoagulant/whole blood ratio. Nonanticoagulated blood samples have no volume limitation. When the sample is obtained from above the site of an intravenous line, dilution may interfere with proper interpretation of the antibody screening test and the crossmatch. Hemolyzed samples generally contain too few intact red blood cells and too much free hemoglobin, which can interfere with interpretation of serologic tests.

3.2.2. Age

If a patient has been pregnant or transfused, because of possible evolving allo-antibody formation, federal regulations *(4)* and the AABB Standards *(1)* require that samples be obtained at least every 72 h (3 d). No compatibility testing should be performed using samples older than this time frame unless an emergency exists.

3.2.3. Label

Every specimen must be labeled with patient's *full* name (first and last) as listed in the facility's database or from other objective sources. A unique identification number must also appear. This number can be a facility-issued number, the patient's social security number, or another number acceptable to the medical director. These data (name and number) *must identically match* the information on the request form. In an *emergency,* a substitute identification may be used as specified in an approved institutional policy.

Other data required on the sample label include the date (and occasionally the time) of collection and some means of identifying the phlebotomist.

Labeling must occur *at the patient's side.*

Recommendation: Every institution should have an administrative policy that requires *objective* identification of every patient receiving a red blood cell transfusion, in or outside of its walls. This identification system must be in place at the time of sample collection and *remain in place* until the crossmatched unit(s) is/are transfused. If the identification is removed from the patient before the crossmatched unit(s) is/are transfused, a system for linking the original identification with the patient must be specifically authorized or a new sample must be obtained and the crossmatch repeated using the new sample. In some situations, a unique blood bank identification system may be prudent. In addition, *strict* adherence to specimen acceptability, including the basic identification elements and the correctly drawn specimen should be required.

4. ABO TESTING

4.1. Current Sample

Both patient and donor ABO testing must be performed using federally approved (or equivalent) reagents. Because of the unique characteristics of the ABO system (antigen-negative persons develop "naturally occurring" antibodies to the missing antigen[s]), the results of both cell and serum testing are used to establish the "true" ABO type of each person. Thus, discrepancies in the expected serologic results must be reconciled before assignment of an ABO type is made. Discrepancies can occur due to illness *(5)*, massive transfusion (with red blood cells, platelets, or plasma of a different ABO type), allogeneic bone marrow/progenitor cell transplantation, presence of auto- or alloantibodies, mistakes or errors, and other reasons.

4.2. Historical Records

An additional safeguard for patients is the requirement to compare prior ABO test records with current ones. When records show a different result than the current typing, no transfusion should occur until this conflict is resolved. In some situations, the historical record is flawed (owing to failure to correctly identify the patient for this or the prior admission or failure to properly merge two records). In others, it is a mistake in collection of the current sample. To minimize the possibility of this error occurring, some institutions obtain a second sample from a patient for whom no historical record exists, and some require a second typing of the first specimen, both of which must type identically with the first sample before a patient ABO assignment is made. Other institutions require that a second person verify the patient identity by signing the sample tube label at the time of collection. Although all of these systems have weaknesses, each has some capacity to catch ABO typing errors.

Recommendation: Because of the importance of correct ABO identification to avoid significant patient morbidity and/or mortality, specific procedures for performing ABO testing should be as detailed as possible. Reconciliation of *any discrepancy* must occur before proceeding.

5. RH TESTING

Testing for Rh antigens differs between patient and donor samples. Only donor cells labeled as "Rh negative" must be reverified to exclude possible weakly reactive D antigens. (Donor cells labeled as "Rh positive" are not retested.) Rh typing for both donor and patient must include use of an Rh control if recommended by the manufacturer (to ensure that reactivity is specific for the D-anti-D reaction). Weak D testing is performed as an option on patient samples in some institutions, whereas other institutions perform no further testing if the D test result is negative.

Recommendation: The institution should have written policies regarding testing of D-negative patient samples to identify possible weak D antigens. Because of its importance in hemolytic disease of the newborn, comprehensive D testing of pregnant women is essential.

6. ANTIBODY SCREENING

Every time a new patient sample is obtained from a patient who has been pregnant or transfused within the past 3 mo, the sample must be screened for the appearance of alloantibodies. This screening consists of mixing appropriate volumes of the patient's serum with reagent red blood cells of defined antigenic types. The choices for transfusion services are to use either a two-cell or a three-cell screen. Reagent screening cells are configured to maximize presence of homozygous antigens in those systems in which dosage of reactivity is documented. Generally, more homozygous antigens are represented in the three-cell reagents than in the two-cell ones. However, detection of clinically significant antibodies occurs in a very high percentage of cases using only the two-cell screen. Cost containment efforts in modern medical care may persuade institutions to use the two-cell screen in preference to the three-cell one. (Purists, on the other hand, may insist on using the three-cell screen exclusively.) If the screen is negative, no alloantibodies are detected and a rapid crossmatch can proceed. However, even if no alloantibodies have been detected serologically, part of the historical check should ensure that there are no prior alloantibodies nor any previously recorded instances of adverse consequences of transfusion. If the historical record documents presence of a prior alloantibody, the units selected for compatibility testing should generally be antigen negative for the offending antigen. Exceptions occur for antigens considered to be *not* "clinically significant."

If screen cells are reactive and the screening test included use of the patient's own (autogeneic) red cells that are also reactive, further testing must be done to establish whether there are both allo- and autoantibodies, and, if an alloantibody is found, to identify it and determine its clinical significance. *Except in emergencies,* no crossmatch should proceed until the identity and characteristics of any autoantibodies or one or more alloantibodies are known. When an emergency exists, the medical director of the transfusion service must determine which units should be used for crossmatching. Units issued during such an emergency generally require completion of a serologic crossmatch, even after the units have been transfused, consistent with institutional guidelines for massive transfusion.

Recommendation: Most facilities may choose to use a two-cell screen as a cost effective strategy that provides a high degree of confidence that significant alloantibodies will be detected. In institutions in which a large number of chronically transfused patients are treated or complex serologic problems are frequently seen, a three-cell screen may be necessary.

7. DIRECT ANTIGLOBULIN TEST

When antibody screening detects the presence of an antibody, testing to exclude possible autoimmunity is indicated. The direct antiglobulin test (DAT) detects presence of autoantibody that has reacted in vivo, coating patient red cells. Such cells can be detected by adding anti-human globulin (AHG) to washed patient red blood cells. The basis for a positive DAT, techniques for defining the identity of the

SERUM TESTING

RBCs	D	C	E	c	e	M	N	S	s	K	Fyᵃ	Fyᵇ	Jkᵃ	Jkᵇ	IS	37	AHG
1	0	+	0	+	+	+	0	0	+	0	+	+	+	+	2+	3+	3+
2	+	+	0	0	+	0	+	0	+	0	+	+	+	+	2+	3+	3+
3	+	+	0	0	+	+	+	0	+	+	+	0	+	0	2+	3+	3+
4	+	0	+	+	0	+	0	+	+	0	0	+	0	+	2+	3+	3+
5	0	0	+	+	+	+	0	+	+	0	+	0	+	+	1+	3+	3+
6	0	0	0	+	+	+	0	0	+	0	+	+	0	+	2+	3+	3+
7	0	0	0	+	+	+	0	0	+	+	0	+	+	0	2+	3+	3+
8	0	0	0	+	+	+	+	+	+	0	0	0	+	0	2+	3+	3+
9	0	0	0	+	+	+	0	+	+	0	0	+	0	+	2+	3+	3+
10	0	0	0	+	+	+	0	+	+	0	+	0	+	+	2+	3+	3+
11	0	+	0	+	+	+	0	0	+	0	+	+	+	0	2+	3+	3+

Fig. 2. Antibody identification: All cells react.

autoantibody and tips for transfusion when the DAT is positive are included in Chapter 4.

Recommendation: Routine DAT is not recommended. Its specific applications are discussed in Chapter 4.

8. ANTIBODY IDENTIFICATION

8.1. Red Cell Panels

When the antibody screen is positive and the DAT is negative, additional testing to establish the identity and characteristics of the alloantibody(ies) is required. Generally, a single 11–16-cell panel of red blood cells whose red blood cell antigen phenotype is known (most transfusion services purchase these from commercial vendors) is tested against screen-reactive patient serum. The conditions for the initial test generally include a room temperature reading followed by a second reading after incubation at 37 °C for 15–30 min, then a final reading after addition of AHG. Check cells (red blood cells coated with human globulin) are added to any negative tube to ensure addition of AHG and proper washing procedure. Occasionally, additional techniques (e.g., ZZAP to dissociate antibodies) or use of specially prepared panels cells (e.g., ficin-treated) are required. (These special methods are performed in reference laboratories and will not be discussed further in this chapter.)

8.2. Reaction Patterns

The identity of the alloantibody is disclosed by interpretation of the reaction strengths and pattern of reactivity of various cells in the panel (*see* Figs. 2–5). The reaction strengths vary from weak to 4+, and may provide clues as to whether one or more alloantibodies are present or whether a dosing pattern should be considered. Three patterns of reaction generally can be seen: All cells react, some cells react, or no cells react.

8.2.1. All Cells React

When all cells react, the patient's serum could contain an antibody to a high-incidence antigen or an autoantibody. This alteration can be inherited (e.g., CAD, HEMPAS, etc.). Because this reaction pattern may obscure the presence of other alloantibodies, further testing may be indicated.

8.2.2. No Cells React

When no cells react, a reassessment of the screening cell results should be made to assure no mistake has occurred. If no mistake has occurred, then use of special identification techniques may be indicated. These are probably best performed in a reference laboratory setting and are not discussed further in this chapter.

8.2.3. Some Cells React

When some cells react and others do not, identification of one or more alloantibodies is usually possible. Reactions seen only at room temperature, regardless of the strength of the reaction at that temperature, are generally considered to be due to alloantibodies that are *"not clinically significant"* and are identified for interest only. Reactions occurring at 37 °C and after addition of AHG are generally considered to be caused by alloantibodies that are clinically significant and must be identified (*see* Chapter 14). The relative strengths of reaction at various temperatures and times of incubation are also helpful in assigning an identity to the alloantibody found.

8.3. Reaction Interpretation

To identify the alloantibody(ies) present, a systematic "cross-off" approach is used. The basic rules for a "cross-off" are as follows.

8.3.1. Presence of a Reaction

If a reagent cell reacted with patient serum, then any antigen *missing* from that cell *cannot* be the reason for the reaction and will not be detected by an alloantibody in the patient serum. Any antigen *not present* on a reacting cell (usually listed across the top of the report form in categories, i.e., Rh antigens, MNSs, Kk, etc.) can be crossed off. Systematic cross-off of missing antigens from all reactive cells may disclose the antigen if only one alloantibody is present (Fig. 3).

8.3.2. Absence of a Reaction

If a reagent cell fails to react with patient serum, then any antigen *present* on that cell *cannot* be responsible for alloimmunization of the patient. Any antigen *present* on a nonreacting cell can be "crossed off" because, if it was responsible for the reaction, a reaction would have occurred. Systematic cross-off of all antigens present on nonreactive cells may disclose a pattern that identifies a single (or multiple) alloantibodies (Fig. 4).

Exception: When both alleles of some antigen systems are present on the reagent red cell, e.g., Jk^a and Jk^b, Fy^a and Fy^b, and so on, the cell may show no or markedly reduced reactivity relative to a cell from an individual homozygous for one of

SERUM TESTING																

RBCs	D	C	E	c	e	M	N	S	s	K	Fyª	Fyᵇ	Jkª	Jkᵇ	IS	37	AHG
1	0	+	0	+	+	+	0	0	+	0	+	+	+	+	0	2+	2+
2	+	+	0	0	+	0	+	0	+	0	+	+	+	+	+	3+	3+
3	+	+	0	0	+	+	+	0	+	+	+	0	+	0	+	2+	2+
4	+	0	+	+	0	+	0	+	+	0	0	+	0	+	0	0	0
5	0	0	+	+	+	+	0	+	+	0	+	0	+	+	0	0	0
6	0	0	0	+	+	+	0	0	+	0	+	+	0	+	0	0	0
7	0	0	0	+	+	+	0	0	+	+	0	+	+	0	0	0	0
8	0	0	0	+	+	+	+	+	+	0	0	0	+	0	0	0	0
9	0	0	0	+	+	+	0	+	+	0	0	+	0	+	0	0	0
10	0	0	0	+	+	+	0	+	+	0	+	0	+	+	0	0	0
11	0	+	0	+	+	+	0	0	+	0	+	+	+	0	+	2+	2+

Fig. 3. Identifying antibodies: Reactive cell cross-out.

SERUM TESTING																

RBCs	D	C	E	c	e	M	N	S	s	K	Fyª	Fyᵇ	Jkª	Jkᵇ	IS	37	AHG
1	0	+	0	+	+	+	0	0	+	0	+	+	+	+	0	2+	2+
2	+	+	0	0	+	0	+	0	+	0	+	+	+	+	+	3+	3+
3	+	+	0	0	+	+	+	0	+	+	+	0	+	0	+	2+	2+
4	+	0	+	+	0	+	0	+	+	0	0	+	0	+	0	0	0
5	0	0	+	+	+	+	0	+	+	0	+	0	+	+	0	0	0
6	0	0	0	+	+	+	0	0	+	0	+	+	0	+	0	0	0
7	0	0	0	+	+	+	0	0	+	+	0	+	+	0	0	0	0
8	0	0	0	+	+	+	+	+	+	0	0	0	+	0	0	0	0
9	0	0	0	+	+	+	0	+	+	0	0	+	0	+	0	0	0
10	0	0	0	+	+	+	0	+	+	0	+	0	+	+	0	0	0
11	0	+	0	+	+	+	0	0	+	0	+	+	+	0	+	2+	2+

Fig. 4. Identifying antibodies: Nonreactive cell cross-out.

SERUM TESTING																

RBCs														IS	37	AHG
1	0	+	0	+	+	+	0	0	+	0	+	+	+	+	0	0	0
2	+	+	0	0	+	0	+	0	+	0	+	+	+	+	0	+/-	1+
3	+	+	0	0	+	+	+	0	+	+	+	0	+	0	0	2+	2+
4	+	0	+	+	0	+	0	+	+	0	0	+	0	+	0	0	0
5	0	0	+	+	+	+	0	+	+	0	+	0	+	+	0	1+	1+
6	0	0	0	+	+	+	0	0	+	0	+	+	0	+	0	0	0
7	0	0	0	+	+	+	0	0	+	+	0	+	+	0	1+	2+	2+
8	0	0	0	+	+	+	+	+	+	0	0	0	+	0	0	1+	2+
9	0	0	0	+	+	+	0	+	+	0	0	+	0	+	0	0	0
10	0	0	0	+	+	+	0	+	+	0	+	0	+	+	0	0	0
11	0	+	0	+	+	+	0	0	+	0	+	+	+	0	+/-	2+	2+

Fig. 5. Identifying antibodies: Dosing pattern.

the alleles. This *dosing* phenomenon must be considered when no apparent pattern of reactivity consistent with a single (or multiple) alloantibodies is discernible after cross off has occurred (Fig. 5).

Generally, for the majority of patients, only a single alloantibody will be found. However, once one antibody has formed, the possibility of additional antibody formation must be kept in mind.

8.4. Phenotyping

Many transfusion facilities will consider performing antigen typing of patient red blood cells when an alloantibody has been identified and the patient is expected to continue to receive red blood cell transfusions. Future transfusions should use red blood cells that lack antigens to which the patient has already formed alloantibodies, both newly detected and historically recorded. For discussion of the use of antigen-negative blood before antibody production, *see* Chapters 1 and 14.

Recommendation:

1. When a single alloantibody reacting only at room temperature (e.g., anti-M, anti-Le[a]) is found, crossmatch-compatible cells can be safely transfused without performing further antigen typing of the donor unit(s).
2. When a single alloantibody reacting at 37°C and/or at AHG is found, donor cells lacking that antigen should be selected (except in emergencies) for crossmatch. Generally single alloantibodies arise against the more common antigens (D, K, E, Jk[a], Fy[a], c), so phenotyping otherwise appropriate units before crossmatching will provide a suitable transfusion. For alloantibodies to antigens that occur in high frequency, e.g., anti-e, antigen-negative units should be requested from a regional blood supplier for crossmatch. Crossmatch-compatible antigen-negative cells should be transfused whenever time permits.

3. In emergencies, when a single or several alloantibodies to common but relatively infrequent antigens (antigens occurring in 50% or less of the population) is found, it may be more efficient (both in time and cost) to crossmatch otherwise suitable units already available in inventory. Any crossmatch-compatible unit will provide a safe transfusion, even though shortened red cell survival may subsequently occur because of an alloantibody that failed to react with sufficient strength to be detectable in crossmatching.

4. When multiple alloantibodies are found, the regional blood supplier should be contacted to provide antigen-negative blood. Sometimes the patient's alloimmunization requires units available only from the frozen rare donor inventory. In these instances, the medical director of the transfusion service should discuss with the ordering clinician the possible delays and requirements to meet this patient's needs. The transfusion service and blood supplier must remain in close contact, particularly for patients requiring intensive repeat transfusions for an acute situation or for patients requiring chronic support.

9. CROSSMATCHING

9.1. Nonemergency Situations

9.1.1. General Strategy

Strategies for crossmatching red blood cells for patients lacking alloantibodies (current or historic) who have or have not been pregnant or transfused during the previous 3 mo include using a serologic crossmatch that consists of only an "immediate spin" reading or, if properly validated according to FDA requirements and AABB Standards, a completely electronic crossmatch.

9.1.1.1. Immediate Spin Crossmatch

An immediate spin crossmatch is intended to detect only gross ABO incompatibility. Procedures include using a low ionic strength solution (LISS) to suspend the donor red blood cells for testing against patient serum in a room temperature, generally tube method. The donor cells and patient serum are added to the same tube, which is spun for a brief time (generally 1 min or less), then read macroscopically for presence of hemolysis or agglutination. Absence of both is interpreted compatibility. Units may be labeled and issued as crossmatch compatible.

9.1.1.2. The Electronic Crossmatch

The electronic crossmatch consists of selecting a unit from an existing inventory of already retyped ABO and Rh (if appropriate) red blood cells that is ABO and Rh identical with the patient. These red cells may also be labeled as compatible if they are electronically ABO (and usually Rh) identical to the patient's ABO and Rh type. For other requirements, see the appropriate section of the AABB Standards *(1)*.

9.1.2. The AHG Crossmatch

Patients with newly detected or historic alloantibodies must receive red blood cells crossmatched using AHG methods. Generally, the units are preselected to be antigen-negative for any known or prior alloantibodies prior to beginning the crossmatch. The antiglobulin method begins the same as the immediate spin method, but the tube is incubated at 37 °C for 15–30 min, then AHG is added and the tube is centrifuged again for 1–2 min before macroscopic reading to detect any degree of agglutination or hemolysis. If no agglutination or hemolysis is seen, the unit is labeled as crossmatch compatible. If any incompatibility is seen, the unit is not labeled or used for this patient.

Recommendation: In nonemergency situations, use immediate spin (or electronic) crossmatch for all patients lacking alloantibodies. Use AHG crossmatch for all patients with historic or current serologic alloantibodies.

9.2. Emergency Situations

9.2.1. Life-Threatening Hemorrhage

In patients who are threatening to exsanguinate (with or without a sample of patient's blood), no crossmatch is required. Group O D-positive red blood cells may be used for all patients except women of childbearing years. For women of childbearing years, use of O D-negative blood is recommended.

If possible, a sample of a patient's blood should be obtained prior to infusing any red cell units, but no delay in transfusion should occur. If a sample of a patient's blood is obtained, as quickly as possible, determine the ABO and D types and issue type-specific (or compatible) units. When time permits, a complete evaluation, including antibody screen, should be performed on the initial patient sample.

Retrospective crossmatch appropriate to the serologic status of the patient prior to transfusion is generally recommended, but not necessary for all units transfused if massive (> 10 units red blood cells) transfusion occurs (*see* Section 9.2.2.).

9.2.2. Urgent Need, Patient Is Not Known To Be Alloimmunized

The following pertains to patients lacking alloantibodies (current or historic), who have or have not been pregnant or transfused during past 3 mo and *who are not exsanguinating.*

If the patient is male or a female not of childbearing years who may have been transfused during the past 3 mo, and there is sufficient time to perform serologic studies (including ABO, D, antibody screen) and a historic check, ABO type identical or compatible but Rh-positive units can be issued, preferably with at least an immediate spin crossmatch. An immediate spin or electronic crossmatch can be used if a reliable history of no transfusion within the past 3 mo is available. These units can be labeled as "crossmatch compatible" and issued. If no history exists or is reliably available, an antiglobulin crossmatch is required. If issuance is urgent and must occur prior to completion of the antiglobulin crossmatch, the units must be labeled as "emergency uncrossmatched." If an antiglobulin crossmatch is performed, the units can be labeled as crossmatch compatible.

If the patient is a woman of childbearing years, the units transfused should be ABO identical or compatible and D type identical or D-negative. At least an immediate spin crossmatch should be performed before issuance, if possible, but the unit(s) must be labeled as "emergency uncrossmatched" if an antiglobulin crossmatch is not completed at the time of issuance.

9.2.3. Urgent Need, Patient Is Alloimmunized

In patients with alloantibodies (current or historic) *and who are not exsanguinating,* complete serologic testing of a fresh patient sample is required. Units selected for crossmatching should, *if at all possible,* lack antigens against which the patient has or is known to have had alloantibodies. When time does not permit phenotyping units (or receipt of antigen negative ones from the blood supplier), AHG crossmatch compatible units can be issued labeled as "crossmatch compatible."

If there is insufficient time to complete the AHG crossmatch, at least an immediate spin crossmatch should show no ABO incompatibility prior to issuance of selected units. These units should be labeled as "emergency uncrossmatched" if issued prior to completion of the AHG crossmatch. All units (or as many as indicated in the massive transfusion protocol) should be completely crossmatched using AHG methods.

9.3. Massive Transfusion

Policies relating to retrospective crossmatch in cases of massive transfusion should be written. Some institutions routinely crossmatch all units transfused. In the current climate of cost constraints, it may be prudent to completely crossmatch only the first 10 units transfused. (Units subsequently given would require repeat collection of new samples because the patient's original blood characteristics would no longer be present.)

9.3.1. No Sample

If no patient sample is available from before the onset of massive transfusion, no crossmatching is possible until a sample can be obtained. Generally, no sample will be required until the massive bleeding is halted. Any sample obtained during the massive bleed will be reflective only of that particular time during the hemorrhage and not necessarily predictive of posthemorrhage serology. Once bleeding is controlled, a new patient sample should be obtained and all subsequent units issued only if compatible using an AHG crossmatch.

Recommendation: In emergency situations, please note the following.

1. Do *not* delay delivery of blood. Issue units labeled as "emergency uncrossmatched."
2. When hemorrhage is life-threatening and until the patient's own blood type is known:
   a. Use O-positive blood for all patients, *except women of childbearing years.*
   b. For women of childbearing years, use O-negative blood.
   c. When patient's type is known, issue type-specific units
3. When time permits:
   a. Perform immediate spin (or electronic) crossmatch before issuing units. Label as "crossmatch compatible."
   b. Select appropriate antigen-negative units for patients with history or evidence of alloimmunization.
   c. Complete an AHG crossmatch after issuance if alloimmunization is discovered.
4. Follow written protocol for massive transfusion situations.

REFERENCES

1. Klein HG, ed. *Standards for Blood Banks and Transfusion Services,* 17th ed. Bethesda, MD: American Association of Blood Banks, 1996.
2. Fuller R, ed. *Technical Manual,* 11th ed. Bethesda, MD: American Association of Blood Banks, 1996.
3. *AABB's Quality Program,* vols. 1 & 2, Bethesda, MD: American Association of Blood Banks, 1995.

4. Title 21, Code of Federal Regulations, Part 606, U. S. Government Printing Office, Washington, D.C., April 1, 1996, and FDA Guideline for Use of Equivalent Procedures for Blood Banks, Bethesda, MD, 1984.
5. Harmening DM, Firestone D. The ABO blood group system. In: Harmening DM, ed. *Modern Blood Banking and Transfusion Practices,* 3rd ed. Philadelphia: F. A. Davis Co., 1994, pp. 102,103.

SUGGESTED READING

Harmening DM, ed. *Modern Blood Banking and Transfusion Practices,* 3rd ed. Philadelphia: F. A. Davis Co., 1994.
Mallory D, ed. *Immunohematology Methods and Procedures,* 1st ed. Rockville, MD: American Red Cross, 1993.
Rudmann SV, ed. *Textbook of Blood Banking and Transfusion Medicine,* Philadelphia, Saunders, 1995.

4

Transfusion in the Face of Autoantibodies

Steven R. Sloan and Leslie E. Silberstein

1. BACKGROUND

It is not unusual for patients to have antibodies directed against their own red blood (RBCs). In many cases, these autoantibodies are totally benign and cause no clinical problems. However, in some instances autoantibodies can cause hemolysis in the patient. If this hemolysis is substantial, an autoimmune hemolytic anemia will develop with significant clinical signs and symptoms. Autoantibodies are readily detected in the Blood Bank laboratory, regardless of whether the autoantibody is pathogenic or benign. This can make it impossible to find compatible blood. In this chapter, the differences between benign and clinically significant autoantibodies are discussed. Next, we discuss the pathophysiology, clinical presentation, laboratory test results, and transfusion therapy for autoimmune hemolytic anemias. Finally, we discuss other situations in which potentially clinically significant autoantibodies can arise.

2. BENIGN AUTOANTIBODIES

Benign autoantibodies (Fig. 1) are often detected in the blood bank when performing a type, screen, or crossmatch (1). Autoantibodies usually are panreactive (i.e., they react with all panel cells tested). The direct antiglobulin test (DAT) will almost always be positive. Several pieces of evidence are used to help determine whether such an antibody is clinically significant. The first and most important step is to determine if the patient has clinical evidence of hemolysis. In addition to obtaining a pertinent history, one should look for laboratory evidence of hemolysis (such as changes on a peripheral blood smear, hemoglobinemia, an increased lactate dehydrogenase (LDH) and bilirubin, and decreased hemoglobinemia). Although there is no perfect test to determine whether an autoantibody is benign or pathogenic, some laboratory tests can help predict the clinical significance of an autoantibody. Autoantibodies that react only at cold temperatures are almost always benign. The higher the temperature at which an autoantibody will react (the higher the "thermal amplitude"), the greater the chance that it will be pathogenic (2). Autoantibodies that react at warm temperatures may be benign, but these autoantibodies are usually present in low titers (2).

From: *Red Cell Transfusion: A Practical Guide*
Edited by: M. E. Reid and S. J. Nance Humana Press Inc., Totowa, NJ

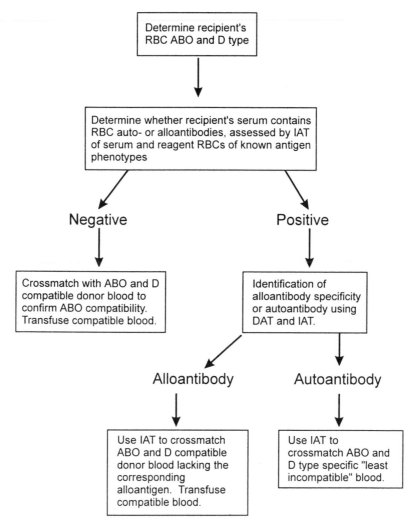

Fig. 1. Algorithm used to determine if allo- or autoantibodies are present in patient's serum.

2.1. Transfusions for Patients with "Benign" Autoantibodies

Benign autoantibodies that are *cold* reactive pose no problem for selection of crossmatch-compatible blood units when all compatibility testing is carried out at 37 °C (e.g., prewarming of both RBCs and the patient's serum).

Patients with seemingly benign *warm* reactive autoantibodies may require transfusions for reasons unrelated to the antibody (bleeding owing to surgery or trauma, for example). If the patient has a history of prior exposure to allogeneic blood (i.e., transfusions or pregnancy), we recommend performing adsorptions to detect alloantibodies that also may be present (*see* Section 3.1. on WAIHA for more details). Clinicians should recognize that this process takes time and should give the blood bank ample warning when patients with autoantibodies will need blood.

3. AUTOIMMUNE HEMOLYTIC ANEMIAS

These are most often chronic disorders that may be primary or secondary to underlying diseases such as B-cell neoplasms or systemic lupus erythematosus (SLE) *(2,3)*. Besides treating the underlying disease, the long-term goal of treatment is to resolve symptoms of the anemia. Although transfusions in these patients can be risky, they are often necessary to treat life-threatening anemias.

3.1. Warm Autoimmune Hemolytic Anemia (WAIHA)

WAIHA is caused by hemolytic autoantibodies directed against RBCs that react at body temperatures. The clinical presentation of WAIHA varies because it can develop gradually or quickly. The principal clinical findings are signs and symptoms generally associated with anemia, jaundice, and an enlarged palpable spleen. Splenomegaly may be the result of an underlying lymphoproliferative disorder or chronic hemolysis. Laboratory findings may include reticulocytosis with microspherocytes, polychromasia, and nucleated erythrocytes on the peripheral smear.

3.2. Laboratory Diagnosis

Laboratory testing in the blood bank provides valuable diagnostic information in cases of WAIHA (Fig. 2). The DAT is usually strongly positive in patients with WAIHA. The titer of the autoantibody does not completely predict the severity of the disease since the pathogenicity of the RBC autoantibody is also influenced by the avidity of the antibody for the RBC autoantigen and the ability of the antibody to fix complement. In WAIHA, IgGs often fix complement. Most WAIHAs are due to immunoglobulins of the IgG1 or IgG3 subclass; these subclasses fix complement better than other IgG subclasses *(4-7)*. If broad-spectrum antiglobulin reagents are initially used in performing the DAT, the laboratory should also use reagents specific for IgG and C3d in cases of suspected WAIHA. If both complement and IgG are detected, a diagnosis of SLE should be considered. IgA and IgM can rarely cause WAIHA and normally do not need to be considered.

The DAT is not specific for WAIHA since a positive DAT is frequently found in the normal population *(1)*. In addition, clotted blood, silicone gel tubes, iv lines containing low ionic strength solution, medications, and hypergammaglobulinemia can all lead to false positive DATs *(8,9)*.

The DAT is also not 100% sensitive in WAIHA (i.e., the DAT can be negative in unusual cases). Even when performed correctly, the DAT may yield a negative result in WAIHA. One reason for this is that the autoantibody may be an IgA or IgM (which is not detected by the antihuman globulin [AHG] reagents normally used). Another reason for a negative DAT in WAIHA is that the autoantibody may be a low affinity IgG. Alternatively, there may be only small numbers of IgG molecules on the erythrocytes, which may still be clinically important.

Manual antiglobulin tests detect 200–500 IgG molecules per cell *(2,10)*. When immune-mediated hemolysis is strongly suspected and the DAT is negative, one can try making a concentrated elute and testing the eluate. This procedure can concentrate the antibody.

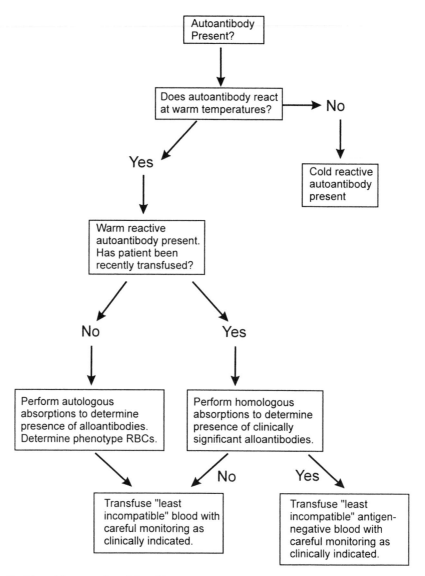

Fig. 2. Algorithm used to identify warm autoantibodies and alloantibodies present in patients with warm autoimmune hemolytic anemia.

3.3. Transfusions for Patients with WAIHA

Transfusing patients with WAIHA can be potentially hazardous, in part because blood bank laboratory testing results can be inconclusive. The autoantibody can interfere with indirect antiglobulin (IAT) tests and RBC phenotype determinations. In addition, even after performing all indicated tests, almost all donor units will be incompatible with the patient's serum.

Because the autoantibody is usually a panagglutinin, screening the patient's serum directly for alloantibodies is usually problematic because the panagglutinin masks the potential existence of an underlying alloantibody *(11)*. The autoantibodies in WAIHA are often directed at an Rh-related molecule since the antibodies often

(50% of the time) react with all cells except Rh_{null} cells *(12,13)*. Such a finding is of no use clinically since Rh_{null} cells are not available for transfusion. In some cases, however, the autoantibody has a relative specificity. Approximately 1–2% of the time, a relative specificity to a particular Rh epitope such as e or D can be identified *(14,15)*. This may be identified by testing the patient's serum directly with a panel of cells; increased reactivity may be seen with cells of a particular Rh phenotype. In some cases, the in vivo survival of transfused RBCs is influenced by the relative specificity of the autoantibody in vitro *(16)*. Some blood banks transfuse random units in these cases, and only transfuse cells lacking the recognized Rh antigen if transfused random units have an unacceptable survival.

3.4. Detecting Alloantibodies in Patients with WAIHA

Alloantibodies will not usually be detected by testing the patient's serum directly. This is important because alloantibodies (usually directed toward antigens Rh or Kell blood group systems) occur in approx 30% of patients with WAIHA and a history of exposure to foreign antigens by pregnancy or previous transfusions. A stronger IAT than a DAT is suggestive that an alloantibody is present.

There are two common methods to detect alloantibodies in patients with auto-antibodies. The first technique involves autogeneic absorptions and the second technique involving allogeneic adsorptions is known as "differential adsorption" test *(17)*. In both techniques, the autoantibody is adsorbed by mixing the patient's serum with red blood cells. The red blood cells bind the autoantibody and the remaining serum has less autoantibody. This usually has to be done multiple times to completely remove detectable levels of autoantibody from the serum.

Autogeneic adsorptions use the patient's own RBCs. All of the RBCs must be from the patient; hence, RBCs collected from patients who have been recently transfused should not be used. If the patient has not been recently transfused, auto-adsorptions are the preferred technique because no alloantibodies will be absorbed onto the patient's own erythrocytes. Prior to the adsorption, the IgG coating the patient's erythrocytes must be eluted from the cells by one of several established techniques *(17)*. The adsorbed serum can then be evaluated for the presence of allo-antibodies using conventional methods.

"Differential adsorption" is more complicated because allogeneic cells can absorb alloantibodies from the serum. Hence, generally one uses three different adsorbing cells of known phenotypes or cells selected to match the patient's phenotype. Knowing the phenotypes allows one to determine which alloantibodies can be adsorbed from the serum. For instance, a cell lacking the K antigen will not absorb anti-K. The adsorbed serum can then be tested against K+ and K− cells to determine if an anti-K is present. Because of the complexities, this is a time intensive and expensive test. Hence, in general one only tests for limited number of alloantibodies using differential adsorptions. The most common clinically significant alloantibodies should be investigated. These include antibodies directed against Rh, Kell, Kidd, and Duffy blood group system antigens.

To determine the phenotype of the erythrocytes in patients with WAIHA, one uses erythrocytes that have been stripped of antibodies by elution techniques. Some elution methods are not recommended for preparing cells for antigen typing. It is useful to determine the phenotype of the patient's erythrocytes when they initially develop WAIHA before they have been transfused. Knowing the phenotype dictates which alloantibodies the patient is capable of producing.

3.5. Selecting RBC Units for Patients with WAIHA

Even after completion of these serologic tests, in most cases no units of RBCs will be compatible with the patient. Hence, there is always a risk in transfusing patients with WAIHA and transfusions should be reserved for patients with life-threatening anemias *(2,3)*. Patients with symptomatic anemia should be placed at bed rest and provided with oxygen. Symptoms requiring transfusions include angina and neurologic disturbances, which often begin as lethargy but can progress to coma. In addition, older patients who are at risk for cerebral vascular accidents and cardiovascular disease should be transfused for symptomatic anemia, even if the hemoglobin is >7 g/dL. In general, blood should be transfused slowly with close monitoring for signs and symptoms of accelerated hemolysis. The goal of the transfusion is to alleviate symptoms. Once symptoms are resolved, the transfusion should be discontinued. As little as 100–200 mL of blood may be sufficient to relieve symptoms in patients with a well-compensated anemia undergoing moderate hemolysis. In rare aggressive cases of WAIHA, hemolysis occurs rapidly and transfusions are not effective. In these cases, aggressive transfusion therapy may be needed, often accompanied by a series of plasmapheresis.

Although transfusions are risky in these patients, failure to transfuse when indicated can be even more hazardous. Any patient with symptoms of a life-threatening anemia should be transfused regardless of the stage of laboratory testing. Although there is greater risk before the blood bank work-up is completed, the risks associated with severe anemia in a patient undergoing hemolysis can be worse.

Patients undergoing transfusion therapy can develop new antibodies and require periodic serologic evaluations. Repeat testing using differential adsorptions should be performed at least weekly and more frequently if there is evidence of a new antibody specificity. An increase in strength of the DAT or IAT suggests that a new antibody may be developing.

4. COLD AGGLUTININ DISEASE

CAD (Fig. 3) is a group of disorders caused by RBC antibodies that bind and agglutinate RBCs at cold temperatures (4–18°C). The major forms of the disease include transient CAD and chronic CAD. Chronic CAD, which is more prevalent than transient CAD, can be idiopathic or secondary to an underlying malignancy.

4.1. Chronic Idiopathic CAD

Chronic idiopathic CAD usually develops in the fifth to eighth decades of life. These patients often have moderately severe, partially compensated anemia and complain of fatigue and malaise. Patients with idiopathic CAD usually have a good long-term survival and may show periods of spontaneous exacerbations and remissions.

The cold agglutinin is usually an IgM autoantibody that transiently binds to erythrocytes and fixes complement in the peripheral circulation. Upon re-entering the central circulation, the antibody elutes off the cells but complement (C3b) remains on the cells. Some of the cells are cleared in the hepatic circulation, where they encounter

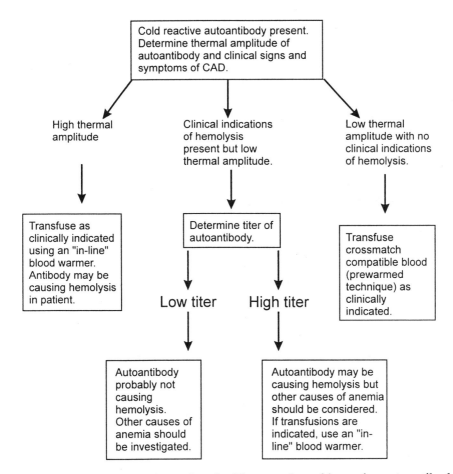

Fig. 3. Algorithm used to determine significance of a cold-reactive autoantibody.

macrophages with receptors specific for C3b. However, many erythrocytes are not coated with enough C3b to activate phagocytosis by macrophages (hepatic clearance of C3b-coated RBCs requires 500–800 C3b molecules per RBC). Hence, these patients usually have only a mild anemia and a DAT performed on blood from these patients will often be positive for complement but not for immunoglobulin (2). The C3b molecules on RBC are subject to breakdown by C3b inactivator enzymes produced by the liver. These enzymes convert C3b into C3c and C3d, although only C3d remains on the RBC. These C3d-coated RBCs have been shown to have a near normal survival.

Some cases of CAD can lead to severe intravascular hemolysis owing to complement-mediated lysis. This can occur if the C3b inactivator proteins are impaired or if the IgM binds at warm temperatures, resulting in efficient complement activation. In these patients, exposure to cold temperatures can accelerate hemolysis resulting in a brisk drop in hematocrit and renal failure.

Patients with CAD may develop ischemic digital infarcts and ulcers, and, on exposure to cold, attacks of acrocyanosis. This is caused by agglutination of the RBCs in the arterioles in the cooler portions of the body. These symptoms may be the patient's chief complaint.

4.2. Chronic Secondary CAD

Chronic secondary CAD is often secondary to B-cell neoplasms such as lymphomas, Waldenström's macroglobulinemia, and chronic lymphocytic leukemia (CLL). Unlike patients with idiopathic CAD, these patients often have lymphadenopathy or splenomegaly. The other signs and symptoms of CAD are identical to those seen in the idiopathic form of the disease.

4.3. Transient CAD

Transient CAD occurs in a younger population. An abrupt onset anemia develops following an infection such as mycoplasma pneumonia or mononucleosis. The anemia can be severe but the disease is usually self-limited.

4.4. Serologic Tests for CAD

Serologic testing in the blood bank contributes to the diagnosis of CAD. Patients always have cold reactive autoantibodies but this is not diagnostic for CAD since such antibodies are commonly found in individuals following some infections and in many healthy individuals. Cold agglutinins causing CAD are usually present in a high titer (>1:1,000). Reactivity at higher temperatures, however, is a better predictor of disease severity. Occasionally reactivity is detected at temperatures as high as 37 °C. Cold agglutinins are IgM antibodies, so the DAT is usually positive for C3d but not IgG. Occasionally, however, low titers of IgG or IgA may accompany the IgM. These antibodies can also precipitate in the cold in approx 25% of cases.

Laboratory testing can also help differentiate the various forms of CAD. In almost all cases, the antibodies found in chronic CAD are IgM x monoclonal proteins directed against the "I" antigen. Antibodies with this specificity are also present in transient CAD following mycoplasma pneumonia but are not monoclonal as defined by immunofixation. The antibodies that develop following infectious mononucleosis are polyclonal and often have anti-i specificity. Whereas CAD caused by both polyclonal and monoclonal antibodies usually express x chain, the rare occurrence of λ light chain is associated with monoclonal secondary to B-cell neoplasms.

4.5. Treatment of CAD

Medical therapy for all forms of the disease is of only limited benefit. Transient CAD usually self-limited and other than keeping the patients warm and at rest, no medical treatment other than transfusions are usually indicated. Whereas chronic CAD does not spontaneously resolve, there are few effective treatments. Corticosteroids are usually ineffective unless there is an IgG component that contributes significantly to the hemolysis. Corticosteroids can be effective in one aggressive variant of CAD in which patients have a low titer antibody with a high thermal amplitude. In some instances of severe cold antibody-induced hemolysis, plasmapheresis may be an effective temporary therapeutic measure. For example, some patients do not respond to RBC transfusions with an expected rise in hemoglobin owing to ongoing intravascular hemolysis. In our experience, these cases often benefit from a short course of plasmapheresis. Long-term, chronic administration of immunosuppressive agents such as Immuran often do not achieve the desired results and are associated with many side-effects. Treatment of secondary CAD consists of treatment of the underlying disease, and the severity of the hemolysis often waxes and wanes in parallel with the underlying process.

4.6. Transfusions for Patients with CAD

Because medical therapy is usually ineffective, patients with chronic CAD may require occasional transfusions and patients with transient CAD may require transfusions during the period of anemia. Unlike WAIHA, identifying alloantibodies and finding crossmatch-compatible units is usually relatively straightforward since the panagglutinin in CAD is usually nonreactive at 37°C and will not mask any underlying alloantibodies. In rare cases, an antibody with reactivity at 37°C will also be present in patients with CAD. If this antibody is an IgM, its reactivity can be removed with 2-mercaptoethanol. If an associated IgG is responsible for the warm reactivity, then strategies similar to those used for WAIHA need to be employed to detect alloantibodies.

Transfusing patients with CAD can be particularly hazardous. The transfused cells are prone to rapid hemolysis because, unlike the patient's own cells, the transfused cells are not protectively coated with C3d,g. "Inline" warmers should be used for transfusions useful for iv solutions to limit the effects of the cold agglutinin.

Patients with CAD may occasionally need surgery for reasons unrelated to their CAD. Caution must be observed if the surgery involves making the patient hypothermic (such as some types of neurosurgery and cardiac surgery). Hypothermia should not be a problem for most patients with cold reactive autoantibodies, but hypothermia should be minimized in patients with CAD. In these cases, the blood bank can determine the thermal amplitude of the antibody to determine the coldest temperature that is safe for the patient. Additionally, if the cold reactive antibody is of high thermal amplitude and clinically significant, a series of plasmapheresis prior to surgery may be helpful to lower the concentration of antibodies.

4.7. Paroxysmal Cold Hemoglobinuria (PCH)

PCH describes a group of two related disorders caused by autoantibodies that bind to erythrocytes at cold temperatures. These antibodies fix complement resulting in hemolysis at warmer temperatures. Currently, the most frequent type of PCH occurs in children and young adults. Following a viral infection, patients develop constitutional symptoms of fulminant intravascular hemolysis including hemoglobinemia, hemoglobinuria, jaundice, severe anemia, and sometimes renal failure. The disease is self-limited, lasting 2–3 wk.

Historically, PCH has also been described in adults with tertiary syphilis and children with congenital syphilis. Patients develop hemolysis on exposure to cold. These patients develop paroxysms of hemoglobinuria and constitutional symptoms such as fever, back and leg pain, abdominal cramps, and rigors followed by hemoglobinuria. Because syphilis is easily treated, this variant is rare.

4.8. Laboratory Testing

To consider a diagnosis of PCH, there should be laboratory evidence of intravascular hemolysis such as increased LDH or bilirubin or a decreased haptoglobin. The next test that is usually performed for most cases of suspected immune-mediated hemolysis is the DAT. However, the DAT performed with anti-IgG will almost always be negative in PCH. Hence, if one has high clinical suspicion of PCH, a Donath-Landsteiner test should be performed. This test detects the Donath-Landsteiner antibody, which binds to RBCs and fixes complement. This leads to complement-mediated hemolysis when the RBCs are brought to warmer temperatures. In performing the test, patient's erythrocytes are mixed with patient's serum. Normal serum is also added to one tube, since patients with PCH often have low levels of complement. Controls include samples that are kept warm, kept cool, and samples that contain patient RBCs but no patient serum. A positive result of the tests requires hemolysis to occur only in the tubes that have been cooled and then warmed and which contain the patient's serum and erythrocytes.

The Donath-Landsteiner test detects the "Donath-Landsteiner antibody." This antibody is often directed against an antigen in the GLOB collection, but rare examples of specificities to I, i, and Pr have been described *(18–20)*.

4.9. Transfusing Patients with PCH

Patients with PCH can develop severe anemia necessitating transfusions. Because the antibody does not have a high thermal amplitude, reagent panel RBCs can be tested and crossmatches performed at 37°C without problem. Significant alloantibodies can be detected and crossmatch-compatible units can usually be identified. Transfusions and administrations of iv fluids should be performed using "in line" blood warmers and patient should be kept warm. Under these conditions, there should not be significant risk of transfusion reaction. If severe intravascular hemolysis occurs with random units, consideration should be given to the transfusion of units negative for the specificity of the antibody.

4.10. Drug-Induced Immune Hemolytic Anemia

Drugs can induce immune hemolytic anemia through a variety of mechanisms. Drug-induced immune hemolytic anemia is unusual now that penicillin is not commonly used in very high doses (>20,000,000 U/d) and α-methyldopa is not frequently used for hypertension *(2)*. Since the late 1980s, however, second- and third-generation cephalosporins have caused immune-mediated hemolysis in several patients *(21)*. Penicillin, α-methyldopa, and other drugs still occasionally induce immune-mediated hemolysis.

In addition to the normal role of the blood bank laboratory in performing antibody screens and finding crossmatch-compatible blood, additional testing can help diagnose a drug-induced immune hemolytic anemia and identify the offending drug. Even if the patient does not require transfusions, this testing can be critical in patient management since the definitive treatment of any drug-induced immune hemolytic anemia is to discontinue administration of the offending drug. The laboratory test results will vary depending on the mechanism by which the drug induces hemolysis.

4.11. Mechanism 1: Opsonization of Membrane with Drug

Antibodies recognize drugs that have attached to the RBC membrane. Penicillin acts by this mechanism and usually only large doses of penicillin cause hemolysis.

Lower doses of penicillin often induce low-avidity antibodies resulting in a positive DAT, but rarely cause hemolysis. Laboratory findings stem from the fact that the antibody is directed against the drug, not the RBCs. The penicillin antibody that causes hemolysis is directed against the benzyl-penicilloyl groups of penicillin; antibodies of this specificity do not typically cause penicillin allergies *(22)*. The DAT is positive because the drug (and antibody) are on the patient's RBCs. The IAT is negative because the erythrocytes used in the IAT are not opsonized. Antibodies eluted from the patient's erythrocytes do not react with other cells because elution removes the antibody and not the drug. Both the eluate and the serum are positive in the IAT when tested with penicillin-coated erythrocytes. Alloantibodies can be identified and crossmatch-compatible blood can usually be found. If the patient develops life-threatening anemia, transfusions may be needed as a temporizing measure.

4.12. Mechanism 2: So-Called "Immune Complex Formation"

Antibodies can recognize complexes of plasma proteins bound to drugs or drug metabolites. The classic example of a drug causing immune complex formation (Fig. 4) is quinidine. This entire antibody:protein:drug complex, also known as an immune complex, can bind to RBCs long enough to activate complement, resulting in intravascular hemolysis, which can lead to hemoglobinemia, hemoglobinuria, and possibly renal failure. Because the antibody component of these complexes are usually of the IgM class, the DAT usually only detects complement. The patient's serum contains few immune complexes because almost all of the complexes are bound to erythrocytes. The IAT is often negative because too few immune complexes are present to coat the test erythrocytes. If a drug (or drug metabolite) is added in vitro, however, additional immune complexes can form and the IAT can be positive. Eluates are also nonreactive in the absence of the drug.

Second- and third-generation cephalosporins usually induce hemolysis by this mechanism in combination with the penicillin type of opsonization *(21)*. Testing for cephalosporin-induced hemolytic anemias is difficult because several cephalosporins modify the RBC membranes so that proteins are adsorbed nonimmunologically to the cell membranes. This can result in false-positive test results. To avoid these false positives, one can dilute the patient's serum (1:20) and/or prepare drug-coated RBCs at low pH (pH 6.0–7.3) *(21)*.

Since the IAT is negative, alloantibodies can be identified and crossmatch-compatible blood can be found using the usual techniques. Whereas transfused blood is as susceptible to immune complexes as patient's blood, immune complexes are not initially bound to transfused blood. If the drug is discontinued, then very few immune complexes may be present to bind to transfused blood and it may have a longer lifespan than the patient's own blood, which is already bound by immune complexes.

4.13. Mechanism 3: Anti-RBC Antibodies Induced by Drugs

Finally, some autoantibodies are induced by drugs. α-methyldopa is the classic drug that induces this type of antibody response. Approximately 20% of patients taking α-methyldopa develop a positive DAT, but only approx 1% develop a

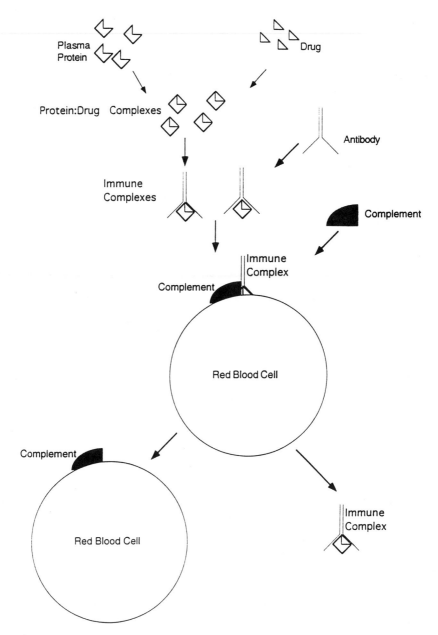

Fig. 4. Diagram depicting drug-induced immune complex formation inducing hemolysis.

hemolytic anemia. The antibodies that are induced are usually only IgG (no complement is detected) and typically have a relative Rh specificity. The serology is identical to that which is found in WAIHA (a positive DAT with a panreactive antibody in the serum).

In these cases, routine screening for alloantibodies will detect the drug-induced autoantibody; no drug needs to be added to detect the antibody in the laboratory. Because these antibodies are usually panagglutinins, crossmatch-compatible blood can almost never be found and transfused blood will be as susceptible to hemolysis as the patient's blood. Transfusion therapy in these patients is directed by the same guidelines as those used in WAIHA.

5. OTHER CASES OF AUTOANTIBODIES

There are a variety of other situations in which serologic testing suggests the presence of erythrocyte autoantibodies. In some cases, these are true autoantibodies; in others, these are passively acquired antibodies that mimic autoantibodies on serologic testing.

5.1. Pregnancy

Pregnant women may have an increased risk of developing autoantibodies and WAIHA *(23)*. The largest study to date suggests that pregnancy increases the risk of WAIHA fourfold *(24)*. Fetal RBCs possess both maternal and paternal antigens and these cells may serve as a stimulus for maternal autosensitized immunocompetent cells. Consistent with this theory is the observation of immune hemolytic disease in some of the neonates from these pregnancies. The severity of the hemolysis in these patients is variable. Some of these patients require medical interventions such as corticosteroids and some may require transfusions. Transfusions are just as risky in these patients as they are in all patients with WAIHA.

5.2. Neonates

Neonates often have IgG coating their erythrocytes, which can be detected by performing a DAT on neonatal (or umbilical cord) blood. These antibodies are almost always maternal antibodies that crossed the placenta. Maternal IgG antibodies directed against the D antigen are classically associated with hemolytic disease of the newborn but this is uncommon now that Rh immune globulin is administered to D– mothers. ABO incompatibilities between mothers and infants can cause many neonates to develop a positive DAT, but very few suffer from significant hemolysis. Hence, we do not feel it is cost effective to routinely perform a DAT on all neonatal blood samples.

If neonatal hemolysis is suspected, a DAT can help identify the etiology of the hemolysis. An eluate from the neonatal cells can be tested by usual techniques to determine the specificity of the antibody. Often, the positive DAT is the result of anti-A,B antibodies produced by type O mothers (we see this in 30% of nontype O babies born to type O mothers); hence, the eluate is often tested against type A and/or type B cells in addition to the type O reagent RBCs. Also, a positive DAT caused by anti-D is sometimes detected in D+ infants born to D– mothers who have been given Rh immune globulin. In these cases, the Rh immune globulin itself coats the infant's erythrocytes, but does not cause significant hemolysis.

Occasionally a baby with a positive DAT requires transfusions, which often are exchange transfusions. The RBCs should be compatible with maternal serum (infant's serum is also acceptable). In some cases, RBCs should be transfused that are not the same phenoype as the infant's. For instance, a maternal anti-K antibody may be responsible for neonatal hemolysis. Even though the infant is K+, he/she should receive K-negative blood. In these situations, the transfused cells may have a longer lifespan than the baby cells.

6. PASSIVE IMMUNIZATIONS

6.1. Platelet Components

Donors and recipients of platelets are not necessarily of the same ABO type. Hence, plasma contained in platelet transfusions may contain anti-A and/or anti-B and cause a positive DAT if the patient's erythrocytes are type A or B. This rarely causes hemolysis but some blood banks make sure that the antibody titer in the donor product is not exceptionally high to avoid potential hemolysis. A positive DAT following a platelet transfusion with the eluate containing anti-A and/or anti-B is normally of no clinical significance. As long as no anti-A and/or anti-B is detected in the serum, RBC units which are the patient's blood type are crossmatched using standard procedures.

6.2. Intravenous Immunoglobulin (IvIg)

IvIg is administered to some patients to modulate the immune response. This product is a concentrate prepared from human plasma and contains antibodies of various specificities. Not surprisingly, anti-RBC antibodies can be a component of these preparations. Anti-A, anti-B, and anti-D have been detected in various lots of IvIg. There are several reports of patients developing positive DATs after receiving these preparations and some of these patients developed immune-mediated hemolysis (25).

Although it is usually unnecessary to consider passively acquired antibodies when transfusing a patient, laboratory tests are used to confirm that the antibody is passively acquired. Any alloantibody that is detected in a patient's serum should not be considered passively acquired; transfused blood should lack the antigen recognized by such an antibody. When a patient who has received IvIg develops a positive DAT, an eluate is performed and the specificity of the antibody determined. The antibody is probably passively acquired if anti-A or anti-B specificity is demonstrated; in these cases, there is no need to transfuse blood of a different ABO blood group than the patient's. Any other antibody detected in the eluate from a patient who has been recently transfused may be passively acquired or may be a newly developing alloantibody being produced by the patient's immune system. In this case, transfused blood should lack the offending antigen. If the patient had not been recently transfused, then any antibody detected in the eluate is probably passively acquired but the patient must still receive IAT-crossmatch compatible blood.

6.3. Anti-Thymocyte Globulin (ATGAM)

ATGAM is an immunoglobulin preparation derived from horse serum that contains reactivity against human T-lymphocytes. Many of these preparations contain antibodies that can adhere to erythrocytes, but these are rarely clinically significant. However, there have been case reports of patients developing hemolysis that was probably caused by RBCs antibodies present in some lots of ATGAM (26).

Serologic testing of specimens from patients receiving ATGAM can be misleading. The DAT may be positive, even though the antibodies from the ATGAM do not lead to hemolysis. Less frequently, the DAT can be negative even though ATGAM is causing hemolysis.

False positive DATs occur because rabbit antihuman globulin reagents often contain antibodies that react with horse immunoglobulin. This reactivity can be neutralized with horse serum *(17)*.

Negative DATs occur because not all AHG reagents recognize horse antibodies. Testing with antihorse immunoglobulin can overcome this problem, but this is not immediately available at most blood banks. In general, detecting the horse immunoglobulins should not be necessary since they do not usually cause hemolysis and they do not usually have specificity toward particular human antigens.

7. SUMMARY

Patients with autoantibodies present challenges to clinicians and blood bank personnel. A patient's clinical condition will influence the blood bank work-up and must considered when interpreting laboratory tests. Communication between the blood bank and the clinicians can facilitate management of these patients.

REFERENCES

1. Gorst DW, Rawlinson VI, Merry AH, Stratton F. Positive direct antiglobulin test in normal individuals. *Vox Sanguinis* 1980;38:99–105.
2. Schwartz RS, Silberstein LE, Berkman EM. Autoimmune hemolytic anemias. In: Hoffman REJ, Benz J, Shattil SJ, Furie B, Cohen HJ, Silberstein LE, eds. *Hematology: Basic Principles and Practice,* 2nd ed. New York: Churchill, 1995, pp. 710–729.
3. Jefferies LC, Transfusion therapy in autoimmune hemolytic anemia. *Hema Onc Clin N Am* 1994:1087–1104.
4. Huber H, Douglas SD, Nusbacher J, Kochwa S, Rosenfield RE. IgG subclass specificity of human monocyte receptor sites. *Nature* 1971;229:419,420.
5. Sokol RJ, Booker DJ, Stamps R. The pathology of autoimmune haemolytic anaemia. *J Clin Path* 1992;45:1047–1052.
6. LoBuglio AF, Cotran RS, Jandl JH. Red cells coated with immunoglobulin G: binding and sphering by mononuclear cells in man. *Science* 1967;158:1582–1585.
7. Abramson N, Gelfand EW, Jandl JH, Rosen FS. The interaction between human monocytes and red cells. Specificity for IgG subclasses and IgG fragments. *J Exp Med* 1970;132:1207–1215.
8. Freedman J, Massey A. Complement components detected on normal red blood cells taken into EDTA and CPD. *Vox Sanguinis* 1979;37:1–8.
9. Molthan L, Reidenberg MM, Eichman MF. Positive direct Coombs tests due to cephalothin. *N Engl J Med* 1967;277:123–125.
10. Merry AH, Thomson EE, Rawlinson VI, Stratton F. The quantification of C3 fragments on erythrocytes: estimation of C3 fragments on normal cells, acquired haemolytic anaemia cases and correlation with agglutination of sensitized cells. *Clin Lab Haematol* 1983;5:387–397.
11. Issitt PD, Pavone BG, Goldfinger D, et al. Anti-Wrb, and other autoantibodies responsible for positive direct antiglobulin tests in 150 individuals. *Br J Haematol* 1976;34:5–18.
12. Weiner W, Vos GH. Serology of acquired hemolytic anemias. *Blood* 1963;22:606.
13. Celano MJ, Levine P. Anti-LW specificity in autoimmune acquired hemolytic anemia. *Transfusion* 1967;7:265–268.
14. Bell CA, Zwicker H, Sacks HJ. Autoimmune hemolytic anemia: routine serologic evaluation in a general hospital population. *Am J Clin Pathol* 1973;60:903–911.

15. Habibi B, Homberg JC, Schaison G, Salmon C. Autoimmune hemolytic anemia children. A review of 80 cases. *Am J Med* 1974;56:61–69.
16. Mollison PL, Engelfriet CP, Contreras M. *Red Cell Antibodies Against Self Antigens, Bound Antigens and Induced Antigens. Blood Transfusion in Clinical Medicine,* 9th ed. Cambridge, MA: Blackwell, 1993, pp. 283–320.
17. Walker RHM, ed. *Technical Manual,* 11th ed. Bethesda, MD: American Association of Blood Banks, 1993.
18. Judd WJ, Wilkinson SL, Issitt PD, Johnson TL, Keren DF, Steiner EA. Donath-Landsteiner hemolytic anemia due to an anti-Pr-like biphasic hemolysin. *Transfusion* 1986;26:423–425.
19. Shirey RS, Park K, Ness PM, et al. An anti-i biphasic hemolysin in chronic paroxysmal cold hemoglobinuria. *Transfusion* 1986;26:62–64.
20. Worlledge SM, Rousso C. Studies on the serology of paroxysmal cold haemoglobinuria (PCH) with special reference to its relationship with the P blood group system. *Vox Sanguinis* 1965;10:293.
21. Garratty G. Review: immune hemolytic anemia and/or positive direct antiglobulin tests caused by drugs. *Immunohematology* 1994;10:41–50.
22. Garratty G, Petz LD. Drug-induced immune hemolytic anemia. *Am J Med* 1975;58: 398–407.
23. Sokol RJ, Hewitt S. Autoimmune hemolysis: a critical review. *Crit Rev Oncol Hematol* 1985;4:125–154.
24. Sokol RJ, Hewitt S, Stamps BK. Erythrocyte autoantibodies, autoimmune haemolysis and pregnancy. *Vox Sanguinis* 1982;43:169–176.
25. Copelan EA, Strohm PL, Kennedy MS, Tutschka PJ. Hemolysis following intravenous immune globulin therapy. *Transfusion* 1986;26:410–412.
26. Prchal JT, Huang ST, Court WS, Poon MC. Immune hemolytic anemia following administration of antithymocyte globulin. *Am J Hematol* 1985;19:95–98.

5

Red Blood Cell Transfusion
of the Immunocompromised Patient

Christopher P. Stowell

1. INTRODUCTION

In this chapter, some of the special problems of red blood cell (RBC) transfusion in immunocompromised patients are discussed. The transfusion therapy of some of these immunocompromised patients is dealt with specifically in later chapters (*see* Chapters 7, 8, and 12 on solid-organ transplant recipients, progenitor-cell transplant recipients, and chronically transfused patients). Immunocompromised patients are obviously at risk for all of the complications of transfusion that may occur in patients with intact immune systems and which are described in Chapter 13. This chapter deals specifically with those complications that are usually limited to patients with congenital or acquired deficiencies of the immune system: Transfusion-associated graft-vs-host disease (TAGVHD), transfusion-transmitted cytomegalovirus (CMV) infection, and anaphylactic or anaphylactoid reactions in patients who are IgA deficient. Patients who are usually considered to be immunocompromised are listed in Table 1. Clearly, the degree of immunodeficiency varies greatly among these groups. Not all of these patients are at equal risk for the transfusion complications discussed here; however, consideration must be given to these particular untoward effects of transfusion in the course of the care of the immunocompromised patient.

2. PASSENGER LEUKOCYTES AND LEUKODEPLETION

2.1. Background

Passenger leukocytes in the transfused unit of RBCs are responsible for two transfusion complications that are particularly serious for immunocompromised recipients, transfusion-associated GVHD and CMV infection, as well as a number of other complications which are seen in immunologically intact recipients. For this reason, a brief discussion of leukocyte-associated transfusion complications and the role of leukodepletion in avoiding them precedes the discussion of transfusion-associated GVHD and CMV infection.

From: *Red Cell Transfusion: A Practical Guide*
Edited by: M. E. Reid and S. J. Nance Humana Press Inc., Totowa, NJ

Table 1
Immunocompromised Patients

Congenital T- and/or B-Cell immunodeficiencies
   (e.g., SCIDS, Wiskott-Aldrich Syndrome, X-linked
   agammaglobulinemia, IgA deficiency)
Acquired immunodeficiency syndrome (AIDS)
Preterm neonates
Fetuses
Hematologic malignancies
Solid tumors (especially with chemo- or radiotherapy)
Transplant recipients
Immunosuppressive medication

Table 2
Leukocyte-Mediated Transfusion
Complications in Immunocompromised Patients

Well-established complications
   Febrile nonhemolytic transfusion reactions
   Alloimmunization
   Transfusion-related acute lung injury (TRALI)
   Graft-vs-host disease
   Infection with CMV, human T-cell lymphotropic virus I
Possible complications
   Immunosuppression
   Infection with Epstein-Barr virus, human herpes virus
     type 6
   Viral activation (HIV, CMV)

2.2. Transfusion Complications Attributed to Leukocytes

Approximately $1–2 \times 10^9$ leukocytes are present in a unit of whole blood or packed RBCs and are responsible for a number of immunologic and infectious complications of transfusion that may be seen in immunocompromised as well as immunocompetent patients (*see* Table 2) *(1)*. The etiologic roles for leukocytes in febrile, nonhemolytic transfusion reactions, alloimmunization, some forms of transfusion-related acute lung injury (TRALI), and TAGVHD are quite well established. Immunosuppressive effects of transfusion have been inferred from animal studies and the correlation between transfusion and the incidence of postoperative infections and tumor recurrence; however, evidence for a causal relationship is incomplete. Leukocytes may also harbor and transmit intracellular organisms such as CMV and human T-cell lymphotropic virus, type I (HTLV-I). The ability of transfused leukocytes to transmit other infectious agents, such as Epstein-Barr virus or human herpes virus type 6, or to activate other latent viruses (such as CMV and HIV) is being studied.

Table 3
Efficacy of Leukodepletion

Indications with clinical evidence of efficacy
    Febrile, nonhemolytic transfusion reactions
    Alloimmunization
    CMV transmission
Indications with experimental evidence of efficacy
    HIV activation
Indications with physiologic rationale
    Immunosuppression
    TAGVHD
    TRALI
    Transmission of other lymphotropic viruses

Table 4
Indications for Leukodepleted RBCs

Patients with febrile, nonhemolytic transfusion reactions
Patients requiring long-term platelet transfusions
    (alloimmunization risk)
Solid-organ or hematopoietic-cell transplant recipients
    (alloimmunization risk)
Patients requiring CMV-safe transfusions

2.3. Leukodepletion

2.3.1. Indications

Removing leukocytes from RBCs has been suggested as a logical means of preventing the complications listed in Table 2. Table 3 summarizes the efficacy of leukodepletion in preventing several complications attributed to leukocytes. Lowering the leukocyte load in a unit of red cells to $< 5 \times 10^8$ prevents most febrile, nonhemolytic transfusion reactions in chronically transfused patients *(2)*. Reducing the residual leukocyte number to $< 5 \times 10^6$ decreases the incidence of alloimmunization, which is most frequently expressed as refractoriness to platelet transfusion *(3)*. The use of third-generation leukodepletion filters is effective in preventing CMV transmission *(4,5)*. The ability of leukodepletion to reduce or prevent other leukocyte-associated transfusion complications has not been proven. Hence, the use of leukodepleted cellular blood components is commonly recommended for the patients listed in Table 4.

2.3.2. Techniques

There are many techniques for reducing the number of leukocytes present in cellular components; however, to comply with the Standards of the American Association of Blood Banks (AABB) *(6)* the method must result in the recovery of at least

Table 5
Routes of CMV Infection

Perinatal
Breast milk
Sexual contact
Body fluids
Blood transfusion
Organ transplantation

80% of the RBCs and reduce the residual leukocyte number to $< 5 \times 10^8$ if the component is to be used to prevent febrile, nonhemolytic transfusion reactions. If leukodepletion is indicated for any other reason, such as the prevention of alloimmunization, the residual leukocytes must number $< 5 \times 10^6$.

A variety of methods have been used to remove leukocytes from RBCs including differential centrifugation and removal of the buffy coat, centrifugation and filtration with a microaggregate filter, washing, or deglycerolizing frozen cells *(7)*. The residual leukocyte number produced by these techniques ranges from slightly $< 10^8$ for frozen, deglycerolized RBCs to nearly 10^9 for several of the simpler differential centrifugation methods. These levels are generally acceptable for reducing febrile, nonhemolytic transfusion reactions, but not for other applications. The leukodepletion filters developed in the past decade reduce the leukocyte content by three logs (99.9% removal) and are capable of producing a component with $< 1 \times 10^6$ residual leukocytes *(8)*. Filter technology continues to improve and even more effective filters are being evaluated. The available filters, which may be used in the blood center for prestorage leukodepletion, in the transfusion service, or at the bedside, are effective for reducing alloimmunization and CMV transmission.

3. TRANSFUSION-TRANSMITTED CMV INFECTION

3.1. Background

Cytomegalovirus is a ubiquitous member of the herpes virus family that is characterized by the ability to remain latent for extended periods of time in infected host cells. Unlike some of the other herpes viruses, it is capable of infecting and residing in a wide range of human tissues, including blood mononuclear cells, most probably T-cells and monocytes, as well as kidney, lung, liver, and brain. It is generally associated with subclinical infection or a mild mononucleosis-like syndrome in immunocompetent individuals. Approximately 30–80% of adults in developed countries have been exposed to CMV as indicated by the presence of antibodies *(9)*. The routes of CMV infection are listed in Table 5. The most frequent routes of infection are thought to be ante/perinatal exposure and sexual contact. Maternal CMV infection is a major source for infants who become infected by passage through a contaminated cervix during birth or by ingestion of breast milk. The presence of CMV in the urine and respiratory tract of infected individuals and the patterns of spread in daycare and home settings suggest that other routes of exposure may also be important, especially from infected children who tend to shed virus for prolonged periods and may infect other susceptible children and adults. Since CMV can infect

Table 6
Patterns of CMV Infection

Primary infection
Reactivation
Reinfection/coinfection

many tissues, including blood mononuclear cells and solid organs, susceptible patients may also become infected by transplantation *(10)* or transfusion *(11)* from infected donors.

Three patterns of CMV infection have been described; primary infection, reactivation, and re- or coinfection (*see* Table 6) *(12)*. Primary infection occurs when a naive individual (CMV seronegative) is exposed to the virus. Primary infection may be marked by seroconversion (IgM followed by IgG), viral shedding (in the urine, typically), fever, and lymphocytosis. Although CMV infection rarely produces serious disease in immunologically intact hosts, it is associated with systemic infection in immunocompromised patients and may be manifested as pneumonitis, enteritis, retinitis, and other infections. CMV infection in immunocompromised patients is also associated with allograft rejection and dysfunction, and superinfection with other organisms. Following recovery, CMV may remain in a latent form in infected cells for years. Replication of latent virus may be triggered by immunosuppression or other unknown stimuli resulting in reactivation. The clinical course of reactivation is much milder than that of primary infection. It is usually marked by an increase in the titer of anti-CMV IgG (though occasionally an IgM response is noted) and viral shedding. Finally, previously infected individuals may become infected with a different strain of CMV. The clinical course of CMV re- or coinfection has been variably reported to be either more severe *(13)* or less severe *(14)* than reactivation. The more general availability of reliable experimental tools for distinguishing between CMV strains may now make it possible to characterize this relatively poorly understood pattern of CMV infection more thoroughly.

3.2. Transfusion-Transmitted CMV Infection

CMV infection may occur as a result of transfusion of blood from a donor whose mononuclear cells carry latent virus. The donor is invariably well at the time of donation, and may have been infected many years before the donation. Once transfused, latent virus may become activated, begin to replicate, and infect the cells of the transfusion recipient. Posttransfusion CMV infection rates of 10–50% were reported in the 1970s and early 1980s. More recently, infection rates of approx 1% have been reported *(15)*. The distinction between CMV infection and disease is seen quite clearly in immunocompetent individuals who are exposed to CMV by transfusion. Whereas many become infected, only a few develop CMV disease. Following infection, most immunocompetent individuals are completely asymptomatic, whereas the remainder develop only a mild, self-limited illness.

The incidence of transfusion-transmitted CMV infection and CMV disease is affected by both donor and host factors. Donor factors affect predominantly CMV infection. Since CMV is transmitted in latent form in passenger leukocytes, only cellular components appear to be capable of transmitting CMV, whereas the acellular

Table 7
Indications for CMV-Safe Components

Seronegative pregnant women (including intrauterine transfusions)
Low birth weight (< 1200 g) neonates who are seronegative or
     whose serological status is unknown
Seronegative recipients of seronegative bone-marrow or solid-
     organ allografts
Seronegative autogeneic bone-marrow transplant recipients
Seronegative AIDS patients

components have not been reported to do so *(16)*. Components containing the largest numbers of leukocytes, such as whole blood and granulocytes, are associated with the highest rates of transmission. Although leukocyte viability would seem to be an important variable, CMV transmission rates by fresher units are not consistently higher, as might be expected. Units from recently infected donors, as identified by the presence of IgM anti-CMV antibodies, appear to be somewhat more likely to transmit CMV than units from donors with latent infection *(17)*, although the correlation is not perfect.

The most important variable in terms of the development of disease following CMV infection appears to be the level of immune competence of the recipient. Recipients with evidence of humoral immunity directed against CMV (i.e., presence of anti-CMV) are generally less susceptible to CMV disease than seronegative recipients. Vaccination or passive antibody transfer in the form of iv immunoglobulin or hyperimmune plasma or globulin preparations have frequently, but not invariably, been shown to attenuate CMV infection and disease *(10)*. A more important factor is the integrity of the host cellular immune system. Patients with defects in T-cell function are much more susceptible to developing significant CMV disease when infected than those with intact cellular immune systems.

3.3. Recommendations for Patients At-Risk

Table 7 lists the groups of immunocompromised patients who have been shown to be particularly susceptible to transfusion-transmitted CMV infection and disease and who benefit from receiving components chosen or prepared to minimize CMV transmission as discussed in Section 3.4. (CMV-Safe Components).

3.3.1. Pregnant Women (Fetuses)

Women who are infected with CMV during pregnancy rarely experience clinically significant disease, but they have about a 50% risk of giving birth to a congenitally infected infant. The fetus, whose immune system is immature, is much more likely to experience serious disease. Intrauterine infection only occurs with a frequency of approx 0.5–2% of live births; however, approx 25% of infected infants present with a spectrum of problems including jaundice, hepatosplenomegaly, thrombocytopenia or a variety of systemic infections. Microcephaly, chorioretinitis, motor disability, and inner ear disease may also be seen. About 20% of affected infants die. There is also a risk for the later development of a variety of neurological problems including deafness. Prudence dictates the provision of CMV-safe components for the transfusion of CMV seronegative pregnant women. Providing CMV-safe com-

Table 8
Patterns of CMV Infection in Transplant Patients

CMV serologic status		Pattern
Recipient	Donor	CMV infection
Positive	Positive	Reactivation
		Reinfection
Positive	Negative	Reactivation
Negative	Positive	Primary Infecton
Negative	Negative	Transfusion

ponents to these patients rarely poses a logistical problem since they so rarely require transfusion. The immaturity of the fetal immune system is also the rationale for providing CMV-safe blood for intrauterine transfusion.

3.3.2. Neonates

CMV infection and disease in neonates was identified as a complication of transfusion by the early 1980s, although the prevalence varied markedly around the country. About half of infants infected perinatally develop a characteristic and usually self-limited syndrome consisting of respiratory compromise, hepatosplenomegaly, gray pallor, and lymphocytosis. Occasionally more serious infections, including pneumonitis, hepatitis, and chorioretinitis occur—resulting in death in some cases. Some late sequelae such as hearing problems and learning and behavior disturbances have also been attributed to perinatal CMV transmission.

Several risk factors for neonatal CMV infection and disease have been identified *(18)*, among them transfusion, which was thought to be the source of infection in many cases. The mother's serologic status is also important, since infants born to CMV-seropositive mothers are less frequently infected and seldom have disease *(19)*. Low birth weight infants are particularly susceptible to infection and disease, perhaps because this variable correlates with prematurity and is a surrogate marker for immaturity of the neonate's immune system. The provision of CMV-safe cellular components has been shown to reduce or eliminate the incidence of perinatal CMV infection, although the background rate of infection also seems to be decreasing. Whereas the infection rate in susceptible infants was reported to be 24–32% in the late 1970s and early 1980s, the rates reported since then have ranged 1–9% *(15)*. Nonetheless, in institutions in which perinatal CMV infection has been observed, or where the incidence has not been studied, transfusion of CMV-safe components is recommended for low birth weight infants born to mothers who are CMV seronegative or whose serologic status is not known.

3.3.3. Bone Marrow Transplant Recipients

CMV infection and disease is a serious complication of allogeneic bone marrow transplantation and is the major infectious cause of death in these patients *(10,20)*. The pattern of CMV infection is determined primarily by the prior exposure of the recipient and the marrow donor. The CMV serologic status of the recipient and donor are used to determine whether or not either is latently infected with CMV. These combinations and the usual patterns of infection are shown in Table 8. Primary infection from a latently infected (seropositive) marrow donor is the major risk factor for uninfected (seronegative) recipients. It is associated with the most severe clinical outcome, which may include interstitial pneumonitis, which has an 85% mortality rate; hepatitis; leukocytosis; and delayed engraftment of platelet and granulocyte lines. Reactivation is the most common manifestation of CMV disease in previously infected transplant recipients and usually has a much milder clinical course consisting of a serologic response and viral shedding. Immunosuppressive drugs are a key factor stimulating reactivation. Cyclophosphamide, azathioprine, cyclosporine, antilymphocyte globulin, and OKT3 are all associated with CMV reactivation, whereas corticosteroids play a subsidiary role. The role of reinfection, from either the allograft or transfusion, is not well delineated.

Transfusion does not contribute measurably to the risk of CMV disease in either the patients who are already infected or who receive an allograft from an infected donor. However, CMV seronegative recipients of allografts from seronegative donors are at risk for severe CMV disease if exposed to units of blood from infected donors. It is generally agreed that these patients should receive CMV-safe components, a measure that has been shown to be effective in markedly reducing transfusion-transmitted CMV infection in this group *(5,21)*.

Previously uninfected autogeneic bone-marrow transplant recipients are also at risk from CMV infection by transfusion, although they are less likely to experience serious disease than newly infected allogeneic graft recipients *(22)*. Transfusion does not appear to be an important source of infection in previously infected recipients, but is a risk factor in seronegative patients. These uninfected individuals should receive CMV-safe components.

3.3.4. Solid-Organ Transplant Recipients

CMV infection and disease are a major cause of morbidity and mortality in solid-organ transplant recipients as well. Reactivation is the major source of morbidity in previously infected allograft recipients, whereas the transplanted organ is the major source of infection in previously uninfected recipients *(23–25)*. Transmission rates of CMV by solid-organ allografts from infected donors ranges from as low as 10–20% for kidneys to virtually 100% for lungs *(15)*. Transfusion plays a minor role in CMV infection in these two groups. However, as in the allogeneic bone-marrow transplant recipients, previously uninfected recipients of solid-organ allografts from CMV seronegative donors are at risk for primary CMV infection from transfusion. Infection occurs in this susceptible population at rates reported from <2–33%, and is associated with significant morbidity. Hence this group also warrants protection from transfusion-transmitted CMV infection.

3.3.5. AIDS Patients

Patients with AIDS have a severe cellular immune deficiency resulting from the infection and obliteration of CD4+ T-cells. Previously uninfected individuals with AIDS may become infected by CMV via transfusion *(26)*. Primary infection in these individuals is associated with considerable morbidity. Retinitis, sometimes resulting in blindness, is a frequent complication, whereas enteritis, pneumonitis, and other infections occur less often. There is experimental evidence that CMV may "transactivate" HIV and thus hasten the course of AIDS *(27)*. Although data from in vitro systems supports this possibility, clinical studies are still needed to confirm the existence of transactivation and determine its significance. The mortality rate for CMV disease in AIDS patients of approx 5% is somewhat lower than in the transplant patient population *(11)*. Previous CMV infection is quite common in AIDS patients who acquired HIV infection through sexual contact or iv drug use. In these patients, reactivation is almost universal, and is the major source of CMV disease. CMV-safe components are commonly provided for seronegative patients with AIDS. The utility of taking this precaution with HIV-infected patients who have not yet progressed to AIDS is debated. As long as adequate numbers of CD4+ cells remain, primary infection with CMV by transfusion is likely to be clinically mild. The greater concern, however, is that, if infected by transfusion, the patient becomes susceptible to reactivation and the clinically significant disease that may accompany it when they later progress to AIDS.

3.3.6. Other Immunocompromised Patients

The morbidity and mortality of CMV infection and disease and the need for CMV-safe components in other immunocompromised patients are not as well studied. Patients with congenital T-cell deficiencies such as Wiskott-Aldrich syndrome and DiGeorge syndrome are particularly susceptible to viral infections; common sense would suggest that the provision of CMV-safe components should be considered for these patients. Patients with malignancies, especially during chemo- and radio-therapy, constitute another group of immunocompromised patients who might be suspected of being susceptible to CMV infection. CMV infection has been documented in this group, but the extent to which transfusion contributes is unknown. Moreover, the morbidity associated with CMV infection in these patients has not been well documented. Although postsurgical CMV infection has been described, morbidity is rare. Significant CMV disease has been reported in a small number of patients following splenectomy *(28)*.

3.4. CMV-Safe Components

CMV-safe blood components have traditionally been obtained from donors who have been screened for the presence of CMV antibody (IgG), an indicator of past exposure and, presumably, latent infection. Although 30–60% of blood donors in the United States are CMV seropositive, <40% of the units drawn from these donors transmit CMV *(29)*. False negative test results are not uncommon, with most of the commercially available test kits for screening donors for antibody to CMV and range from 1% *(30)* to considerably worse *(11,31)*. As an alternative to choosing CMV-seronegative blood components, leukocytes can be removed effectively from RBCs by the process of freezing and deglycerolizing *(32)*. More recently, filtration with high performance leukodepletion filters has been shown to prevent CMV infection in neonates and bone-marrow transplant recipients *(4,5)*. There continues to be some debate about the relative efficacy of screening and filtering, although both approaches are highly effective in preventing CMV infection *(11)*. The decision to rely on one method or the other, or to use them both interchangeably should not be made based entirely on published experience. Consideration must be given to local factors that could affect the application and outcome of these two approaches,

Table 9
Comparision of GVHD and TAGVHD

Parameter	GVHD	TAGVHD
Rash	+	+
Fever	+	+
GI Disease	+	+
Cytopenia	–	+
Course		
acute	+	+
chronic	+	(Rare)
Therapy	Yes	No
Mortality	Variable	>95%

e.g., CMV antibody test technique, whether the test is done routinely by a fixed staff or as needed by available personnel, site and timing of leukodepletion, training or experience of personnel performing filtration, quality control practices, and so on.

4. TAGVHD

4.1. Background

Passenger lymphocytes present in cellular blood components can initiate GVHD when transfused into an immunocompromised host *(33)*. Upon exposure to the alloantigens of the transfusion recipient (host), transfused T-cells (graft) become activated and mount an immune response that targets susceptible host tissues. Ordinarily, donor T-cells would be recognized and eliminated by the recipient's immune system. However, recipients with T-cell defects are unable to respond to the presence of donor T-cells and allow them to circulate and proliferate.

TAGVHD is compared to conventional GVHD in Table 9. In common with patients with marrow-transplant-associated GVHD, patients with TAGVHD present with fever, rash, and gastrointestinal disturbances including anorexia, nausea, vomiting, and diarrhea that may be accompanied by abnormalities in liver function tests. The feature that distinguishes TAGVHD is bone marrow involvement resulting in pancytopenia. It is this characteristic that contributes to the almost universally fatal outcome of TAGVHD. No successful therapy has been found to treat TAGVHD, and patients usually succumb within a month.

4.2. Patients at Risk and Recommendations

Over 200 cases of TAGVHD have been reported in the literature, almost all in patients with defects in cellular immunity *(see* Table 10) *(34)*. The list of reported cases is dominated by patients with congenital T-cell immunodeficiencies, but also includes neonates and patients with hematologic malignancies. TAGVHD has occasionally been reported in autogeneic marrow transplant patients and rarely in patients with solid tumors and solid-organ allografts.

A small number of cases have also been described in immunocompetent patients, often receiving transfusions from relatives *(35)*. In almost all cases studied, the related donors were found to be homozygous for an HLA haplotype shared with

Table 10
Patient Diagnosis
in Reported Cases of TAGVHD

Congenital T-cell immunodeficiencies
Hematologic malignancies
Intrauterine transfusion
Premature neonates
Neonatal exchange transfusion
Autologous bone-marrow transplants
Solid tumors
Solid organ transplants
Related donors
Immunocompetent patients

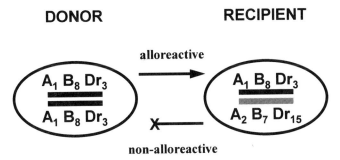

Fig. 1. Transfusion-associated graft-vs-host disease: haplotype constellation in the immunocompetent transfusion recipient.

the recipient (*see* Fig. 1). In this situation, the transfused lymphocytes are perceived as "self" by the host immune system and escape immune surveillance, but they are themselves capable of attacking host tissues, which bear a "foreign" haplotype, resulting in TAGVHD. This entity is quite rare in the United States but has been reported more frequently in Japan, reflecting the greater degree of HLA homogeneity of that population.

This scenario occurs even more rarely with unrelated donors. Calculations based on the frequency of HLA haplotypes in the U.S. population indicate that the probability of this constellation occurring in unrelated donor/recipient pairs ranges from approx 1 in 2000 transfusions (using serologically determined specificities only) to 1 in nearly 40,000 transfusions using HLA specificities determined by both serology and DNA sequence information *(36)*. These calculations predict a much larger number cases of TAGVHD than have been reported. Although failure to recognize TAGVHD and underreporting may explain some of the discrepancy, is also suggests that, whereas the haplotype constellation described is necessary for TAGVHD in immunocompetent hosts, it is not sufficient. Other as yet undefined host factors must influence the development of this devastating complication of transfusion.

Exposure of blood components to gamma irradiation has been shown to prevent TAGVHD. Based on the reported experience and our understanding of the pathophysiology of TAGVHD, irradiated cellular blood components are frequently pro-

Table 11
Indications for Irradiated RBCs

Bone marrow and peripheral blood progenitor cell transplant recipients[a]
Congenital T-cell immunodeficiency syndromes,
   e.g., SCIDS, Wiskott-Aldrich, DiGeorge
Intrauterine transfusion[a]
Neonatal exchange transfusion
Premature neonates weighing <1200 g
Transfusions from blood relatives[a]
Patients with some hematologic malignancies (Hodgkin's, Non-Hodgkins
   Lymphoma, acute leukemias) and neuroblastoma while they are being
   treated with marrow-ablative chemotherapy

[a] Listed in *AABB Standards,* 17th ed.

vided in the situations listed in Table 11 *(37,38)*. Low birthweight neonates and fetuses appear to be susceptible to TAGVHD because their immune system is immature. TAGVHD has been described following exchange transfusion in neonates, although it is not clear if it is the transfusion itself, or the disorder being treated by exchange (usually hemolytic disease of the newborn) that predisposes the infant to TAGVHD. TAGVHD has also been reported in patients with congenital T-cell defects, patients with hematologic malignancies, and bone-marrow transplant recipients, hence the recommendation to provide them with irradiated blood. Interestingly, TAGVHD has not been reported in patients with one of the most profound defects of T-cell immunity, AIDS. TAGVHD may be underrecognized in this patient population in which rashes and gastrointestinal dysfunction are common, or perhaps the donor T-cells become infected by HIV once transfused into the host. The necessity of irradiating blood components for patients with other malignancies or who are recipients of solid-organ allografts is debated.

The situations in which the AABB Standards specifically recommends the irradiation of blood components are indicated by the footnote in Table 11. Note that the AABB Standards also recommends the irradiation of cellular components for "selected immunoincompetent or immunocompromised recipients" intending for individual institutions to evaluate the risk of TAGVHD in other patient groups in which this complication is less well defined but has been reported.

4.3. Irradiation

Gamma irradiation of cellular blood components eliminates the ability of lymphocytes to proliferate, thereby preventing them from mounting an effective immunological response to host tissues. A radiation dose of 2500 rads (25 Gy) has been shown to ablate the ability of lymphocytes in blood to replicate in response to allogeneic stimulation *(39)*. To ensure that irradiation is effective, both the AABB *(6)* and the Food and Drug Administration *(40)* require a minimum dose of 25 Gy delivered to the midplane of the irradiation chamber with no less than 15 Gy delivered to all parts of the chamber. Irradiation of blood components at this level is effective in preventing TAGVHD in susceptible patients. Irradiation does not remove lymphocytes from the blood component, hence alloimmunization and febrile transfusion reactions in response to leukocyte antigens may still occur. At these levels, irradiation also has no effect on the transmission of infectious diseases.

Irradiated red blood cells show increased leakage of K^+ into the plasma *(41)*. For this reason, they may not be stored as long as unirradiated red cells. Although unirradiated red cells may be stored for 35–42 d, depending on the anticoagulant-preservative solution, irradiated red blood cells are assigned an expiration date that is the earlier date of either the originally assigned outdate or 28 d from the date of irradiation.

The elevated plasma K^+ levels found in units of irradiated red cells are rarely clinically significant. Once the irradiated red cells are transfused, they immediately begin to replete their ATP levels and, within minutes to hours, replace the lost K^+. Even from units stored for the maximum time permitted, the amount of plasma K^+ infused would not exceed 5–10 mEq/unit, a quantity that is readily removed by the kidneys. Patients who might be put at risk by the K^+ load include those with severe renal insufficiency, patients who are already hyperkalemic and have a susceptible dysrhythmia, or those receiving high volume transfusions. Consideration should be given to providing washed cells or recently irradiated units to these patients to minimize the K^+ load.

Irradiated blood components do not pose a radiation hazard to patients or healthcare workers. Noncellular components do not require irradiation.

5. TRANSFUSION OF THE IgA DEFICIENT PATIENT

5.1 Background

Selective IgA deficiency is the most common humoral immunodeficiency with a frequency of approx 1:700 in the Caucasian population *(42)*. This syndrome is characterized by a serum IgA level < 0.05 mg/dL, no deficiencies in other immunoglobulins, and no defects of cellular immunity. Most affected individuals are clinically well, but some have histories of multiple infections of the upper respiratory tract or the gastrointestinal tract. They are not otherwise considered to be significantly immunocompromised and are not susceptible to the complications of transfusion discussed previously in this chapter. Upon exposure to IgA through transfusion or pregnancy, approximately one-third of IgA deficient individuals make IgG and/or IgE antibody to IgA *(42,43)*. Uncommonly, an individual may produce anti-IgA in the absence of known immune stimulation.

IgA-deficient patients with anti-IgA are at risk for anaphylactoid or frank anaphylactic reactions when transfused with blood components that contain even trace amounts of plasma. These reactions are quite rare occurring from 1 in 20,000 transfusions *(44)* to 1 in 47,000 transfusions *(45)*. Although it is the test for IgG anti-IgA that is commonly available, it is in fact IgE anti-IgA in the plasma and on the surface of mast cells that is responsible for mediating the acute hypersensitivity reaction. IgA–anti-IgA complexes activate complement, generating the anaphylatoxins C3a and C5a, and bind to mast cells inducing degranulation and histamine release. These mediators produce increased vascular permeability, smooth muscle contraction, and vasodilatation. Within minutes, patients experience flushing, laryngeal edema and/or bronchospasm, hypotension (often accompanied by tachycardia) that may lead to loss of consciousness or shock, and a variety of gastrointestinal symptoms including cramps, nausea, vomiting, and diarrhea.

5.2. Management of IgA-Deficient Patients

The diagnosis of selective IgA deficiency is only known before transfusion in the small fraction of affected patients who present with recurrent infections. For most IgA-deficient patients who experience an anaphylactoid or anaphylactic transfusion reaction, the diagnosis is made after the unfortunate event. Although most patients experiencing this type of transfusion reaction will not be found to be IgA deficient, they must be evaluated for this deficiency by obtaining an IgA level and testing for the presence of anti-IgA. Both tests are recommended since patients who lack only one of the two subclasses of IgA (IgA1 or IgA2) may have a normal or only slightly reduced level of IgA, yet they may develop antibody to the missing subclass of IgA and be at risk for an anaphylactoid reaction *(46)*. It is, however, the presence or absence of the anti-IgA that determines the subsequent transfusion management of the IgA-deficient patient according to the protocol of Vamvakas and Pineda *(47)* as described in Sections 5.2.1. and 5.2.2.

5.2.1 Management of IgA-Deficient Patients without Anti-IgA

If an IgA-deficient patient who has experienced an anaphylactoid transfusion reaction is found not to have anti-IgA, alternative explanations for the reaction should be sought. Whereas the discovery of a reasonable alternative explanation is comforting, it is reasonable in any case to proceed with the transfusion of standard components. These components should be administered slowly, under close supervision with emergency facilities at hand. If the patient does not react to the transfusion, then standard components may be transfused in the future with no special precautions. If an anaphylactoid reaction occurs again, then the patient should receive washed RBCs and platelets. Transfusion of plasma and cryoprecipitated antihemophilic factor (AHF) should only be attempted if absolutely necessary and following appropriate premedication with diphenhydramine and corticosteroids.

5.2.2. Management of Patients with Anti-IgA Antibody

If anti-IgA can be demonstrated, then the patient should receive IgA-deficient blood components as listed in Table 12. Red cells may be rendered suitably IgA deficient by washing in an automated device using 2 L of wash saline *(48)*. Alternatively, frozen, deglycerolized red cells may be used *(49)*. Obtaining red cells from IgA-deficient donors is the most cumbersome option, but is feasible in an elective transfusion situation. It is important that the IgA levels of donors in such a registry be checked periodically, as there is variation in an individual's IgA levels over time *(50)*. Only donors with IgA levels shown to be < 0.02 mg/dL using an assay with adequate sensitivity should be chosen for an IgA-deficient registry. IgA-deficient patients planning elective surgery for which transfusion is likely, should undertake autogeneic blood donation.

The optimal platelet products for these patients are obtained by pheresis either from the patient or from an IgA-deficient donor. Alternatively, platelets may be washed on automated devices using saline or buffered saline *(51)*. Fresh frozen plasma and cryoprecipitated AHF should be obtained from IgA-deficient donors,

Table 12
Management of IgA-Deficient
Patient With Anti-IgA

Red cells
    Washed
    Frozen, deglycerolized
    IgA-deficient donor
    Autogeneic blood
Platelets
    IgA-deficient pheresis donor
    Autogeneic plateletpheresis
    Washed
Fresh, frozen plasma and cryoprecipitated AHF
    IgA-deficient donor
    Autogeneic plasmapheresis
Plasma derivatives
    Check IgA level of each lot

---

or from the patient, if the circumstances permit. Plasma derivatives should be chosen on the basis of the IgA content determined for the specific lot of product which is to be infused. Lot-to-lot variation is such that assumptions should not be made about the amount of residual IgA in plasma derivatives.

REFERENCES

1. Klein HG. Wolf in wolf's clothing: is it time to raise the bounty on the passenger leukocyte? editorial, *Blood* 1992;80:1865–1868.
2. Reverbere R, Menini C. Clinical efficacy of five filters specific for leukocyte removal. *Vox Sanguinis* 1990;58:188–191.
3. Heddle NM. The efficacy of leukodepletion to improve platelet transfusion response: a critical appraisal of clinical studies. *Transf Med Rev* 1994;8:15.
4. Eisenfeld L, Silver H, McLaughlin J, et al. Prevention of transfusion-associated Cytomegalovirus infection in neonatal patients by the removal of white cells from blood. *Transfusion* 1992;32:205–209.
5. Bowden RA, Slichter SJ, Sayers M, et al. A comparison of filtered leukocyte-reduced and cytomegalovirus (CMV) seronegative blood products for the prevention of transfusion-associated CMV infection after marrow transplant. *Blood* 1995;86:3598–3603.
6. American Association of Blood Banks. *Standards for Blood Banks and Transfusion Services,* 17th ed., Bethesda, MD, 1996.
7. Meryman HT, Hornblower M. The preparation of red cells depleted of leukocytes. Review and evaluation. *Transfusion* 1986;26:101–106.
8. Dzik S. Leukodepletion blood filters: Filter design and mechanisms of leukocyte removal. *Transf Med Rev* 1993;7:65.
9. Ho M. Epidemiology of cytomegalovirus infections. *Rev Infec Dis* 1990;12:S701–710.
10. Winston DJ, Ho WG, Champlin RE. Cytomegalovirus infection after allogeneic bone marrow transplantation. *Rev Infec Dis* 1990;12:S76–792.
11. Bowden RA. Transfusion-transmitted cytomegalovirus infection. *Hematol Oncol Clin N Amer* 1995;9:155–156.
12. Luban NLC. Cytomegalovirus. In: Anderson KC, Ness PM, eds. *Scientific Basis of Transfusion Medicine: Implications for Clinical Practice.* Philadelphia: WB Saunders, 1994.

13. Manez R, Kusne S, Martin M, et al. The impact of blood transfusion on the occurrence of pneumonitis in primary cytomegalovirus infection after liver transplantation. *Transfusion* 1993;33:594–597.
14. Grob JP, Prentice HG, Hoffbrand AV, et al. Immune donors can protect marrow transplant recipients from severe Cytomegalovirus infections. *Lancet* 1987;i:774.
15. Preiksaitis JK. Indications for the use of cytomegalovirus-seronegative blood products. *Transf Med Rev* 1991;5:1–17.
16. Bowden RA, Sayers M. The risk of transmitting cytomegalovirus infection by fresh frozen plasma. *Transfusion* 1990;30:762–763.
17. Lamberson HV, McMillan JA, Weiner LB, et al. Prevention of transfusion associated Cytomegalovirus (CMV) infection in neonates by screening blood donors for IgM to CMV. *J Infec Dis* 1988;157:820–823.
18. Yeager AS, Grumet FC, Hafleigh EB, et al. Prevention of transfusion-acquired Cytomegalovirus infections in newborn infants. *J Pediatr* 1981;98:281–287.
19. Cheung KS, Lang DJ. Activation of Cytomegalovirus with blood transfusion: a mouse model. *J Infect Dis* 1977;135:841–845.
20. Hillyer CD, Snydman DR, Berkman EM. The risk of cytomegalovirus infection in solid organ and bone marrow transplant recipients: transfusion of blood products. *Transfusion* 1990;30:659–666.
21. Wingard JT, Chen DYH, Burns WH, et al. Cytomegalovirus infection after autologous bone marrow transplantation with comparison to infection after allogeneic bone marrow transplantation. *Blood* 1988;71:1432–1437.
22. MacKinnon S, Burnett AK, Crawford RJ, Cameron S, Leask BGS, Somerville RC. Seronegative blood products prevent primary Cytomegalovirus infection after bone marrow transplantation. *J Clin Path* 1988;41:948–950.
23. Chou S. Acquisition of donor strains of Cytomegalovirus by renal-transplant recipients. *N Engl J Med* 1986;314:1418–1423.
24. Dummler JS. Cytomegalovirus infection after liver transplantation: clinical manifestations and strategies for prevention. *Rev Infec Dis* 1990;12:S767–775.
25. Preiksaitis JK, Rosno S, Grumet C, Merigan TC. Infections due to herpesviruses in cardiac transplant recipients: Role of the donor heart and immunosuppressive therapy. *J Infec Dis* 1983;147:974–981.
26. Drew WL. Cytomegalovirus infection in patients with AIDS. *J Infec Dis* 1988;158:449–456.
27. Skolnik PR, Kosloff BR, Hirsch M. Bidirecional interactions between Human Immunodeficiency Virus, Type 1 and CMV. *J Infec Dis* 1988;157:508–514.
28. Sayers MH, Anderson KC, Goodnough LT, et al. Reducing the risk for transfusion-transmitted Cytomegalovirus infection. *Ann Int Med* 1992;116:55–62.
29. Preiksaitis JK, Brown L, MacKenzie M. The risk of Cytomegalovirus injection in seronegative transfusion recipients not receiving exogenous immunosuppression. *J Infec Dis* 1988;157:523–529.
30. Bowden RA, Sayers M, Gleaves CA, et al. Cytomegalovirus-seronegative blood components for the prevention of primary cytomegalovirus infection after marrow transplantation. *Transfusion* 1987;27:478–481.
31. Beckwith DG, Halstead DC, Alpaugh K, et al. Comparison of a latex agglutination test with five other methods for determining the presence of antibody against Cytomegalovirus. *J Clin Microbiol* 1985;21:328–331.
32. Brady MT, Milam JP, Anderson DC, et al. Use of deglycerolized red blood cells to prevent post-transfusion infection with Cytomegalovirus in neonates. *J Infec Dis* 1984;150:334–339.
33. Anderson KC, Weinstein HJ. Transfusion-associated graft-versus-host diseases. *N Engl J Med* 1990;323:315–321.

34. Greenbaum BH. Transfusion-associated graft-versus-host disease: historical perspectives, incidence, and current use of irradiated blood products. *J Clin Oncol* 1991;9: 1889–1902.

35. Ohto H, Anderson KC. Survey of transfusion-associated graft-versus-host disease in immunocompetent recipients. *Transf Med Rev* 1996;10:31–43.

36. Wagner FF, Flegel WA. Transfusion-associated graft-versus-host disease: risk due to homozygous HLA haplotypes. *Transfusion* 1995;35:284–291.

37. Anderson KC, Goodnough LT, Sayers M, et al. Variations in blood component irradiation practice: implications for prevention of transfusion-associated graft-versus-host disease. *Blood* 1991;77:2096–2102.

38. Anderson KC. Clinical indicaitons for blood component irradiation. In: Baldwin ML, Jeffries LC, eds. *Irradiation of Blood Components*. Bethesda, MD: American Association of Blood Banks, 1992, pp. 31–49.

39. Pelszynski MM, Moroff G, Luban NLC, Taylor BJ, Quinones RR. Effect of γ irradiation of red blood cell units on T-cell inactivation as assessed by limiting dilution analysis: implications for preventing transfusion-associated graft-versus-host disease. *Blood* 1994;83:1683–1689.

40. Recommendations regarding license amendments and procedures for gamma irradiation of blood products. Memorandum, 7/22/93, Food and Drug Administration, Center for Biologics Evaluation and Research.

41. Davey RJ, McCoy NC, Yu M, Sullivan DM, Speigel DM, Leitman SF. The effect of prestorage irradiation on posttransfusion red cell survival. *Transfusion* 1992;32: 525–528.

42. Clark JA, Callicoat PA, Brenner NA, Bradley NA, Smith DM. Selective IgA deficiency in blood donors. *J Lab Clin Med* 1983;80:210–213.

43. Sandler SG, Eckrich R, Mamamut D, Mallory D. Hemagglutination assays for the diagnosis and prevention of IgA anaphylactic transfusion reactions. *Blood* 1994;84: 2031–2035.

44. Bjerrum OJ, Jersild C. Class-specific anti-IgA associated with severe anaphylactic transfusion reactions in a patient with pernicious anemia. *Vox Sanguinis* 1971;21: 411–424.

45. Pineda AA, Taswell H F. Transfusion reactions associated with anti-IgA antibodies: report of four cases and review of the literature. *Transfusion* 1975;15:10–15.

46. Koistinen J, Leikola J. Weak anti-IgA antibodies with limited specificity and non-hemolytic transfusion reactions. *Vox Sanguinis* 1977;32:77–81.

47. Vamvakas EC, Pineda AA. Allergic and anaphylactic reactions. In: Popovsky M, ed. *Transfusion Reactions*. Bethesda, MD: American Association of Blood Banks, 1996, pp. 81–123.

48. Fox SM, Stavely-Haiber LM. Immunoglobulin A (IgA) levels in blood products and plasma derivatives. *Immunohematology* 1988;4:5–9.

49. Yap PL, Pryde EAD, McClelland DBL. IgA content of frozen-thawed-washed red blood cells and blood products measured by radioimmunoassay. *Transfusion* 1982; 22:26–28.

50. Laschinger C, Gauthier D, Valet JP, Naylor DH. Fluctuating levels of serum IgA in individuals with selective IgA deficiency. *Vox Sanguinis* 1984;47:60–67.

51. Pineda AA, Zylstra VW, Clare DE, Dewanjee MK, Forstrom LA. Viability and functional integrity of washed platelets. *Transfusion* 1989;29:524–527.

6

Red Blood Cell Transfusions for Selected Neonatal and Pediatric Patients

Elaine K. Jeter and Mary Ann Spivey

1. INTRODUCTION

Neonatal and pediatric transfusion practice includes consideration of the neonate's immature immunologic, renal, and hepatic function; and it encompasses new technologies and innovative programs that limit donor exposures and infectious disease risks. Neonatal and pediatric transfusion practice is not merely the transfusion of small volumes of blood to small people.

2. RED BLOOD CELL (RBC) TRANSFUSIONS FOR NEONATES

RBC transfusions are an integral and essential component of modern therapy for the sick and premature neonate. Most RBC transfusions are given to replace phlebotomy losses owing to laboratory monitoring or to treat anemia of prematurity. In many infants, the quantity of blood removed for laboratory testing relative to their circulating blood volume represents 2% of their total circulating RBC volume per day. Generally, these losses are empirically replaced when 5–10% of the neonate's total blood volume has been removed *(1)*. Historically, in neonatal intensive care practice, replacement transfusions accounted for 8–12 donor exposures per neonate *(2)*. The potential risk of infectious disease transmission with each transfusion has led to a concerted effort to reduce donor exposures by use of laboratory testing microtechnology, elimination of redundant compatibility testing during the neonatal period which is defined as the first 4 mo of life, and by establishment of better neonatal transfusion guidelines. Implementation of sterile connecting device technology and preparation of multiple aliquots from a dedicated unit of RBCs for individual neonates have markedly reduced donor exposures.

Most RBC transfusions administered to neonates are of small volume (10–15 mL/kg) and are repeated frequently. Precise guidelines for the use of RBCs to replace phlebotomy losses and to treat significant clinical problems in infants with anemia of prematurity are not well defined scientifically or physiologically. Infants requiring ventilatory support and/or oxygen support, or infants with congenital heart disease may be transfused to maintain a hematocrit of >40%. Infants who

From: *Red Cell Transfusion: A Practical Guide*
Edited by: M. E. Reid and S. J. Nance Humana Press Inc., Totowa, NJ

are relatively stable but exhibit clinical symptoms of apnea, bradycardia, and tachypnea may be transfused to maintain a hematocrit of > 30%. These symptoms have been attributed to decreased oxygen delivery to the respiratory center of the brain *(3)*. However, there are studies that both support *(4,5)* and refute *(6)* the effects of transfusion on these clinical symptoms. Failure to thrive is considered by some neonatologists as an indication for RBC transfusion, particularly in infants with a hematocrit of < 30% *(6)*. Acute blood loss exceeding 10% of an infant's total blood volume is also an indication for RBC transfusion.

2.1. Testing for Antibodies and Compatibility

When RBCs are initially needed for transfusion, a cord blood sample can be used to determine the ABO and D typings. Either serum or plasma from the infant (peditube), or from the mother, if available, may be used to perform an antibody screen for clinically significant antibodies. Because neonates rarely form RBC antibodies *(7)*, it is not necessary to crossmatch donor RBCs for initial or subsequent transfusions if the initial antibody screen is negative and group O Rh-compatible red cells are used for transfusions *(8)*. The elimination of repeat testing during an infant's singular hospitalization and the use of group O RBCs, a matter of convenience for many hospital transfusion services, have had a dramatic impact on decreasing blood loss.

When the initial antibody screen is positive for clinically significant antibodies, antigen-negative RBCs should be selected for transfusion or compatibility testing may be limited to the antiglobulin crossmatch until the antibody is no longer demonstrated. When donor RBCs are not group O, the neonate's serum must be tested for the presence of anti-A and/or anti-B. Only when anti-A and/or anti-B are not detected, can subsequent antiglobulin crossmatching be eliminated *(8)*.

2.2. Special Considerations for Neonatal Transfusions

There are a number of special considerations for neonatal transfusions that take into consideration the neonate's physiological and immunological limitations. Furthermore, strategies to limit donor exposures and pharmacologic alternatives to RBC transfusions have reduced the number of donor exposures in this population group as a whole during recent years.

2.2.1. Anticoagulants, Additives, and Storage Limits

Neonatologists have traditionally preferred to use RBCs stored for <5–7 d, presumably to ensure oxygen off-loading prior to loss of red cell 2,3-DPG, and to avoid hyperkalemia and low pH that occur during extended storage. However, although 2,3-DPG concentration is neglible after 21 d of storage, the p50 of 2,3-DPG-depleted blood is comparable to the p50 of blood from many premature newborns *(9)*, and offers the transfused infant a distinct advantage as 2,3-DPG is readily regenerated within hours following transfusion, unlike the neonate's own red cells.

Another concern raised by many neonatologists is the transfusion of blood stored in additive solutions. The small concentration of adenine in RBCs collected in CPDA-1 extends red cell viability to 35 d, and is not known to cause untoward transfusion-related effects. Additive solutions, also known as extended storage

Table 1
Comparison of CPDA-1 Anticoagulant-Preservation Solution,
and AS-1 and AS-3 Extended Storage Media[a]

Constituent	CPDA-1	CPD	AS-1 (Adsol)	CP2D	AS-3 (Nutricel)
Sodium citrate hydrous (mg)	1657	1657	0	1657	588
Citric acid hydrous (mg)	206	206	0	206	42
Phosphate hydrous (mg)	140	140	0	140	276
Dextrose (mg)	2000	1607	2200	3220	1100
Adenine (mg)	17	0	27	0	30
Mannitol (mg)	0	0	750	0	0
Sodium chloride (mg)	0	0	900	0	410
Volume (mL)	63	63	100	63	100

[a]Approximately 450 mL of donor blood is drawn into 63 mL of CPDA-1. When AS-1 and AS-3 is used, 450 mL of blood is drawn into CPD and CP2D, respectively. After centrifugation, the plasma-anticoagulant is removed, and the red cells are suspended in 100 mL of AS-1 and AS-3, respectively.

media, such as AS-1 (Adsol™) and AS-3 (Nutricel™), consist of different concentrations of dextrose, adenine and mannitol which maintain red cell survival and extend storage to 42 d (Table 1).

Neonatologists are concerned about neonatal exposure to very high concentrations of additive constituents (dextrose, adenine, mannitol) and the cumulative effect of these additives in neonates who require multiple transfusions during relatively short intervals. Renal toxicity is the main concern with adenine and mannitol in the additive solutions. In a double cross-over comparison of CPDA-1 and AS-1 solutions stored for < 5 d, there was no evidence by clinical observation or laboratory values in 16 neonates that simple transfusion was deleterious (10). In a more recent report, it was shown that RBCs in Adsol stored 5–21 d are also acceptable (11).

Potassium load in RBCs during extended storage has also been a concern of many neonatologists. After 35 d of storage, supernatant K^+ concentrations in CPDA-1 RBCs are approx 70 mmol/L, whereas AS-1 RBCs stored for 42 d have a K^+ concentration of 50 mmol/L (12). It is estimated that a 1-kg infant, with a potassium requirement of 2–3 mmol/L/kg/d, who receives a slow infusion of 10 mL/kg of 3–5 d stored CPDA-1 RBCs will receive approx 0.1 mmol/L of potassium (9). The safety of extended storage blood is supported by recent studies using CPDA-1 whole blood stored for 28 d (13) and CPDA-1 RBCs stored for 30 d (14) and 35 d (15).

From a theoretical prospective, storage in AS-1 should not present problems when used as small volume transfusions (16). Because data are not available on the toxicity, or lack thereof, of exposure to extended-storage solutions in massive transfusion settings, the authors suggest removal of the additive solution by washing or centrifugation with resuspension of RBCs in normal saline or balanced electrolyte solutions. In support of the theoretical calculations, recent studies demonstrate the safety and efficacy of small volume transfusion of RBCs stored in Adsol up to 21 d (17) and 42 d (18,19). This trend toward transfusion of RBCs in extended storage additive solutions is borne out in nearly 20% of 437 institutions responding to an

American Association of Blood Banks (AABB) neonatal transfusion practice survey *(20)* and is primarily the result of an effort to limit neonatal donor exposure.

2.2.2. Strategies to Limit Donor Exposures

In the past, in an effort to maximize blood usage and minimize wastage, many aliquots were prepared from a single unit of blood. For infants requiring multiple, small-volume transfusions within a short period of time, this approach maximized donor exposure and the risk of transfusion-related disease. In one situation, this led to disastrous results *(21)*. A variety of approaches to limit donor exposures have been reported: increasing the transfusion dose volume from 10–15 mL/kg *(22)*; assigning a dedicated unit of RBCs per neonate for use up to 24 d *(23)* or 35 d *(24,25)*; assigning three patients per unit of RBCs *(24,26)*; sequential consignment of a unit to multiple infants for up to 30 d of storage *(27)*; and collection of half-volume units from dedicated parents at 14-d intervals.

Programs to limit donor exposure to neonates undergoing extracorporeal membrane oxygenation (ECMO) have included use of sequential aliquots utilizing the sterile connecting device from dedicated RBCs in extended storage media *(28)*. Other programs have increased dose volumes from 10–15 mL/kg and eliminated exchange transfusions, and prophylactic use of fresh frozen plasma (FFP) and cryoprecipitate during ECMO *(22)*. In a recent report, four dedicated donors were able to provide all the RBC and platelet components for a neonate undergoing bone marrow transplantation *(29)*.

2.2.3. Erythropoietin (EPO) and Other Strategies to Decrease RBC Transfusion in the Neonate

There have been a number of controlled studies to establish the effects of recombinant human EPO on the neonate. In general, these have shown that EPO-treated neonates were less likely to receive RBC transfusions than the controls, and success has been most evident in treatment of the anemia of prematurity that occurs 4–10 wk postnatally *(30)*. The data are not as promising in very low birth weight (VLBW) neonates (>1.0 kg, >30 wk gestation) with early iatrogenic blood loss. Although the U.S. EPO Study Group *(31)* showed a statistically significant difference in the number (1.1 ± 1.5 in the EPO group versus 1.6 ± 1.7 in the placebo group) and volume of RBC transfusions in VLBW neonates (16.5 ± 23.0 mL compared to 23.9 ± 25.7 mL in the controls), the difference was only modest.

The prospects for preventing transfusion during the first 2 wk are poor, since an appreciable increase in hematocrit is not evident for nearly 1 wk after beginning EPO, and iatrogenic blood loss may approach one half of the infant's blood volume in the first week. In a large European multicenter study *(32)*, 23% of study and 14% of control infants received RBCs before the 3rd d of life. Infants require higher doses of EPO (200–1400 U/kg/wk) than adults and concurrent iron supplementation (2–6 mg/kg). Questions regarding cost-effectiveness and the risk–benefit ratio need to be addressed more fully before EPO becomes standard medical practice for the preterm neonate. Although large studies support the safety of EPO in the neonatal population *(30,32)*, potential risks include sudden infant death syndrome, hypertension, thrombosis, neutropenia, and sepsis.

In addition to EPO administration, other strategies to decrease RBC transfusion in the neonate include decreasing the amount of blood drawn for laboratory tests by developing noninvasive monitoring methods and microtechniques, and delaying umbilical cord clamping, which has been shown to result in a significantly larger red cell mass *(33)*. Autologous blood has also been transfused to the neonate by collecting placental blood after delivery and storing it for later transfusion, but adequate anticoagulation and ensuring sterility have been perceived as problems. In a study of 31 placental collections from term infants, all blood cultures remained negative during a 4-wk storage period *(34)*. Adequate anticoagulation was obtained in only 15 specimens (APTT > 90 s at collection), though no clots were apparent. The majority of the volumes yielded 30–50 mL of RBCs adjusted to a hematocrit of 80%. Delayed cord clamping may not be safe in VLBW premature infants owing to sudden intravascular volume increase, and placental collection may not yield adequate volume to significantly offset iatrogenic need.

2.2.4. Infectious Disease Risks

The risk of cytomegalovirus (CMV) transmission and the risk of transfusion-associated graft-vs-host disease (TAGVHD) are two potential complications (*see* Chapter 5) that require special consideration when transfusing RBCs to neonates.

2.2.4.1. CYTOMEGALOVIRUS

VLBW infants born to CMV-seronegative mothers are at an increased risk of transfusion-associated CMV (TACMV) disease because they have not received protective maternal CMV antibodies *(35)*. When there is no attempt to reduce the number of leukocytes that are presumed to be the vehicle of transmission or to provide CMV-seronegative blood, the incidence of TACMV infection has been reported as high as 32% *(35)* with a mortality rate of 38% *(36)*. In the VLBW setting, the use of CMV-seronegative cellular blood components or frozen deglycerolized RBCs have significantly reduced TACMV *(37,38)*. In more recent studies, these high infection rates have not been confirmed and the use of CMV-seronegative blood components *(39)*, extended to include all neonatal patients in many hospitals, has been challenged as it may place premature infants of seropositive mothers at risk to maternally acquired CMV infection and disease *(40)*.

There has been intense interest in the prevention of CMV transmission by white blood cell (WBC) reduction. Whereas the absolute number of infected WBCs to cause CMV transmission is unknown, there is much evidence that CMV transmission can be reduced by the use of leukocyte-reducing filters. A few studies have specifically focused on CMV transmission during the neonatal period *(41,42)*. To provide blood components to neonates with the least risk of CMV transmission, it is prudent to follow the current recommendations from the Standards of the AABB *(8)*. It recommends that cellular components should be selected or processed to reduce the risk of CMV transmission to infants weighing < 1200 g at birth, when either the infant or the mother is CMV seronegative or when the CMV serostatus is unknown. For the practicing physician, the routine use of leukocyte-reduced cellular blood components provides a practical and reasonable approach for preventing

TACMV infection in the VLBW neonate and does not appear to be justified for other routine neonatal patients.

2.2.4.2. TRANSFUSION-ASSOCIATED GRAFT-VS-HOST DISEASE

Fetuses, premature neonates, and infant patients with congenital immune deficiencies are at increased risk of TAGVHD *(43)*. This disease was first recognized in immunodeficient children who had received blood transfusions *(44)* and has been described in premature newborns *(45,46)* and those with hemolytic disease of the newborn *(47–49)*. TAGVHD can also occur in immunocompetent individuals when a human leukocyte antigen (HLA) haploidentical recipient receives a cellular blood component from a donor who is homozygous for the HLA haplotype *(50,51)*. The probability of this occurring is greater among family members *(51)*, and the pediatric population occasionally receives directed transfusions from family members.

Cellular blood products are implicated in the transmission of this disease. Viable lymphocytes have not been identified in fresh-frozen plasma or cryoprecipitate. Gamma irradiation is the only effective method for preventing TAGVHD. Leukocyte-reduction filters are not an alternative method *(52)*. The role of gamma irradiation is to destroy the ability of donor lymphocytes to undergo blast transformation, and at the same time to preserve the functional activities of the blood product. Currently, the AABB requires a minimum of 25 Gy (J8.430) to blood products administered to fetuses receiving intrauterine transfusions, selected immunoincompetent or immunocompromised recipients, recipients of donor units known to be from a blood relative, and recipients of bone marrow or peripheral stem-cell transplantation (J8.410) *(8)*.

2.3. Small Volume RBC Transfusions

RBC concentrates are the product of choice for small volume transfusions since most neonates require approx 10–20 mL of RBCs per transfusion. In a recent survey of neonatal transfusion practice, RBC components for neonates included use without further modification (73%), RBCs modified by leukocyte-reduction (4%), washed (13%), and frozen, deglycerolized (9%) cells *(53)*. Primary reasons for washing RBCs were to remove metabolic toxins such as potassium and hemoglobin (50%), and to remove leukocytes (27%) and additive solutions (10%) *(53)*.

Multipack (quad) collection systems, dispensing of blood in syringes, and the use of a sterile connecting device are approaches that allow easy dispensing of red cells as small aliquots. A quad bag collection system consists of a main collection bag and three attached transfer bags. Whole blood is collected into the main storage bag and centrifuged. The supernatant plasma is expressed into one of the transfer bags and used as FFP or for production of plasma derivatives. The RBCs may be stored in the original collection bag with attached empty transfer bags until needed for transfusion, or they may be distributed equally using the remaining two transfer bags yielding a volume in each bag of approx 80–90 mL.

Red blood cells in a quad transfer bag can be aliquoted into even smaller volumes by using a blood coupler and transfer pack sets, or a blood coupler with an in-line blood filter for preparation of syringes. A major disadvantage of this system is that both the blood bag and all aliquots prepared from the blood product expire 24 h after initial entry into the blood product. Sterile connecting devices have now made

Table 2
Guidelines for Treatment of Hyperbilirubinemia
in Low Birth Weight Infants >3-d-Old

Birth weight	Bilirubin concentrations, mg/dL	
	Photopherapy	ET
<1500	5–8	13–16
1500–1999	8–12	16–18
2000–2499	11–14	18–20

it possible to aseptically weld blood bag tubing to single or multiple bag transfer packs or syringes without changing the original expiration date of the blood.

2.4. Intrauterine Transfusion (IUT)

IUT is primarily performed in cases of severe hemolytic disease of the fetus to prevent hydrops fetalis resulting from fetal anemia. The intraperitoneal transfusion (IPT) technique developed by Liley *(54)* in 1963 has been replaced in many centers by intravascular transfusion (IVT) in which transfusion is performed by umbilical venous puncture under ultrasound guidance *(55)*. Since a more rapid rise but wider swings in hematocrit are seen after IVT, Moise and colleagues *(56)* examined IUT techniques and found that a combined IVT/IPT resulted in a more stable hematocrit and longer intervals between transfusion. RBCs are administered by IVT to achieve a hematocrit of 35–40%. IPT is performed to serve as a reservoir with the volume transfused based on gestational age.

Group O D-negative allogeneic, CMV-negative, Hgb S-negative irradiated RBCs <5-d-old traditionally have been used for IUT; but more recently some workers have been using washed, irradiated, leukocyte-reduced maternal RBCs in order to decrease infectious disease and alloimmunization risk *(57)*. The washing removes the offending maternal antibody and leukoreduction renders the blood CMV-safe.

2.5. Exchange Transfusion (ET)

ET is the postnatal treatment of choice for the neonate with severe hemolytic disease of the newborn (HDN) and it is occasionally done in the intrauterine setting as well. In addition, it may be performed for other causes of severe hyperbilirubinemia, removal of toxic substances, polycythemia, severe anemia, respiratory distress syndrome (to substitute HgbA for HgbF), and neonatal sepsis (particularly if in conjunction with desseminated intravascular coagulation).

The decision to treat the hyperbilirubinemic neonate with ET rather than a less invasive technique such as phototherapy should depend on bilirubin level and rate of rise, degree of anemia, and the birth weight and clinical condition of the neonate (Table 2).

Blood used for ET is frequently <1-wk-old whole blood, partially packed RBCs, or RBCs suspended in fresh frozen plasma. The donor RBCs should be compatible with maternal hemolytic antibody (if the ET is for HDN), and the plasma should be compatible with the neonate's RBCs. The volume to be exchanged should be based on the blood volume of the neonate (85 mL/kg for full-term, 100 mL/kg for premature) and the reason for the exchange. For bilirubin removal, a two-volume exchange is generally performed; a single volume exchange may be sufficient for other causes. A final hematocrit of 50% is usually desired. Small aliquots (5–20 mL) are exchanged using multiple stopcock assemblies usually via the umbilical vessels.

Hazards of ET include cardiac arrythmias; vessel perforation; air embolism; infections; and hematologic, immunologic, and metabolic complications. Since TAGVHD has been reported in some infants following IUT and multiple ETs *(46)*, it is prudent to irradiate blood for ET. Most blood currently used for ET is collected in CPDA-1. If it is necessary to use blood with an additive solution, the additive solution should be removed just before the transfusion *(16)*.

2.6. Extracorporeal Membrane Oxygenation

ECMO is used to support full-term infants with reversable life-threatening respiratory failure. It can be thought of as a type of prolonged cardiopulmonary bypass (CPB). Either the right internal jugular vein and right common carotid artery are catheterized (venoarterial ECMO) or, alternatively, the return line is via a central venous catheter (venovenous ECMO), thus sparing the carotid artery. The catheters are connected to the circuit primed with an albumin–blood mixture. Two units of RBCs are needed initially for the circuit with another unit immediately available. Though most infants receiving ECMO are full-term and should not be at risk for CMV infection, over half of ECMO centers use CMV-seronegative cellular products. This is based on one case where a 3-kg infant developed disseminated CMV infection after over 100 donor exposures during ECMO *(58)*. Graft-vs-host disease has also been reported in a term infant leading the investigators to recommend irradiation of blood used for ECMO *(59)*. Platelet, FFP, and cryoprecipitate support varies and should be adapted to individual need. As with other CPB surgery, one sees ECMO circuit-induced thrombocytopenia as well as platelet dysfunction, so adequate platelet support is necessary.

3. RBC TRANSFUSIONS FOR INFANTS AND CHILDREN

Most red cell transfusions administered to infants (>4 mo and <2 yr) and children are associated with surgical procedures or in response to anemia of chronic disease and hematologic malignancies.

3.1. Compatibility Testing and Selection of RBC Components

All pediatric patients over 4 mo of age must be tested for ABO and D type, and for the presence of clinically significant antibodies. In addition, if the patient may have been exposed to allogeneic red cells, antibody screening must be performed within 3 d of the scheduled transfusion. If the antibody screen is negative, a crossmatch with donor RBCs and recipient serum or plasma may be limited to the immediate spin reaction phase. If the antibody screen is positive, RBCs lacking the antigen against which the recipient antibody is directed should be selected for transfusion, and the crossmatch must include an antiglobulin test phase *(see* Chapters 3 and 14).

3.2. RBC Tranfusions in Selected Hematologic Disorders

The major hematologic disorders requiring transfusion in pediatric patients are sickle cell disease (SCD), hematologic malignancies, and thalessemia. Although a small number of pediatric sickle cell anemia patients have been cured by bone mar-row transplantation, medical management of this disorder continues to be based on symptomatic and supportive care, with transfusion therapy remaining a mainstay of treatment. Because of the presence of hemoglobin F during the neonatal period, problems are not present at birth. Clinical manifestations generally begin at 6–12 mo of age, and are characterized by variable severity among patients as well as within individuals during childhood.

Similar to the SCD patient, transfusion therapy for patients with thalassemia is mainly supportive. Hypertransfusion, designed to maintain the hemoglobin >90 g/L by infusion of RBCs every 3–4 wk, and supertransfusion protocols, designed to maintain the hemoglobin <115–120 g/L, have attempted to limit the effect of chronic anemia and to contribute to normal growth and development in these chil-dren. However, aggressive transfusion therapy protocols increase the frequency and severity of problems from iron overload. In the past, the life expectancy of patients with secondary hemachromatosis was dramatically reduced. Their prognosis has improved with the introduction of deferoxamine as an iron-chelation therapy, but this presents additional problems, such as compliance, particularly in teenagers *(60)*. For additional information on hemoglobinopathies *see* Chapter 12.

3.2.1. SCD Patients

Absolute indications for RBC transfusion in SCD include sequestration crises, aplastic crises, acute chest syndrome, and stroke. Relative indications for RBC transfusions include pain crises and priapism when symptoms are severe and pro-tracted, pregnancy, and preparation for surgery. Because hypotensive shock occurs during acute splenic sequestration crises, treatment strategies must include restora-tion of blood volume and oxygen-carrying capacity. During aplastic crises, the need for transfusion depends on the severity of the anemia. Red cell replacement therapy may acutely prevent congestive heart failure or may provide maintenance support in patients with prolonged aplasia. Simple RBC transfusion therapy is beneficial in patients with acute chest syndrome with anemia and hypoxemia *(61)*. When hypox-emia is progressive and the patient's clinical condition is deteriorating, RBC exchange transfusions can reduce the HbS concentration to 20–30% and ameliorate the pulmonary vaso-occlusion *(62)*. Stroke is a major complication of cerebral vaso-occlusive disease in children with SCD. Exchange transfusion is essential in the management of children with acute or impending cerebrovascular episodes to reduce the HbS concentration to <30% *(63)*. Most of these patients go on to require a chronic transfusion program designed to maintain HbS <30% *(64)*.

3.2.1.1. COMPLICATIONS OF RBC TRANSFUSIONS IN SCD

Alloimmunization, although not limited to patients with SCD, is a frequent com-plication of RBC transfusion therapy. For SCD patients an incidence rate of 20% is generally cited *(65)*, although reports range from 8% in children *(66)* to 50% in adults *(67)*. The risk of alloimmunization increases with increasing numbers of RBC transfusions, frequently involves antigens in the Rh, Kell, Duffy, and Kidd blood group systems *(68)*, and is a result of RBC antigenic differences from a largely Caucasian donor pool, into recipients who do not possess these antigens *(69)*. Since many patients develop multiple alloantibodies *(70)*, and may develop autoanti-bodies as well *(71)*, it may be difficult to find compatible blood. Furthermore, because some antibodies become undetectable over time, SCD patients who are recipients of blood components at hospitals where their previous transfusion history is not known are at increased risk of severe delayed transfusion reactions *(72)*.

3.2.1.2. Selection of Blood Components for Children with SCD

Prophylactic use of phenotypically matched RBCs is increasingly used to meet the transfusion requirements of SCD patients *(71,73)*. A variety of approaches have been advocated: use of partial phenotypical matching after formation of two allo-antibodies *(74)*, partial phenotypic matching prior to antibody formation, full pheno-type matching *(73)*, and blood selected from random black blood donors *(75)*. The degree of antigen-matching for transfusion has, to a large part, been dictated by the frequency of occurrence of antibodies in the local population. Furthermore, the suc-cess of transfusion programs for SCD patients has depended heavily on collection of antigen compatible blood largely from African-American donors, and requires the cooperation of local blood collection centers. One such program is designed to limit antigen exposure as well as to limit donor exposure *(76)*.

3.2.2. Pediatric Oncology Patients

Hematologic and nonhematologic malignancies of children frequently require transfusion support either as a result of the underlying malignancy or as a result of intensive chemotherapy and/or radiotherapy. In many hospitals, pediatric hematolo-gists insist that blood products are irradiated to prevent TAGVHD and leukocyte-reduced by filtration to prevent febrile transfusion reactions, CMV transmission and HLA alloimmunization.

3.3. RBC Transfusions in Pediatric Surgery

Transfusion therapy is often indicated in the management of four groups of pediatric surgical procedures: congenital abnormalities such as complex heart and orthopedic defects, burns and accidental trauma, vascular malformations, and trans-plantation. Since these patients are likely to experience significant blood loss, a total blood conservation program should include consideration of pre-operative donation programs, as well as intraoperative and/or pharmacologic techniques to limit allo-geneic exposure.

3.3.1. Autologous and Directed Donations

Autologous donations should be discouraged for surgical procedures during which transfusion is rarely utilized. Autologous donation requests that comply with maxi-mum surgical blood ordering schedules are likely to reflect the true transfusion needs for pediatric surgical patients. The collection of autologous blood in these patients is limited by their vascular access and their ability to cooperate with the phlebotomy. Generally, children aged 8–16 yr can contribute the majority of their blood require-ments *(77,78)*. Both the amount of anticoagulant and the whole blood collection volume must be reduced for children weighing < 50 kg. The volume of blood to draw is determined by the following calculation:

$$\text{Blood volume to draw} = (\text{Donor's weight in kg}/50) \times 450 \text{ mL}$$

Many pediatric patients are either too small or suffer from conditions that preclude autologous donation. Directed donations, particularly from parental donors, may be offered as a substitute. Whether parental donations offer an advantage over allogeneic blood has not been determined, but it does allay parental fears of infectious disease transmission and allow parents to have a direct role in the medical care of their small child. One such program has focused on a committed family member to provide all the anticipated blood components for a cardiac surgery patient *(79,80)*. In another program, all blood components are provided by a dedicated-directed donor *(81)*. Whereas the frequency of donation for routine allogeneic donors is every 56 d, dedicated-directed donor programs require the full cooperation of blood centers to draw all the required components at more frequent intervals *(82)*.

3.3.2. Perioperative Techniques to Limit Allogeneic Transfusion

Blood salvage and infusion procedures are frequently employed in children undergoing cardiac and spinal surgery, as well as in orthotopic liver transplantation *(83)*. Generally, blood is aspirated from the surgical field and is washed with saline prior to infusion. Cellular debris, platelets, white blood cells, and plasma proteins including the coagulation factors, are eliminated prior to direct RBC infusion or temporary intraoperative storage.

Acute normovolemic hemodilution is a technique in which whole blood is removed immediately prior to or after induction of anesthesia. Crystalloid and/or colloid are infused during the phlebotomy. This technique effectively reduces the patient's hematocrit, which increases blood flow, and decreases the amount of red cell mass that is lost. It has been used in cardiac and spinal procedures, in hepatic resection and in major cancer surgery *(84)*.

Pharmacologic agents, such as the administration of aprotinin, have been associated with reductions in perioperative blood loss *(85)*. Deamino-D-arginine vasopressin has also been shown to reduce operative blood loss and allogeneic transfusion replacement in spinal, orthopedic, and cardiac surgery *(86)*. It is also effective in managing the uremic surgical patient *(87)*.

3.3.3. Selection of Blood Components for Surgical Patients

Perioperative transfusion requirements in infants and children can be met by use of routine RBC components. Children with congenital or acquired immunosuppression will benefit from leukocyte-reduced, irradiated blood components to reduce the risk of CMV transmission and the risk of TAGVHD. In addition, blood from blood relatives of recipients must be irradiated to prevent TAGVHD.

Traditionally, fresh RBCs, stored in either CPDA-1 or extended storage solutions (AS-1/AS-3) for < 5–7 d, have been the product of choice for oxygen-carrying capacity in pediatric open heart surgery cases. More recently, the use of < 48-h-old whole blood has found favor with pediatric cardiovascular surgeons because postoperative hemorrhage is significantly reduced *(88)*. It has been hypothesized that improved hemostasis results from better functioning larger platelets *(89)*.

In the setting of massive transfusion, including cardiopulmonary bypass, it is desirable to use the freshest blood available. Blood that is stored in excess of 21 d is depleted of 2,3-DPG, and although 2,3-DPG is regenerated within hours after transfusion, delivery of oxygen to the tissues may be impeded temporarily. Furthermore, cardiac arrest and death have resulted from high potassium concentrations in older blood *(90,91)*.

REFERENCES

1. Sacher RA, Luban NLC, Strauss RG. Current practice and guidelines for the transfusion of cellular blood components in the newborn. *Transfus Med Rev* 1989;3:39–54.
2. Donowitz LG, Turner RB, Searcy MA, et al. The high rate of blood donor exposure for critically ill neonates. *Infect Control Hosp Epidemiol* 1989;10:509–510.
3. Kattwinkel J. Neonatal apnea: pathogenesis and therapy. *J Pediatr* 1977;90:342–347.
4. Joshi A, Gerhardt T. Shandloff D, Bancalari E. Blood transfusion effects on the respiratory pattern of preterm infants. *Pediatrics* 1987;80:79–84.
5. DeMaio JG, Harris NC, Deubner C, Spitzer AR. Effect of blood transfusion on apnea frequency in growing premature infants. *J Pediatr* 1989;14:1039–1041.
6. Stockman JA, Clark DA. Weight gain: a response to transfusion in selected preterm infants. *Am J Dis Child* 1984;738:828–830.
7. Ludvigsen C, Swanson JL, Thompson TR, McCullough J. The failure of neonates to form red cell alloantibodies in response to multiple transfusion. *Am J Clin Pathol* 1987;87:250–251.
8. *Standards for Blood Banks and Transfusion Services,* 17th ed. Bethesda, MD: American Association of Blood Banks, 1996.
9. Strauss RG, Sacher RA, Blazina JF, et al. Commentary on small-volume red cell transfusion for neonatal patients. *Transfusion* 1990;30:565–570.
10. Goodstein MH, Locke RG, Wlodarczyk D, et al. Comparison of two preservation solutions for erythrocyte transfusions in newborn infants. *J Pediatr* 1993;123:783–788.
11. Goodstein MH, Smith J. Herman JH, Rubenstein SD. Use of Adsol (AS-1) preserved packed red blood cells (PRBCS) greater than 5 days (D) of age in the transfusion (TX) of neonates. *Soc Pediatr Res* 1995;37:206A.
12. Jeter EK, Gadsden RH, Cate J. Effects of irradiation on red cells stored in CPDA-1 and CPD-Adsol (AS-1). *Ann Clin Lab Sci* 1991;21:177–186.
13. Patten E, Robbins M, Vincent J, et al. Use of red blood cells older than five days for neonatal transfusion. *J Perinatol* 1991;11:37–40.
14. Batton DG, Goodrow D, Walker RH. Reducing neonatal transfusions. *J Perinatol* 1992;12:15–25.
15. Liu EA, Mannino FL, Lane TA. Prospective, randomized trial of the safety and efficacy of a limited donor exposure transfusion program for premature neonates. *J Pediatr* 1994;125:92–96.
16. Luban NLC, Strauss RG, Hume HA. Commentary on the safety of red cells preserved in extended-storage media for neonatal transfusions. *Transfusion* 1991;31:229–235.
17. Smith JF, Ness PM. Adsol preserved red blood cells greater than five days of age are acceptable for neonatal transfusion (abstract). *Transfusion* 1995;35:16S.
18. Strauss RG, Burmeister L, James T. et al. A randomized trial of fresh versus stored RBCS for neonatal transfusions (abstract). *Transfusion* 1994;34:65S.
19. Lee DA, Slagle TA, Jackson TM. A safe and practical approach to reducing donor exposures in premature infants (abstract). *Transfusion* 1993;33:76S.
20. Levy GJ, Strauss RG, Hume H. et al. National survey of neonatal transfusion practices: I. red blood cell therapy. *Pediatrics* 1993;91:523–529.
21. Van den Berg H. Gerritsen EJA, van Tol MJD, et al. Ten years after acquiring an HIV-1 infection: a study in a cohort of eleven neonates infected by aliquots from a single plasma donation. *Acta Paediatr* 1994;83:173–178.
22. Minifee PK, Daeschner CW, Griffin MP, et al. Decreasing blood donor exposure in neonates on extracorporeal membrane oxygenation. *J Ped Surg* 1990;25:38–42.
23. Humphrey MJ, Harrel-Bean HA, Eskelson C, Corrigan JJ. Blood transfusion in the neonate; effects of dilution and age of blood on hemolysis. *J Pediatr* 1982;101:605–607.

24. Wang-Rodriguez J. Mannino F. Lane T. Limitation of donor exposure in premature neonates and elimination of blood wastage using a novel transfusion strategy (abstract). *Transfusion* 1994;34:32S.

25. Eshleman JR, Akinbi H. Pleasure J. et al. Prospective doubleblind study of small volume neonatal transfusion with RBCs up to 35 days old (abstract). *Transfusion* 1994;34:32S.

26. Cook S. Gunter J. Wissel M. Effective use of a strategy using assigned red cell units to limit donor exposure for neonatal patients. *Transfusion* 1993;33:379–383.

27. Pothiawaka M, Azeem S. Minimizing donor exposure to infants using consigned units (abstract). *Transfusion* 1993;33:14S.

28. Rosenberg EM, Chambers LA, Gunter JM, Good JA. A program to limit donor exposures to neonates undergoing extracorporeal membrane exygenation. *Pediatrics* 1994;94:341–346.

29. Karandish S. DePalma L, Quinones RR, Luban NLC. Minimal allogeneic donor exposure with the use of dedicated donors and a sterile connecting device in a newborn undergoing bone marrow transplantation. *Am J Pediatr Hematol Oncol* 1994; 16:90–93.

30. Meyer MP, Meyer JH, Commerford A, et al. Recombinant human erythropoietin in the treatment of the anemia of prematurity: results of a double-blind, placebo-controlled study. *Pediatrics* 1994;93:918–923.

31. Shannon KM, Keith JF, Mentzer WC, et al. Recombinant human erythropoietin stimulates erythropolesis and reduces erythrocyte transfusions in very low birth weight preterm infants. *Pediatrics* 1995;95:1–10.

32. Maier RF, Obladen M, Scigalla P. et al. The effect of epoetin beta (recombinant human erythropoietin) on the need for transfusion in very-low-birth weight infants. *N Eng J Med* 1994; 330:1173–1178.

33. Yao AC, Lind J. Tiisala R. Michelsson K. Placental transfusion in the premature infant with observation on clinical course and outcome. *Acta Paediat Scand* 1969;58: 561–566.

34. Bifano EM, Dracker RA, Lorah K, Palit A. Collection and 28-day storage of human placental blood. *Pediatr Res* 1994;36:90–94.

35. Yeager AS, Grummet FC, Hafleigh EB, et al. Prevention of transfusion-acquired cytomegalovirus infections in newborn infants. *J Pediatr* 1981; 98:281–287.

36. Alder SP, Chaddrika T. Lawrence L, Baggett J. Cytomegalovirus infections in neonates acquired by blood transfusion. *Pediatr Infect Dis* 1983;2:114–118.

37. Taylors BJ, Jacovs RF, Baker RL, et al. Frozen deglyceroized blood prevents transfusion-acquired cytomegalovirus infection in neonates. *Pediatr Infect Dis* 1986;5: 188–191.

38. Brady MT, Milam JD, Anderson DC, et al. Use of deglycerolized red blood cells to prevent post transfusion infection with cytomegalovirus in neonates. *J Infect Dis* 1984;150:334–339.

39. Preiksaitis JK, Brown L, McKenzie M. Transfusion-acquired cytomegalovirus infection in neonates: a prospective study. *Transfusion* 1988;28:205–213.

40. Tegtmeier GE. The use of cytomegalovirus-screened blood in neonates. *Transfusion* 1988;28:201–203.

41. Eisenfeld L, Silver H. McLaughlin J. et al. Prevention of transfusion-associated cytomegalovirus infection in neonatal patients by the removal of white cells from blood. *Transfusion* 1992;32:205–209.

42. Gilbert GL, Hayes K, Hudson IL, James J. Prevention of transfusion-acquired cytomegalovirus infection in infants by blood filtration to remove leukocytes. *Lancet* 1989;2:1228–1231.

43. Brubaker DB. Transfusion-associated graft-versus-host disease. In: Anderson KC, Ness PM, eds. Scientific Basis of Transfusion Medicine. Philadelphia: Saunders, 1994, pp. 557–558.

44. Hathoway WE, Githens JA, Blackburn JR, et al. Aplastic anemia, histiocytosis, and erythroderma in immunologically deficient children. *N Engl J Med* 1965;273:953–955.

45. Funkhouser AW, Vogelsang G. Zehnbauer B. et al. Graft versus host disease after blood transfusion in a premature infant. *Pediatrics* 1991;87:247–250.

46. Sanders MR, Graeber JE. Posttransfusion graft-versus-host disease in infancy. *J Pediatr* 1990;117:159–163.

47. Berger RS, Dixon SL. Fulminant transfusion-associated graft-versus-host disease in a premature infant. *J Am Acad Dermatol* 1989;20:945–950.

48. Bohm N. Kleine N. Enzel U. Graft-versus-host disease in two newborns after repeated blood transfusions because of Rhesus incompatibility. *Beitr Pathol* 1977;160:381–400.

49. Naiman JL, Punnett HH, Lischner HW, et al. Possible graft-versus-host reaction after intrauterine transfusion for Rh erythroblastosis fetalis. *N Engl J Med* 1969;281:697–701.

50. Otsuka S. Kunieda K, Kitamura F. et al. The critical role of blood from HLA-homozygous donors in fatal transfusion-associated graft-versus-host disease in immunocompetent patients. *Transfusion* 1991;31:260–264.

51. Thaler M, Shamiss A, Orgad S. et al. The role of blood from HLA-homozygous donors in fatal transfusion-associated graft-versus-host disease after open-heart surgery. *N Engl J Med* 1989;321:25–8.

52. Akahoshi M, Takanashi M, Masuda M, et al. A case of transfusion-associated graft-versus-host disease not prevented by white cell-reduction filters. *Transfusion* 1992;32:169–172.

53. Levy GJ, Strauss RG, Hume H. et al. National survey of neonatal transfusion practices: I. red blood cell therapy. *Pediatrics* 1993;91:523–529.

54. Liley AW. Intrauterine transfusion of foetus in haemolytic disease. *Br Med J* 1963;2:1107–1109.

55. Bang J. Bock JE, Trolle D. Ultrasound-guided fetal intravenous transfusion for severe Rhesus haemolytic disease. *Br Med J* 1982;284:373–374.

56. Moise KJ, Carpenter RJ, Kirshon B. et al. Comparison of four types of intrauterine transfusion: effect on fetal hamatocrit. *Fetal Ther* 1989;4:126–137.

57. Gonsulin WJ, Moise KJ, Milam JD, et al. Serial maternal blood donations for intrauterine transfusion. *Obstet Gynecol* 1990;75:158–162.

58. Tierney AJ, Higa TE, Finer NN. Disseminated cytomegalovirus infection after extracorporeal membrane oxygenation. *Pediatr Infect Dis J* 1992;11:241–243.

59. Hatley RM, Reynolds M, Paller AS, Chou P. Graft-versus-host disease following ECMO. *J Pediatr Surg* 1991;26:317–319.

60. Olivieri NF, Koren G. St. Louis P. et al. Studies of the oral chelator 1,2-dimethyl-3-hydroxypyrid-4-one in thalassemia patients. *Semin Hematol* 1990;27:101–104.

61. Haynes J. Kirkpatrick MB. The acute chest syndrome of sickle cell disease. *Am J Med Sci* 1993;305:326–30.

62. Kirkpatrick MB, Bass JB. Pulmonary complication in adults with sickle cell disease. *Pulmonary Perspectives* 1989;6:6–10.

63. Wayne AS, Kevy SV, Nathan DG. Transfusion management of sickle cell disease. *Blood* 1993;81:1109–1123.

64. Russell MO, Goldberg Hl, Hodson A, et al. Effect of transfusion therapy on arteriographic abnormalities and on occurrence of stroke in sickle cell disease. *Blood* 1984;63:162–169.

65. Rosse WF, Gallager D, Kinney TR, et al. The cooperative study of sickle cell disease: Transfusion and alloimmunization in sickle cell disease. *Blood* 1990;76:1431–1437.

66. Sarnaik S. Schornack J. Lusher JM. The incidence of development of irregular red cell antibodies in patients with sickle cell anemia. *Transfusion* 1986;26:249–252.

67. Reisner KG, Kostyu DD, Phillips G. et al. Alloantibody responses in multiply transfused sickle cell patients. *Tissue Antigens* 1987;30:161–166.

68. Patten E, Patel SN, Soto B. Gayle RA. Prevalence of certain clinically significant alloantibodies in sickle cell disease patients. *Ann NY Acad Sci* 1989;565:443–445.

69. Giblett ER. A critique of the theoretical hazard of inter- vs intraracial transfusion. *Transfusion* 1961;1:233–238.

70. Orlina AR, Sosler SD, Koshy M. Problems of chronic transfusion in sickle cell disease. *J Clin Apheresis* 1991;6:234–240.

71. Vichinsky EP, Earles A, Johnson RA, et al. Alloimmunization in sickle cell anemia and transfusion of racially unmatched blood. *N Engl J Med* 1990;322:1617–1621.

72. Salama A, Mueller-Eckhardt C. Delayed hemolytic transfusion reactions. Evidence for complement activation involving allogenic and autologous red cells. *Transfusion* 1984;24:188–193.

73. Ambruso DR, Githern JH, Alcorn R. et al. Experience with donors matched for minor blood group antigens in patients with sickle cell anemia who are receiving chronic transfusion therapy. *Transfusion* 1987;27:94–98.

74. Orlina AR, Unger PJ, Koshy M. Post-transfusion alloimmunization in patients with sickle cell disease. *Am J Hematol* 1978;5:101–106.

75. Sosler SD, Jilly BJ, Saporito C, Koshy M. A simple, practical model for reducing alloimmunization in patients with sickle cell disease. *Am J Hematol* 1993;43:103–106.

76. Hare VW, Liles BA, Crandall LW, Nufer CN. "Partners for Life"—A safer therapy for chronically transfused children (abstract). *Transfusion* 1994;34:92S.

77. Silvergleid AJ. Safety and effectiveness of predeposit autologous transfusion in preteen and adolescent children. *JAMA* 1987;257:3403,3404.

78. Novak RW. Autologous blood transfusion in a pediatric population. *Clin Pediatr* 1988;27:184–187.

79. Brecher ME, Taswell HF, Clare DE, et al. Minimal-exposure transfusion and the committed donor. *Transfusion* 1990;30:599–604.

80. Brecher ME, Moore SB, Taswell HF. Minimal-exposure transfusion: a new approach to homologous blood transfusion. *Mayo Clin Proc* 1988;63:903–905.

81. Strauss RG, Wieland MR, Randels MJ, Koerner TAW. Feasibility and success of a single-donor red cell program for pediatric elective surgery patients. *Transfusion* 1992;32:747–749.

82. Becker LM, Weitekamp LA, Kleis DG, McFarland JG. Minimal donor exposure: low risk/high benefit (abstract). *Transfusion* 1993;33(Suppl):80S.

83. Kruger LM, Colbert JM. Intraoperative autologous transfusion in children undergoing spinal surgery. *J Pediatr Orthop* 1985;5:330–332.

84. Schaller RT, Schaller J. Furman EB. The advantages of hemodilution anethesia for major liver resection in children. *J Pediatr Surg* 1984;19:705–710.

85. Kawaguchi A, Bergeland J. Subramanian S. Total bloodless open heart surgery in the pediatric age group. *Circulation* 1984;70(suppl):30–37.

86. Kobrinsky NL, Letts M, Gatel LR, et al. DDAVP (desmopressin) decreases operative blood loss in patients having Harrington rod spinal fusion surgery. *Ann Intern Med* 1987;107:446–450.

87. Mannuccio PM, Remuzzi G. Pusineri F. et al. Deamino-8-D-arginine vasopressin shortens the bleeding time in uremia. *N Engl J Med* 1983;308:8–12.

88. Manno CS, Hedberg KW, Kim HC, et al. Comparison of the hemostatic effects of fresh whole blood, stored whole blood, and components after open heart surgery in children. *Blood* 1991;77:930–936.
89. Mohr R. Martinowitz U. Lavee J. et al. The hemostatic effect of transfusing fresh whole blood versus platelet concentrates after cardiac operations. *J Thorac Cardiovasc Surg* 1988;96:530–534.
90. Stoops CM. Acute hyperkalemia associated with massive blood replacement (letter). *Anesth Analg* 1983;62:1044.
91. Batton DG, Maisels MJ, Shulman G. Serum potassium changes following packed red cell transfusions in newborn infants. *Transfusion* 1982;23,163–164.

7
Transfusion Support
in Solid-Organ Transplantation

Darrell J. Triulzi

1. INTRODUCTION

Solid-organ transplantation continues to grow as a treatment modality in this country, limited only by the availability of organs. Total transplants in the United States were up 3.6% in 1995 with liver, lung, and kidney accounting for the majority of the increase (*see* Table 1). Transfusion support remains an integral part of solid-organ transplantation, imparting demands on the transfusion service not only quantitatively in terms of blood product support, but also qualitatively with respect to consultation for increasingly complex clinical issues. Aside from the well-known problems associated with massive transfusion, transplant recipients present unique challenges in terms of requirements for specialized blood components, serologic problems, and immunologic effects of transfusion on both the allograft and the recipient. This chapter explores the laboratory and clinical issues involved in transfusion support of solid-organ transplantation.

2. BLOOD COMPONENT UTILIZATION

The typical requirements for blood components for each type of organ transplant in adults at the University of Pittsburgh are shown in Table 2. It is clear from the table that liver transplant procedures use the most blood components despite the fact that blood use in liver transplantation has declined dramatically over the last decade. In a study of 70 liver transplants performed between 1981 and 1983 at the University of Pittsburgh, the mean component usage was 43 red cells, 40 fresh frozen plasma, and 21 units of platelets *(1)*. Eighty-six percent of patients required 10 or more units of red cells. Today, in the same center, the median component usage for an adult primary liver transplant procedure is 12 U of red cells, 13 U of fresh frozen plasma (FFP), and 10 U of platelets. Seventy-one percent of patients required 10 U or more of red cells. The factors contributing to the reduction in blood usage are multiple and include: improved surgical technique, organ preservation, and anesthetic management, and better intraoperative monitoring of coagulation status and pharmacologic treatment of fibrinolysis *(2)*. Heart–lung transplant

From: *Red Cell Transfusion: A Practical Guide*
Edited by: M. E. Reid and S. J. Nance Humana Press Inc., Totowa, NJ

Table 1
Organ Transplant Volumes in the United States[a]

Year	Kidney	Liver	Heart	Lung	Heart–Lung
1994	10,644	3652	2340	722	70
1995	10,793	3915	2358	863	69

[a]UNOS Scientific Registry, Research Department Richmond, VA.

Table 2
Median Blood Use (Units) in Organ Transplantation Procedures at the University of Pittsburgh

Organ	Red cells	Plasma	Platelets	Cryoprecipitate
Liver ($n = 118$)	12	13	10	—
Heart ($n = 51$)	4	5	10	—
Lung				
Single ($n = 46$)	0–2	—	—	—
Double ($n = 30$)	7	2	8	—
Heart–lung ($n = 14$)	4	7	20	4
Kidney	0–2	—	—	—

surgery can also use substantial amounts of blood components, but remains an uncommon procedure with only 69 performed in the United States in 1995. As compared to heart–lung transplantation, heart transplantation is associated with lower blood requirements that approximate blood usage observed in complex cardiopulmonary bypass procedures. Blood usage in lung transplantation varies by the type of lung transplant procedure. Over two-thirds of single-lung transplant recipients do not require any transfusions. Double-lung transplant procedures typically require more red cells than heart or heart–lung transplant procedures, but slightly fewer plasma products. The majority of patients receiving kidney or kidney/pancreas transplants do not require blood.

3. STRATEGIES FOR SELECTION OF COMPATIBLE COMPONENTS

For solid-organ transplant procedures other than liver, transfusion requirements are generally not sufficient to require deviation from traditional selection criteria of ABO identical/compatible red cells that are antigen negative in patients with potentially clinically significant alloantibodies. However, in liver transplantation, the majority of cases still require a large number of transfusions and meet the accepted definition of massive transfusion: one blood volume transfused within a 24-h period. Transfusion volumes in this range frequently exceed the available supply of ABO identical red cells, antigen-negative red cells, or compatible plasma, and thus warrant the development of protocols to optimally use available resources in terms of components and blood bank staffing.

3.1. Group A Patients

Group A patients are rarely switched since group A blood is generally plentiful and group O blood, the only alternative, is frequently in short supply. In patients who receive more than 6–8 group O CPDA-1 red cells, a crossmatch with A cells should be performed to ensure compatibility before switching back to A red cells. A crossmatch does not appear to be necessary if group O additive red cells are used, since they contain less then half of the 60 mL of incompatible plasma found in CPDA-1 red cells *(3)*.

3.2. Group B Patients

Group B patients may need to be switched to group O blood when their transfusion requirements exceed the available group B supply. Since only 10% of donors are group B, this occurs frequently when transfusion requirements exceed 1–2 blood volumes (10–20 U of red cells). The guidelines described in Section 3.1. should be used to switch back to B red cells.

3.3. Group AB Patients

Since group AB patients can receive red cells of any ABO group, available outdating AB red cells should be used and then the patient can be switched to group A cells since these are typically in greatest supply. Group O cells are generally not required but can be used if A red cells are not available. Group A red cells and 10 AB FFP are routinely set up for liver transplantation procedures. The advantage of this approach is that after approx 10 group A FFP red cells are transfused, the patient can then be switched to group A FFP thereby conserving AB FFP. Group AB patients who receive group A or O red cells can be switched back to AB red cells following the guidelines outlined in Section 3.1.

3.4. Group O Patients

Group O patients should not be switched to other red cell groups but can receive any ABO group FFP. The FFP ABO choice is mainly determined by inventory availability.

3.5. Rh_o (D) Selection

Rh negative (D−) patients should be provided with D− red cells as supply allows. D− women over age 45 and adult men may be switched to D+ red cells when their transfusion requirement exceeds 1 blood volume. Greater effort should be made to maintain D− women of childbearing age and children on D− blood, although the risk of D alloimmunization in liver transplantation is low. A recent study reported 0/17 developing anti-D *(4)*. The major clinical significance of an anti-D is that it may limit the ability to switch to D+ red cells if retransplantation is required or massive bleeding is encountered postoperatively. Hemolytic disease of the newborn is a minor concern although pregnancy has been reported following liver transplantation *(5)*.

3.6. Patients with Clinically Significant Alloantibodies

Pre-existing potentially clinically significant red cell alloantibodies are found in approx 6% of liver transplant candidates *(6)*. Usually at least 8–10 U of antigen-compatible blood can be found for surgery. In order to minimize the risk of hemolysis, these patients are ideally managed by using antigen-negative units for the first 5–10 U, switching to antigen-unscreened units in the middle of the case, and then

Table 3
Recommendations for Use of Specialized
Blood Components in Solid-Organ Transplantation

Organ	CMV negative	Filtered	Irradiated
Kidney	Yes[a]	Yes[b]	No
Heart	Yes[a]	Yes[b]	No
Lung	Yes[a]	Yes[b]	No
Liver	Yes[a]	No	No

[a] CMV-negative pairs only. Components rendered CMV-safe by filtration are a reasonable substitute.
[b] Transfusions to transplant candidates only. Not for intraoperative or postoperative transfusions.

switching back to antigen-negative units for the last 5–10 U transfused. This strategy requires close cooperation between the anesthesiologist and blood bank, and has been used successfully in our institution numerous times; only rarely complicated by delayed hemolysis *(6,7)*.

4. INDICATIONS FOR SPECIALIZED BLOOD COMPONENTS

Patients undergoing solid-organ transplantation receive immunosuppressive agents to prevent allograft rejection. One complication of immmunosuppressive therapy is that the patient may be more susceptible to infectious or immunologic complications of transfusion such as cytomegalovirus (CMV) infection or transfusion-associated graft-vs-host disease (TAGVHD). Other immunologic consequences of transfusion such as alloimmunization may also be severe, resulting in acute or chronic graft rejection. The transfusion specialist must recommend the most cost-effective approach to reducing the risk of these complications in organ transplant recipients. Table 3 summarizes the recommendations for use of specialized blood components in these patients.

4.1. CMV-Negative Blood Components

CMV infection is the most frequent infectious complication following solid-organ transplantation *(8)*. In seropositive solid-organ recipients, reactivation of latent virus represents the major risk for CMV infection *(9)*. Although superinfection with a second strain of CMV has been reported from an organ donor *(10)*, this has not been reported from a blood component. Thus, there is no documented benefit to providing blood components that have reduced risk for transmitting CMV to patients who are CMV seropositive. In seronegative patients, the major source for primary CMV infection is the seropositive transplanted organ and, to a lesser extent, transfused blood components. The most severe infections are seen in CMV-negative recipients of a CMV-positive organ *(8)*. The magnitude of the risk of CMV transmission by transfusion can be determined by studying CMV-negative recipients of a CMV-negative organ who receive unscreened blood components. A summary of published data is shown in Table 4 *(10–18)*. Although the overall rate of CMV transmission is low (5–15%), the morbidity associated with this complication would support the use of methods to prevent CMV transmission from blood components.

Table 4
**Incidence of Transfusion-Transmitted CMV Infections
in Seronegative Recipients of Seronegative Organs**

Organ	Total patients	Patients with infection (%)
Kidney *(10–12)*	289	18 (6%)
Heart *(11,13–15)*	87	13 (15%)
Lung *(15)*	3	0 (0%)
Heart–lung *(11,16)*	40	5 (13%)
Liver *(11,17,18)*	34	3 (9%)

Historically, this was accomplished by using blood components from donors who lack antibodies to CMV. Recent data in allogeneic bone marrow transplant recipients demonstrate that leukocyte reduction by filtration is equally effective in reducing the risk of CMV transmission from a blood component *(19)*. It is likely that this method would also be effective in solid-organ transplant recipients although similar data are not available. The volumes of blood used in organ transplant procedures other than liver transplantation generally do not pose supply problems when restricted to CMV-negative pairs. In the liver transplant setting, the choice of using CMV-seronegative blood or filtered blood should be based on inventory availability and cost considerations comparing CMV-serologic screening to filtration.

4.2. Irradiated Blood Components

GVHD occurs much less commonly following solid-organ transplantation compared to bone marrow transplantation. This is a function of a smaller dose of lymphocytes in the lymphoid tissue accompanying the allograft and the less intense recipient immunosuppression. GVHD has been reported following liver *(20–22)*, heart *(23,24)*, heart–lung *(25)*, kidney *(26,27)*, and pancreas–spleen *(28)* transplantation. The organ donor was suspected or proven to be the source of cytotoxic T-cells in all but four cases, liver *(22)*, heart *(23)*, and kidney *(26,27)*. The latter four cases were reported as transfusion-related GVH; however, one was not confirmed by human leukocyte antigen (HLA) or DNA typing of the lymphocytes *(26)*. Although underreporting undoubtedly occurs, the paucity of cases of GVHD derived from the donor organ and only three confirmed cases of TAGVHD would not support routinely providing irradiated blood components to these patients. A national survey conducted by the American Association of Blood Banks (AABB) found that 60% (201/337) of institutions, including the author's, do not provided irradiated components for solid-organ transplant recipients *(29)*.

4.3. Leukocyte-Reduced Blood Components:
Alloimmunization vs the Transfusion Effect

Alloimmunization to HLA antigens is of considerable importance to patients considered for organ transplantation. A sensitized patient presents problems in identifying a crossmatch-compatible donor and, for some organs, the outcome of transplantation is inferior. However, white cells in blood components may be beneficial in inducing tolerance and prolonging allograft survival *(30)*. Thus, the decision to provide leukocyte-reduced components must weigh the risks and benefits of the constituent white cells.

4.3.1. Alloimmunization vs the Transfusion Effect in Renal Transplantation

It has been recognized for almost three decades that patients with preformed lymphocytotoxic antibodies are at risk for hyperacute kidney rejection *(31)*. Patients who become sensitized through transfusion, pregnancy, or previous transplantation are less likely to find a crossmatch-compatible donor. Although it is clearly desirable to avoid sensitization by leukocytes, these same leukocytes have been shown to prolong allograft survival *(31,32)*. Studies of renal transplant candidates receiving pretransplant nonleukocyte-reduced transfusions have reported alloimmunization rates of 29% with donor-specific transfusions (DST) *(33)* and 19% with random donor transfusions *(34)*. These rates can be substantially reduced by giving concommitant azothiaprine *(35)* or cyclosporine (CsA) *(36)*, or using HLA haploidentical transfusions *(34,37)*. In the 1980s clinicians accordingly gave renal transplant candidates conditioning with azothiaprine or CsA when giving nonleukocyte-reduced transfusions. By the early 1990s, the widespread use of CsA largely mitigated any advantage to pretransplant transfusions *(38)* and the concern over the residual risk of sensitization from transfusion resulted in a decline in this practice. If the transfusion effect is not a concern, then leukocyte reduction makes sense to reduce the risk of alloimmunization. The efficacy of leukocyte reduction in preventing alloimmunization in this setting has not been established, but supportive data do exist *(39)*. It is not clear whether leukocyte reduction is necessary for intra- or postoperative transfusions since the patient is immunosuppressed and will be exposed to the alloantigens on the organ regardless of whether the blood is leukocyte reduced. There is a theoretical risk that nonleukocyte-reduced transfusions may sensitize the patient to additional HLA antigens that may interfere with crossmatching and graft survival if another transplant is required.

More recently, pretransplant transfusions have regained some favor as longer term follow up has revealed a survival advantage *(40)*. Additionally, the transfusion effect appears to be enhanced and alloimmunization minimized by using blood from HLA haplo-identical donors *(34,37,41)*. The transfusion service must thus determine how transfusions are used for renal transplant candidates in their institution. If they are used to prolong allograft survival, then filtration is contraindicated. If not used for this purpose, then filtration is indicated, at least preoperatively, to reduce the risk of allosensitization.

4.3.2. Alloimmunization vs the Transfusion Effect in Cardiac Transplantation

Humoral alloimmunization in cardiac transplant candidates has been shown to correlate with lower cardiac allograft survival *(42,43)*. Patients with lymphocytotoxicity panel reactive antibodies (PRA) of 0–10%, 11–25%, and >25% had 5-yr actuarial freedom from death owing to acute and chronic rejection of 85, 68, and 57% respectively *(42)*. There was no correlation between hyperacute rejection and %PRA. These data indicate that HLA alloimmunization is a risk factor for acute and/or chronic cardiac allograft rejection.

The transfusion effect and the role of DST in cardiac transplantation has not been well documented in human studies although animal studies have demonstrated a graft prolongation effect *(44)*. Retrospective single-center clinical data have demonstrated a transfusion effect *(45–49)*, however, the Collaborative Transplant Study Group reported no cardiac graft survival advantage in 419 transfused vs 2195 untransfused cardiac allograft recipients *(50)*. An explanation for this discrepancy may be found in a small study looking at the effect of random pretransplant transfusions *(37)*. Patients who had received blood matched for one HLA-DR antigen had a lower rate of alloimmunization and fewer rejection episodes than those receiving blood mismatched for both DR antigens, however a difference in survival could not be demonstrated. Thus, in the absence of prospective clinical data indicating a transfusion effect, the risk of alloimmunization seems to be of greater clinical concern. It would seem prudent therefore to provide leukocyte-reduced blood components to cardiac transplant candidates to reduce the risk of alloimmunization. For the reasons discussed in renal transplant recipients, the value of leukocyte-reduced products intra- or postoperatively is unclear. Cardiac retransplantation is uncommon, acounting for only 2 of 40 heart transplant procedures in 1995 at the University of Pittsburgh.

4.3.3. Alloimmunization vs the Transfusion Effect in Lung Transplantation

Hyperacute rejection after lung transplantation is rare; suspected in only 2 cases among 359 lung transplants performed in Pittsburgh and felt to be the result of pre-existing alloantibodies to vascular endothelium *(51)*. However, a limited amount of data have implicated HLA antibodies in mediating acute rejection *(52)* and chronic rejection characterized by obliterative bronchiolitis *(53)*. There are no published clinical data demonstrating a transfusion effect in lung transplantation. Thus, providing leukocyte-reduced blood components to lung transplant candidates appears warranted, given the potential serious clinical consequences of HLA alloimmunization in lung transplant recipients. It is unclear whether leukocyte-reduced products would be of benefit perioperatively. Lung retransplantation is uncommon, accounting for none of the 48 lung transplant procedures performed in 1995 at the University of Pittsburgh.

4.3.4. Alloimmunization vs the Transfusion Effect in Liver Transplantation

The role of humoral alloimmunization in liver transplantation is unclear. Hyperacute rejection in a patient with donor-specific lymphocytotoxic antibodies has been described but is uncommon *(54)*. There are conflicting data regarding the long-term effects of liver transplantation in the presence of lymphocytotoxic antibodies. Data from Pittsburgh showed lower 1-yr graft survival of approx 56% in patients with donor-specifc antibody compared to 82% in patients without antibody *(55)*. In contrast, Lobo et al. *(56)* recently reported that pre-existing donor-specific lymphocytotoxic antibodies had no effect on 1-yr graft survival. The deleterious effect of pretransplant alloimmunization on liver allograft survival appears to be less than that observed in renal or cardiac transplantation. Initial studies suggested that alloimmunized patients require more transfusions during their liver transplant procedure presumably owing to shortened survival of transfused platelets and more bleeding *(57)*. This has not been found in a recent study *(56)*. Given the lack of clear clinical significance of alloimmunization in liver transplantation, and the practical considerations (cost and logistics) of providing large numbers of transfusions to these patients, leukoreduction of blood components is not warranted.

The role of pretransplant transfusions in mediating the transfusion effect in liver transplantation is poorly defined. Animal models have suggested that a transfusion effect exists *(58)*, but clinical data are sparse and equivocal *(59,60)*. Available data are insufficient to recommend intentional pretransplant transfusions in liver transplantation at this time.

5. ABO BLOOD GROUP SYSTEM IN ORGAN TRANSPLANTATION

The ABO system is clinically important in two areas involving solid-organ transplantation: first, as a transplantation antigen important in graft survival, and second as an antigen–antibody system implicated in immune hemolytic anemias in ABO nonidentical organ transplant recipients.

5.1. ABO Blood Group System as a Transplantation Antigen

The importance of the ABO system in organ transplantation was recognized over 30 yr ago when rapid rejection of ABO-incompatible kidney transplants was observed *(61)*. Preformed recipient isohemagglutinins bind to ABO antigens on endothelial surfaces in the organ, resulting in complement activation, endothelial damage, ischemic necrosis, and rapid (hyperacute) graft loss *(62)*. Transplantation across ABO lines will typically cause hyperacute rejection of kidney *(63)* and heart transplants *(64)*, although exceptions do exist *(65,66)*. Successful transplantation of kidneys and hearts across ABO lines has been accomplished by removing ABO antibodies in the recipient *(65,67)* or by taking advantage of the variable expression of ABO antigens on endothelial surfaces such as in A2 individuals *(68)*. For the most part, ABO-incompatible organs are avoided in kidney and heart transplantation.

ABO incompatible (major mismatch) liver allografts are used in 6.9% of pediatric and 2.4% of adult liver recipients due to organ shortages *(69)*. Liver allografts are felt to be resistent to hyperacute rejection when transplanted across ABO barriers *(70)* however reports of hyperacute rejection do exist *(71,72)*. ABO-incompatible liver transplants are commonly associated with acute graft failure with a 46% graft failure rate reported within 30 d of the transplant *(72)*. Long-term results in adults demonstrate that 1-yr graft survival is lower compared to ABO compatible transplants 30% *(72)* vs 80% *(69)*, however 1-yr patient survival (52%) did not differ from recipients of ABO-compatible grafts matched for medical urgency and indication *(72)*. Pediatric recipients of ABO-incompatible livers appear to fare better with a recent study reporting 1- and 3-yr patient and graft survival rates comparable to recipients of ABO-identical livers *(73)*. Plasmapheresis to remove recipient isohemagglutinins may be of benefit *(74,75)*. Currently, ABO-incompatible liver allografts are reserved for patients with fulminant liver failure in whom death is imminent without transplantation and when an ABO-compatible organ is not available *(76)*.

ABO compatible but nonidentical (minor mismatch) liver transplants are associated with a modest reductions in 1- and 3-yr survival; however, the factor of urgency may account for some of the observed difference *(77)*. Approximately 15% of liver transplants performed at our institution are ABO minor mismatches and are also at risk for immunohematologic complications described in Section 5.2.

5.2. *Immunohematologic Complications of ABO Minor Mismatch Organ Transplants*

Unexpected antibodies of A and B specificity have been reported in recipients of ABO minor mismatch (O donors to non-O recipients, A or B donors to AB recipients) solid organs *(78)*. Isohemagglutinins are produced by the viable donor lymphocytes passively transferred with the organ at the time of transplantation. The donor origin of the antibody has been confirmed using immunoglobulin allotyping *(79)*. Over 100 cases have been described involving transplantation of the liver *(78,80)*, kidney *(78,81)*, pancreas *(78)*, spleen *(78)*, heart *(78)*, lung *(78,82,83)*, and heart–lung *(78,84,85)*. Unexpected ABO antibodies can also develop in minor ABO-mismatched bone marrow transplant recipients *(86)*. A recent review *(78)* found that the frequency of antibodies and hemolysis was 70% (for both) in heart-lung transplant recipients, 40 and 29%, respectively, in liver transplant recipients, and 17 and 9% in kidney transplant recipients. It has been suggested that the amount of lymphoid tissue transplanted with the organ accounts for these differences. Rarely, antibodies to red-cell antigens outside the ABO system (i.e., anti-D, Kell) have been reported in association with transplanted kidneys *(78)*, livers *(78)*, and heart–lungs *(85)*.

Donor-derived ABO antibody (DDAb) typically develops 7–14 d after transplantation with a time-course independent of the type of organ transplanted. The appearance of DDAb in the serum and the development of a positive DAT are generally concurrent. Serum antibody is predominantly IgG, but may also be IgM. Red cell eluates will reveal anti-A, anti-B, or anti-A,B. DDAbs are short-lived antibodies that persist for a median of 5 wk in kidney transplant recipients and 2–3 wk in liver transplant recipients. It is not clear why the antibody disappears, whether it is related to elimination or downregulation of donor lymphocytes.

DDAbs are associated with hemolysis in a variable proportion of ABO minor mismatched organ transplant recipients. Among kidney transplant recipients with DDAb, approx 50% developed hemolysis, and most required transfusion of red cells *(78)*. Hemolysis was complicated by acute renal failure requiring hemodialysis in several patients and one patient died.

In liver transplant recipients, the incidence of hemolysis in those with DDAb is higher than in renal transplantation. Sixty-eight *(78)* to 100% *(80)* of liver transplant patients with DDAb develop hemolysis. Although the hemolysis is usually mild and self-limited, substantial morbidity associated with hemolysis including acute renal failure, disseminated intravascular coagulation, hypotension, and multiorgan failure has been reported *(78,80)*.

Currently there are no reliable factors that can predict which recipients of ABO unmatched organs will develop DDAb or hemolysis. However, it is more likely in group A recipients of group O organs who receive CsA or tacrolimus immunosuppression *(78,80,87)*. In most cases, the hemolysis associated with DDAb is mild and can be treated with transfusions. Transfused red cells should be of *organ donor* ABO group to replace susceptible red cells with cells that will not be hemolyzed. Plasma products should be of *recipient* ABO group to reduce the risk of hemolysis by providing soluble ABO antigen capable of neutralizing DDAb. Patients who develop severe hemolysis can be treated with plasmapheresis or red cell exchange with donor type red cells. Although there are anecdotal reports of success with these therapies *(78,80)*, their efficacy remains unproven. Steroids have not been shown to be of benefit in treating hemolysis in this setting. Prophylactic use of O red cells in CsA-treated group A recipients of O livers may be of benefit *(80)*.

6. FUTURE CONSIDERATIONS

The field of organ transplantation is rapidly evolving. The persistent shortage of human organs for transplantation has prompted use of animal sources. Recently performed baboon liver xenotransplants have raised new challenges for transfusion medicine specialists *(88,89)*. The demonstration of microchimerism in long-term allograft survivors *(90)* have prompted clinical trials of organ donor bone-marrow infusion to enhance the establishment of chimerism and prolong graft survival *(91)*. Donor peripheral blood lymphocytes collected by apheresis have been used successfully to treat post-bone marrow transplant lymphoproliferative disorders *(92)* and are under investigation in the solid-organ transplant setting. These emerging trends in solid-organ transplantation ensure the continuing role and critical need for transfusion medicine expertise and support.

REFERENCES

1. Bontempo FA, Lewis JH, Van Thiel DH, Spero JA, Ragni MV, Butler P, Israel L, Starzl TE. The relation of preoperative coagulation findings to diagnosis, blood usage, and survival in adult liver transplantation. *Transplantation* 1985;39:532–536.
2. Kang Y, Lewis JH, Navalgund A, Russell MW, Bontempo FA, Niren LS, Starzl TE: ε-aminocaproic acid for treatment of fibrinolysis during liver transplantation. *Anesthesiology* 1987; 66:766–773.
3. Nicol SL, Shirey RS, Banez-Sese GC, Ness PM. Significance of residual plasma from group O additive solution RBC transfusions (abstract). *Transfusion* 1995;35(Suppl): S247.
4. Casanueva M, Valdes MD, Ribera MC. Lack of allo-immunization to D antigen in D-negative immunosuppressed liver transplant recipients. *Transfusion* 1994;34:570–572.
5. Jain A, Venkataramanan R, Lever J, Warty V, Fung J, Todo S, Starzl T. FK506 and pregnancy in liver transplant patients (letter). *Transplantation* 1993;56:751.
6. Ramsey G, Cornell FW, Hahn LF, Larson P, Issitt LB, Starzl TE. Red cell antibody problems in 1000 liver transplants. *Transfusion* 1989;29:396–399.
7. Ramsey G, Cornell FW, Hahn LF, Fonzi F, Starzl TE. Incompatible blood transfusions in liver transplant patients with significant red cell alloantibodies. *Transplant Proc* 1989;21:3531.
8. Rubin RH. Impact of cytomegalovirus infection on organ transplant recipients. *Rev Infect Dis* 1990;12(Suppl):S754–S766.
9. Ho M. Epidemiology of cytomegalovirus infections. *Rev Infect Dis* 1990;12(Suppl): S701–S710.
10. Grundy JE, Super M, Sweny P, Moorhead J, Lui SF, Berry NJ, Fernando ON, Griffiths PD. Symptomatic cyto-megalovirus infection in seropositive kidney recipients: reinfection with donor virus rather than reactivation of recipient virus. *Lancet* 1988;371:132–135.
11. Preiksaitis JK. Indications for the use of cytomeglovirus seronegative blood products. *Transfusion Med Rev* 1991;5:1–17.
12. Fryd DS, Peterson PK, Ferguson RM, Simmons RL, Balfour HH, Najarian JS: Cytomegalovirus as a risk factor in renal transplantation. *Transplantation* 1980;30:436–439.

13. Laske A, Gallino A, Carrel T, Niederhauser U, von Segesser LK, Turina MI: Cytomegalovirus infection and prophylaxis in heart transplantation. *Transplant Proc* 1993; 25:1427–1428.

14. Grossi P, Minoli L, Percivalle E, Irish W, Vigano M, Gerna G. Clinical and virological monitoring of human cytomegalovirus infection in 294 heart transplant recipients. *Transplantation* 1995;59:847–851.

15. Egan JJ, Barber L, Lomax J, Fox A, Yonan N, Rahman AN, Campbell CS, Deiraniya AK, Carroll KB, Craske J, Turner A, Woodcock AA. Detection of human cytomegalovirus antigenaemia: a rapid diagnostic technique for predicting cytomegalovirus infection/pneumonitis in lung and heart transplant recipients. *Thorax* 1995;50:9–13.

16. Smyth RL, Scott JP, Borysiewicz LK, Sharples LD, Stewart S, Wreghitt TG, Gray JJ, Higenbottam TW, Wallwork J. Cytomegalovirus infection in heart-lung transplant recipients: risk factors, clinical associations, and response to treatment. *J Infect Dis* 1991;164:1045–1050.

17. Winston DJ, Wirin D, Shaked A, Busuttil RW. Randomised comparison of ganciclovir and high-dose acyclovir for long-term cytomegalovirus prophylaxis in liver-transplant recipients. *Lancet* 1995;346:69–74.

18. Rakela J, Wiesner RH, Taswell HF, Hermans PE, Smith TF, Perkins JD, Krom RAF. Incidence of cytomegalovirus infection and its relationship to donor-recipient serologic status in liver transplantation. *Transplant Proc* 1987;19:2399–2402.

19. Bowden RA, Slichter SJ, Sayers M, Weisdorf D, Cays M, Schoch G, Banaji M, Haake R, Welk K, Fisher L, McCullough J, Miller W. A comparison of filtered leukocyte-reduced and cytomegalovirus (CMV) seronegative blood products for the prevention of transfusion-associated CMV infection after marrow transplant. *Blood* 1995;86:3598–3603.

20. Burdick JF, Vogelsang GB, Smith WJ, Farmer ER, Bias WB, Kaufmann SH, Horn J, Colombani PM, Pitt HA, Perler BA, Merritt WT, Williams GM, Boitnott JK, Herlong HF. Severe graft-vs host disease in a liver transplant recipient. *N Engl J Med* 1988;318:689–691.

21. Roberts JP, Ascher NL, Lake J, Capper J, Purohit S, Garovoy M, Lynch R, Ferrell L, Wright T. Graft-vs-host disease after liver transplantation in humans: a report of four cases. *Hepatology* 1991; 14:274–281.

22. Wisecarver JL, Cattral MS, Langnas AN, Shaw BW, Fox IJ, Heffron TG, Rubocki RJ. Transfusion-induced graft-versus-host disease after liver transplantation. *Transplantation* 1994;58:269–271.

23. Sola MA, Espana A, Redondo P, Idoate MA, Fernandez AL, Llorens R, Quintanilla E. Transfusion-associated acute graft-versus-host disease in a heart transplant recipient. *Br J Dermatol* 1995;132:626–630.

24. Sliman GA, Beschorner WG, Baughman KL, et al. Graft-versus-host-like disease in a heart allograft recipient: a possible autoimmune phenomenon. *Transplantation* 1988; 45:253–256.

25. Wood H, Higenbottam T, Joysey V, Wallwork J. Graft-versus-host disease after human heart-lung transplantation. *International Congress of the Transplantation Society* (abstract) 1990;364.

26. Andany MA, Martinez W, Arnal F, Yebra T, Falcon TG, Lozano IR, Lorenzo D, Alonso A. Transfusion-associated graft-versus-host disease in a renal transplant recipient. *Nephrol Dial Transplant* 1994;9:196–198.

27. Andersen CB, Ladefoged SD, Taaning E. Transfusion-associated graft-versus-graft and potential graft-versus-host disease in a renal allotransplanted patient. *Hum Pathol* 1992;23:831–834.

28. Deierhoi MH, Sollinger HW, Bozdech MJ, Belzer FO. Lethal graft-vs-host disease in a recipient of a pancreas-spleen transplant. *Transplantation* 1986;41:544–546.

29. Anderson KC, Goodnough LT, Sayers M, Pisciotto PT, Kurtz SR, Lane TA, Anderson CS, Silberstein LE. Variation in blood component irradiation practice: implications for prevention of transfusion-associated graft-versus-host disease. *Blood* 1991;77: 2096-2102.
30. Opelz G, Sengar DPS, Mickey MR, et al. Effect of blood transfusions on subsequent kidney transplants. *Transplant Proc* 1973;5:253-259.
31. Kissmeyer-Nielsen F, Olsen S, Petersen VP, Fjeldborg O. Hyperacute rejection of kidney allografts, associated with pre-existing humoral antibodies against donor cells. *Lancet* 1966;2:662-665.
32. Horimi T, Terasaki PI, Chia D, Sasaki N. Factors influencing the paradoxical effect of transfusions on kidney transplants. *Transplantation* 1983;35:320-323.
33. Colombe BW, Lou CD, Salvatierra O, Jr, Garovoy MR. Two patterns of sensitization demonstrated by recipients of donor-specific transfusion: limitations to control by Imuran. *Transplantation* 1987;44:509.
34. Bayle F, Masson D, Zaoui P, Vialtel P, Janbon B, Bensa JC, Cordonnier DJ. Beneficial effect of one HLA haplo- or semi-identical transfusion versus three untyped blood units on alloimmunization and acute rejection episodes in first renal allograft recipients. *Transplantation* 1995;59:719-723.
35. Radvany RM, Patel KM. Donor-specific transfusions. Donor-recipient HLA compatibility, recipient HLA haplotype, and antibody production. *Transfusion* 1988;28: 137-141.
36. Cheigh JS, Suthanthiran M, Fotino M, et al. Minimal sensitization and excellent renal allograft outcome following donor-specific blood transfusion with a short course of cyclosporine. *Transplantation* 1991;51:378-381.
37. Lagaaij EL, Hennemann IPH, Ruigrok M, de Haan MW, Persijn GG, Termijtelen A, Hendriks GFJ, Weimar W, Claas FHJ, van Rood JJ. Effect of one-HLA-DR-antigen-matched and completely HLA-DR-mismatched blood transfusions on survival of heart and kidney allografts. *N Engl J Med* 1989;321:701-705.
38. Ahmed Z, Terasaki PI. Effect of transfusion. In: Terasaki PI, ed. *Clinical Transplants*. Los Angeles: UCLA Tissue Typing Laboratory, 1991, pp. 305-312.
39. Fisher M, Chapman JR, Ting A, Morris PJ. Alloimmunization to HLA antigens following transfusion with leukocyte-poor and purified platelet suspensions. *Vox Sanguinis* 1985;49:331-335.
40. Flye MW, Burton K, Mohanakumar T, Brennan D, Keller C, Goss JA, Sicard GA, Anderson CB. Donor-specific transfusions have long-term beneficial effects for human renal allografts. *Transplantation* 1995;60:1395-1401.
41. Bayle F, Masson D, Zaoui P, Janbon B, Bensa JC, Vialtel P. One HLA haplo-identical transfusion in first renal allo-graft recipients: effect on alloimmunisation, acute rejection episodes, and graft survival. *Transplant Proc* 1995;27:2457-2458.
42. Lavee J, Kormos RL, Duquesnoy RJ, Zerbe TR, Armitage JM, Vanek M, Hardesty RL, Griffith BP. Influence of panel reactive antibody and positive lymphocytotoxic crossmatch on cardiac transplant survival. *J Heart Lung Transplant* 1991;10(6): 921-929.
43. Sucui-Foca N, Reed E, Marboe C. The role of anti-HLA antibodies in heart transplantation. *Transplantation* 1993;51:716-724.
44. Johnson CP, Munda R, Alexander JW, Balakrishnan K, Blanton M. The effect of donor-specific transfusions on rat heart allograft survival. *Transplantation* 1984;38: 575-578.
45. Dong E, Stinson EB, Griepp RB, Coulson AS, Shumway NE. Cardiac transplantation following failure of previous cardiac surgery. *Surg Forum* 1973;24:150-152.
46. Cooper DKC, Boyd ST, Lanza RP, Barnard CN. Factors influencing survival following heart transplantation. *Heart Transplant* 1983;3:86-91.

47. Katz MR, Barnhart GR, Goldman MH, Rider S, Hastillo A, Szentpetery S, Wolfgang TC, Hess ML, Mohanakumar T, Lower RR. Pretransplant transfusions in cardiac allograft recipients. *Transplantation* 1987;43:499–501.
48. Kerman RH, Van Buren CT, Lewis RM, Frazier OH, Cooley D, Kahan BD. The impact of HLA A, B, and DR blood transfusions and immune responder status on cardiac allograft recipients treated with cyclosporine. *Transplantation* 1988;45:333–337.
49. Keogh A, Baron D, Chang V. The effect of blood pretransfusion on orthotopic cardiac transplantation. *Transplant Proc* 1987;19:2503.
50. Opelz G. Factors affecting the outcome of kidney and heart transplants today. 8th Scientific Meeting of the Transplantation Society of Australia and New Zealand, March 1990.
51. Keenan RJ, Zeevi A. Immunologic consequences of transplantation. *Basic Biol Thorac Surg* 1995;5:107–120.
52. Nelson KA, Albert RK, Davies C, et al. Association of antibody to donor HLA class I antigens with early acute lung rejections in lung transplant recipients. *Am J Respir Crit Care Med* 1994;149:A1097.
53. Bando K, Paradis IL, Similo S, Konishi H, Komatsu K, Zullo TG, Yousem SA, Close JM, Zeevi A, Duquesnoy RJ, Manzetti J, Keenan RJ, Armitage JM, Hardesty RL, Griffith BP. Obliterative bronchiolitis after lung and heart-lung transplantation. An analysis of risk factors and management. *J Thorac Cardiovasc Surg* 1995;110:4–13.
54. Bird G, Friend P, Donaldson P, O'Grady J, Portmann B, Calne R, Williams R. Hyperacute rejection in liver transplantation: a case report. *Transplant Proc* 1989;21: 3742–3744.
55. Takaya S, Bronsther O, Iwaki Y, Nakamura K, Abu-Elmagd K, Yagihashi A, Demetris AJ, Kobayashi M, Todo S, Tzakis AG, Fung JJ, Starzl TE. The adverse impact on liver transplantation of using positive cytotoxic crossmatch donors. *Transplantation* 1992;53:400–406.
56. Lobo PI, Spencer C, Douglas MT, Stevenson WC, Pruett TL. The lack of long-term detrimental effects on liver allografts caused by donor-specific anti-HLA antibodies. *Transplantation* 1993; 55:1063–1066.
57. Weber T, Marino IR, Kang YG, Esquivel CO, Starzl TE, Duquesnoy RJ. Intraoperative blood transfusions in highly alloimmunized patients undergoing orthotopic liver transplantation. *Transplantation* 1989;47:797–801.
58. Yokoi Y, Yamaguchi A, Kimura H, Nakamura S, Baba S, Amemiya H. Donor-specific transfusion: critical role of class I antigen presenting molecules in rat liver transplantation. *Transplant Proc* 1995;27:1558–1559.
59. Rouch DA, Thistlethwaite JR, Lichtor L, Emond JC, Broelsch CE. Effect of massive transfusion during liver transplantation on rejection and infection. *Transplant Proc* 1988;20:1135–1137.
60. Palomo JC, Jiminez C, Moreno E, Garcia MA, Bercedo J, Loinaz C, Palma F, Ibanez J, Corral MA. Effects of intraoperative blood transfusion on rejection and survival after orthotopic liver transplantation. *Transplant Proc* 1995;27:2326–2327.
61. Starzl TE, Marchioro TL, Holmes JH, Waddell WR. The incidence, cause and significance of immediate and delayed oliguria or anuria after human renal transplantation. *Surg Gynecol Obstet* 1964;188:819–827.
62. Demetris AJ, Murase N, Nakamura K, Iwaki Y, Yagihashi A, Valdivia L, Todo S, Iwatsuki S, Takaya S, Fung JJ. Immunopathology of antibodies as effectors of orthotopic liver allograft rejection. *Semin Liver Dis* 1992;12:51–59.
63. Cook DJ, Graver B, Terasaki PI. ABO incompatibility in cadaver donor kidney allografts. *Transplant Proc* 1987;19:4549–4552.
64. Cooper DKC. Clinical survey of heart transplantation between ABO blood group-incompatible recipients and donors. *J Heart Transplant* 1990;9:376–381.

65. Alexandre GPJ, Squifflet JP, De Bruyere M, Latinne D, Reding R, Gianello P, Carlier M, Pirson Y. Present experiences in a series of 26 ABO-incompatible living donor renal allografts. *Transplant Proc* 1987;19:4538–4542.

66. Carvana RJ, Zumbro GL Jr, Hoff RG, Rao RN, Daspit SA. Successful cardiac transplantation across an ABO blood group barrier. *Transplantation* 1988;46:472–474.

67. Cooper DKC, Ye Y, Kehoe M, Niekrasz M, Rolf LL Jr, Martin M, Baker J, Kosanke S, Zuhdi N, Worsley G, Romano E. A novel approach to "neutralization" of preformed antibodies: cardiac allotransplantation across the ABO blood group barrier as a paradigm of discordant transplantation. *Transplant Proc* 1992;24:566571.

68. Nelson PW, Helling TS, Shield CF, Becj M, Bryan CF. Current experience with renal transplantation across the ABO barrier. *Am J Surg* 1992;164:541–544.

69. Belle SH, Beringer KC, Murphy JB, Detre KM. The Pitt-Unos liver transplant registry. In: Terasaki PI and Cecka JM, eds. *Clinical Transplants 1992*. Los Angeles, CA: UCLA Tissue Typing Laboratory, 1992, p. 7.

70. Demetris AJ, Jaffe R, Tzakis A, Ramsey G, Todo S, Belle S, Esquivel C, Shapiro R, Zjako A, Markus B, Morozec E, Van Thiel DH, Sysyn G, Gordon R, Makowka L, Starzl TE. Antibody mediated rejection of human liver allografts: transplantation across ABO blood group barriers. *Transplant Proc* 1989;21:2217–2220.

71. Gugenheim J, Samuel D, Fabiani B, Saliba F, Castaing D, Reynes M, Bismuth H. Rejection of ABO incompatible liver allografts in man. *Transplant Proc* 1989;21: 2223–2224.

72. Farges O, Kalil AN, Samuel D, Saliba F, Arulnaden JL, Debat P, Bismuth A, Castaing D, Bismuth H. The use of ABO-incompatible grafts in liver transplantation: a lifesaving procedure in highly selected patients. *Transplantation* 1995; 59:1124–1133.

73. Cacciarelli TV, So SKS, Lim J, Concepcion W, Cox K, Esquivel CO: A reassessment of ABO incompatibility in pediatric liver transplantation. *Transplantation* 1995;60: 757–768.

74. Mor E, Skerrett D, Manzarbeitia C, Sheiner PA, Schwartz ME, Emre S, Thung SN, Miller CM: Successful use of an enhanced immunosuppressive protocol with plasmapheresis for ABO-incompatible mismatched grafts in liver transplant recipients. *Transplantation* 1995;59:986–990.

75. Renard TH, Andrews WS: An approach to ABO-incompatible liver transplantation in children. *Transplantation* 1992;53:116–121.

76. Conference of the Consensus on the indications of liver transplantation. *Hepatology* 1994;20(1 pt 2).

77. Gordon RD, Iwatsuki S, Esquivel CO, Tzakis A, Todo S, Starzl TE. Liver transplantation across ABO blood groups. *Surgery* 1986;100:342–348.

78. Ramsey G. Red cell antibodies arising from solid organ transplants. *Transfusion* 1991;31:77–86.

79. Swanson JL, Sastamoinen RM, Steeper TA, Sebring ES. Gm allotyping to determine the origin of red cell antibodies in recipients of solid organ transplants. *Vox Sanguinis* 1987;52:75–78.

80. Triulzi DJ, Shirey RS, Ness PM, Klein AS. Immunohematologic complications of ABO unmatched liver transplants. *Transfusion* 1992;32:829–833.

81. Orchard J, Young NT, Smith C, Thomas S, Darke C. Severe intravascular haemolysis in a renal transplant recipient due to anti-B of donor origin. *Vox Sanguinis* 1990; 59:172–175.

82. Magrin GT, Street AM, Williams TJ, Esmore DS. Clinically significant anti-A derived from B lymphocytes after single lung transplantation. *Transplantation* 1993;56: 466–467.

83. Taaning E, Morling N, Mortensen SA, Pettersson G, Simonsen AC. Hemolytic anemia due to graft-derived anti-B production after lung transplantation. *Transplant Proc* 1994;26:1739.

84. Perlman EJ, Shirey RS, Farkosh M, Kickler TS, Ness PM. Immune hemolytic anemia following heart-lung transplantation. *Immunohematology* 1992;8:38–40.

85. Knoop C, Andrien M, Antoine M, Lambermont M, Yernault JC, Dupont E, Goldman M, Estenne M. Severe hemolysis due to a donor anti-D antibody after heart-lung transplantation. Association with lung and blood chimerism. *Am Rev Respir Dis* 1993;148:504–506.

86. Lasky LC, Warkentin PI, Kersey JH, Ramsay NKC, McGlare PB, McCullough J. Hemotherapy in patients undergoing blood group incompatible bone marrow transplantation. *Transfusion* 1983;23:277–285.

87. Bradley R, Triulzi DJ, Starzl TE. Donor derived red cell antibodies in liver transplant recipients treated with FK-506 (abstract). *Transfusion* 1993;33(Suppl):S163.

88. Triulzi DJ, Jochum EE. Red cell compatibility testing in baboon xenotransplantation. *Transfusion* 1995;35:756–759.

89. Triulzi DJ, Jochum EA, Marino IR, Starzl TE. Heteroagglutinins and their significance in baboon hepatic xenotransplantation. *Transplantation* 1995;60:127–131.

90. Starzl TE, Demetris AJ, Murase N, Ildstad S, Ricordi C, Trucco M. Cell migration, chimerism, and graft acceptance. *Lancet* 1992;339:1579–1582.

91. Fontes P, Rao AS, Demetris AJ, Zeevi A, Trucco M, Carroll P, Rybka W, Rudert WA, Ricordi C, Dodson F, Shapiro R, Tzakis A, Todo S, Abu-Elmagd K, Jordan M, Fung JJ, Starzl TE. Bone marrow augmentation of donor-cell chimerism in kidney, liver, heart, and pancreas islet transplantation. *Lancet* 1994;344:151–155.

92. Papadopoulos EB, Ladanyi M, Emmanuel D. Infusions of donor leukocytes to treat Epstein-Barr virus associated lymphoproliferative disorders after allogeneic bone marrow transplantation. *N Engl J Med* 1994;330:1185–1191.

8

Hematopoietic Stem Cell
Processing and Transplantation

Patricia L. Kotula, Ellen M. Areman, and Ronald A. Sacher

1. INTRODUCTION

Transplantation of hematopoietic stem cells (HSCs) is an accepted treatment for hematological diseases such as severe aplastic anemia and most leukemias. In this setting, the HSC are used to replace the diseased or damaged bone marrow (BM) *(13)*. More recently, HSC have been used to restore BM function following treatment with high dose chemotherapy and/or radiation in patients with lymphomas and some solid tumors *(4,5)*. With the use of recombinant colony-stimulating factors (CSFs) with or without the addition of cytotoxic drugs, it is possible to mobilize large numbers of stem and progenitor cells into the peripheral blood for collection by apheresis. These peripheral blood stem cells (PBSCs) can be used alone or in combination with BM to regenerate hematopoiesis. Advances in cell separation have made it possible to refine BM and PBSC grafts so that specific cell populations may be isolated and infused *(6–8)*. Incubation with certain cytokines and pharmacologic agents can also induce in vitro proliferation of some cell populations while inhibiting others. These manipulated cells can then be used for adoptive immunotherapy *(9,10)*, as vehicles for gene therapy *(11)*, and perhaps even to induce tolerance of an organ transplant from the same donor *(12)*.

2. TYPES OF HSC TRANSPLANTATION

There are three basic types of HSC transplants. In an *allogeneic transplant,* the donor is phenotypically compatible with the recipient at certain loci of the major histocompatibility complex (MHC). These human leukocyte antigens (HLAs) must be closely matched in order to prevent graft rejection or graft-vs-host disease (GVHD). Until recently, allogeneic donors were usually siblings matching at least five of the six antigens of the HLA-A, B, and DR loci. In the last few years, a large unrelated donor pool has developed, providing many patients who lack a matched sibling the opportunity to receive a phenotypically matched allogeneic graft *(13)*. In some instances, such as for leukemia in remission or in patients with solid tumors, the patient may be used as his or her own donor. In these *autologous transplants,* the cells must be collected prior to conditioning therapy and stored until the patient

From: *Red Cell Transfusion: A Practical Guide*
Edited by: M. E. Reid and S. J. Nance Humana Press Inc., Totowa, NJ

is ready for the cell infusion. Because the autologous cells may be contaminated with tumor cells, these grafts may require special treatment before they can be used (*see* Section 5.). The third and rarest type of HSC transplant is the *syngeneic* or identical twin transplant, in which the donor cells are genotypically identical to those of the recipient. Because of this genetic identity, the patient is not at risk for the GVHD often experienced by recipients of allogeneic transplants, nor is there the possibility of tumor cell contamination.

3. SOURCES OF HSC

3.1. Bone Marrow

There are a several sources of HSC. The original and, until very recently, the principal source of these cells has been BM, which can be used for both allogeneic and autologous transplantation. The marrow is harvested in the operating room with the patient receiving either general or regional anesthesia *(14)*. Multiple aspirations of 2–5 mL are usually taken from the posterior iliac crest by means of stainless steel beveled harvesting needles and glass or plastic syringes, but marrow may in rare instances also be collected from other bones such as the anterior iliac crest or sternum *(15)*. In the original technique developed by Thomas and Storb *(16)*, the marrow is placed in stainless-steel beakers containing tissue culture medium and heparin. At the end of the harvest, the marrow is pressed through two stainless steel mesh screens, of 300 and 200-μm mesh size, to filter out most of the bone chips, clots, fat, and fibrin. The mixture is then transferred to one or more sterile blood transfer packs and transported to the laboratory. This procedure has been modernized with the introduction of the disposable collection kit (Baxter Biotech, Deerfield, IL), which contains a filtered and capped plastic collection container with interlocking filters and transfer bags. The use of this kit has probably decreased the risk of bacterial contamination from that encountered with the open beaker system. At least 1 L of marrow must usually be collected to yield sufficient nucleated cells for an adult allogeneic recipient, especially if further processing is required *(15)*.

3.2. Peripheral Blood Stem Cells

PBSC are collected by apheresis, a process that does not require hospitalization or anesthesia. As with BM, PBSC can be used in both the allogeneic and autologous settings. In most cases, an adequate number of progenitor cells can be collected in 1–3 apheresis procedures *(17)*. The autologous cells are then cryopreserved, to be thawed and infused after the patient has undergone myeloablative therapy. PBSC from allogeneic donors, either freshly collected or frozen/thawed, are also used for transplantation.

Although adequate stem cells for marrow reconstitution can be collected with one BM harvest from most allogeneic and autologous donors, the percentage of circulating progenitor cells in normal donors and untreated patients is extremely low. In this "steady state," unacceptably large numbers of leukapheresis procedures are required for collection of adequate PBSC for engraftment in either the autologous or allogeneic situation. Patients and donors are usually "primed" for PBSC collection with mobilizing therapy, which consists of CSFs for the allogeneic donor and CSF with or without cytotoxic therapy for the autologous donor. When a patient is treated with myelotoxic drugs with or without CSF, and their cells collected during the rebound period following the chemotherapy-induced cytopenic nadir, large numbers of HSC can be obtained; however, the period of maximum progenitor production is short and unpredictable *(18,19)*. Depending on the dose and type of drugs administered, as well as previous treatment, patients may recover their white blood cell counts in as few as 10 d or only after several weeks. This uncertainty can cause difficulties in scheduling the apheresis procedures.

When allogeneic and autologous PBSC donors are mobilized or "primed" with only CSFs, scheduling can be much more exact because there is no marrow suppression limiting recovery. The apheresis procedures can be scheduled to begin on a specific day after the start of CSF administration and continued until either a target number of progenitor cells has been collected or for a predetermined number of days *(7,8)*. A number of different criteria are used to evaluate the quality of the apheresis collection. Quantitation of nucleated cells (NCs), mononuclear cells (MNCs), colony-forming units granulocyte-macrophage (CFU-GM) or CD34+ cells are most commonly used, with CFU-GM and CD34+ probably representing the most predictive parameters of engraftment potential *(20)*. Of course, all of these are surrogate measurements for the true stem cell, which has not yet been identified or quantitated by any reliable assay. One problem encountered when priming with CSFs alone is the generation of large numbers of granulocytes, most of which do not survive the stresses of freezing and thawing. The intracellular materials released from these lysed cells have been implicated in transplant-related toxicity *(21)*.

In order to collect an optimal number of HSC, volumes of 7 to >20 L of blood may be processed using one of the commercially available cell separation devices originally developed for leukapheresis and platelet pheresis. Some centers have reported an increase in the percentage of CD34+ cells collected after 10 L or more of blood have been processed *(22)*. Although this may result in higher numbers of progenitor cells being collected per procedure and, therefore, reducing costs by requiring fewer number of collections, some patients may not be able to tolerate the longer procedure.

3.3. Umbilical Cord Placental Blood (UCB)

The collection of UCB is the least invasive and most versatile of all HSC collection techniques. At present, this source of HSC is being used in both related and unrelated allogeneic transplants *(23)*. For optimal collection, the cord is clamped and drained into a sterile collection vessel containing an anticoagulant, usually ACD-A or CPD-A. After delivery of the placenta, additional fetal blood can be aspirated from placental vessels *(24,25)*. Care must be taken to avoid collecting maternal blood, because this would expose the recipient to cells with mismatched HLA antigens and the risk of severe GVHD. The cells are cryopreserved and stored until needed. Testing of the fetal blood and maternal blood is necessary to ensure that no infectious disease will be transmitted by the UCB transplant.

4. STEM CELL PROCESSING

Once HSC have been collected, a variety of processing techniques may be performed (Table 1). Bone marrow and UCB and, to a lesser extent, PBSC, are heter-

Table 1
Processing of HSC Components

Procedure	Components processed	Purpose(s)
Centrifugation	BM	Plasma removal
	PBSC	Volume reduction
	UCB	Removal of donor antibodies
		Platelet depletion
Sedimentation	BM	Red cell depletion
	UCB	
Semiautomated processing	BM	Red cell depletion
		Buffy coat for cryopreservation
Automated processing	BM	Red cell depletion
		Mononuclear cell concentrate for cryopreservation
		Density-gradient purified mononuclear cells

ogeneous collections of cellular and noncellular components. Varying degrees of separation and purification of these components can be achieved, depending on the procedure or combination of procedures applied.

4.1. Centrifugation

As with preparation of red blood cell (RBC) components, centrifugation of the HSC product results in concentration of the RBCs, which have the highest density, at the bottom of the container. The white blood cells (WBCs), which are less dense, distribute to the top of the cellular pellet, whereas the lightest elements, plasma and platelets, locate at the top of the container. Plasma removal by centrifugation may be necessary when the donor plasma contains one or more antibodies to recipient RBC antigen(s), a "minor" incompatibility *(26)*. Plasma removal may also be necessary to reduce the volume of a graft collected for a pediatric patient *(27)*.

Centrifugation can be used to further fractionate the bone marrow by making it possible to collect the WBC layer, or "buffy coat," at the plasma and RBC interface *(28)*. A buffy coat preparation can be used to provide a component reduced in RBC for an allogeneic ABO-incompatible transplant in which the recipient has circulating antibody to one or more donor RBC antigens. This technique may also be used to prepare a marrow or UCB graft for cryopreservation. A buffy coat preparation can substantially reduce the volume of a BM harvest from > 1000 to approx 200 mL, with expected recovery of 75–80% of the original WBC *(28)*.

4.2. Sedimentation

An alternative processing technique for RBC removal is sedimentation. If hydroxyethyl starch (HES) is added to the marrow and the mixture allowed to stand for 0.5–3 h, the RBCs will sediment by gravity and can then be removed. This technique has been reported to remove up to 99% of the erythrocytes *(29–32)*.

4.3. Semiautomated and Automated Processing

Semiautomated and automated procedures have been developed using equipment designed for washing of RBC components and for apheresis. A concentration

Table 2
Purging of HSC

Type of purging	Purging agent(s)	Target	Purpose
Pharmacologic	Chemotherapeutic drugs	Tumor cells	Removal of residual tumor in the graft
	Corticosteroids	T-cells	Prevention of GVHD
Immunologic			
Complement	MAbs	Tumor cells	Removal of residual tumor in the graft
Magnetic Immunotoxins		T-cells or T-cell subsets	Prevention of GVHD
E-rosetting	Lectin	T-cells	
Mechanical	None	Lymphocytes	Prevention of GVHD
Immunotherapy	Activated cells (autologous or allogeneic)	Tumor cells	In vivo killing; induction of GVT[a] effect

[a]GVL, graft vs tumor.

technique using the Cobe 2991 (Cobe, Lakewood, CO) blood bank cell washer in manual mode produces a buffy coat preparation containing approx 75% of the starting nucleated cells *(33)*. This product can be further processed by a density-gradient technique using the same instrument, yielding a final component enriched for mononuclear cells (MNCs) *(34)*. An MNC product can also be produced using modified apheresis procedures on the CS3000 Plus (Baxter, Deerfield, IL) and Cobe Spectra *(35,36)*. These instruments use differential centrifugation without density gradient materials to remove 95% of the RBC while recovering up to 80% of the MNC and at least 75% of the CFU-GM. Granulocyte contamination is greatly reduced by this technique. For greater purification, a density-gradient step can be added to these procedures *(37)*.

5. PURGING

Purging, the depletion of unnecessary or undesirable cell populations from the graft before storage or infusion, may be necessary to prevent either immediate or delayed adverse responses to the transplant. Techniques have been developed which exploit antigenic surface phenotypic chacteristics and functional differences to isolate and remove specific cell types from both autologous and allogeneic BM and PBSC (Table 2).

5.1. Purging of Autologous BM and PBSC

Autologous BM and, to a lesser extent, PBSC of cancer patients may be contaminated with clonogenic tumor cells which could potentially reintroduce metastatic disease if not removed. Brenner and coworkers *(38)*, using ex vivo gene marking, demonstrated the presence of marked autologous cells in recurrent neuroblastoma *(38)*. A variety of techniques have been developed for removal of these contaminating cells.

5.1.1. Pharmacologic Purging

Pharmacologic purging uses cytotoxic drugs similar to those used in cancer chemotherapy for in vitro removal or destruction of rapidly dividing tumor cells. The agents most commonly used are cyclophosphamide derivatives such as 4-hydroperoxycyclophosphamide (4-HC), mafosfamide and ASTA-Z, with other chemotherapeutic drugs used, both singly and in combination *(39–43)*. After an incubation period, the chemical is washed from the cell suspension, after which the cells are cryopreserved. This type of purging is relatively nonspecific and can also cause lethal damage to committed progenitor cells, often resulting in prolonged periods of neutropenia and thrombocytopenia *(44)*.

5.1.2. Immunologic Purging

Immunologic purging is more specific than the pharmacologic technique because it uses monoclonal antibodies (MAbs) directed against cell surface markers found predominantly on certain tumor cells. These antibodies are bound to assorted molecules which damage or allow removal of the targeted cells using a number of different systems. In complement-mediated immunologic purging, antibody-sensitized target cells are lysed following multiple incubations with complement *(45)*. Howell and coworkers *(46)* developed an automated method of complement lysis using a cell separator to constantly introduce fresh complement into the cell suspension, with a single complement treatment usually sufficient to remove three logs of tumor cells.

MAbs can also be linked to toxins such as the A chain of the ricin molecule or pseudomonas exotoxin. The antibody binds to the target cell, which is then poisoned by the attached toxin *(47)*. An efficient technique for removal of targeted cells that does not adversely affect HSC, involves the use of magnetic polymer microspheres bound to one or more MAbs. The antibody-coated beads attach to the cells of interest during an incubation period, after which the cell suspension is exposed to a strong magnet. The magnet holds the cells that have bound to the beads, allowing the unbound cells to be removed from the suspension *(48–50)*.

5.1.3. Positive Selection

MAbs to CD34, a surface marker on immature progenitor cells that is gradually lost as hematopoietic cells mature and differentiate *(51)*, can be used to select these cells for infusion. If the patient's tumor cells are negative for this antigen, this may provide a more efficient method of preventing tumor reinfusion than is possible with the negative selection methods described above. CD34-positive cells selected using devices such as the Ceprate® avidin–biotin immunoadsorption column (Cellpro, Bothell, WA) or Isolex 300 (Baxter) can be used *(52,53)*. The CD34-positive cells are captured, whereas the CD34-negative cells run through. The positive cells are then collected and cryopreserved and the CD34-negative cells discarded. However, because the purity of the selected cells is < 100%, there is no assurance that all tumor cells have been removed.

5.1.4. Other Autologous Purging Techniques

Techniques for generation of a graft-vs-tumor (GVT) effect in the autologous setting have also been developed. Areman and coworkers *(9,10)* showed that BM and PBSC when incubated with interleukin-2 (IL-2) for 24 h, can generate effecter cells which have a potent antitumor effect in vitro and in vivo *(9,10)*. The in vitro data suggests that these activated natural killer cells may preferentially suppress or kill malignant committed leukemic progenitors while sparing normal hematopoietic progenitors. Clinical trials are currently underway to determine whether infusion of these cells followed by a course of iv IL-2 can increase disease-free survival in patients with solid tumors and hematologic malignancies. Other studies by this group have also shown that long-term culture with IL-2 can completely eliminate leukemia cells in vitro *(54)*. Because normal hematopoietic cells seem to be less sensitive to temperature extremes than tumor cells, freezing alone may, in some cases, preferentially preserve normal cells and damage some tumor cells *(55,56)*.

Long-term incubation of BM in various culture systems has been explored as yet another method of autologous purging. When BM from patients with chronic myelogenous leukemia (CML) is placed in culture for 7 d or longer, a decrease in the number of Philadelphia chromosome-positive (Ph$_1$) cells is seen. However, approx 30% of these Ph$_1$ cells may survive and contaminate the graft *(57)*.

Whether any of the purging methods currently in use or under investigation is capable of removing all clonogenic tumor cells from autologous grafts is not yet known. Until recently, there were no methods available for detection and measurement of minimal residual disease in vivo nor occult tumor cell contamination in vitro. Tumor cells in grafts of patients with leukemia, lymphoma, and even breast cancer can now be detected using sophisticated cell culture and molecular or immunochemical techniques. When these assays are standardized and widely available, investigators will be able to measure the efficacy of various purging techniques and determine which are most effective at removing tumor cells *(58)*.

5.2. Allogeneic Purging and T-Cell Depletion

In the allogeneic setting, the purpose of purging is to either remove RBCs from the graft when the recipient has antibody to red cell antigens of the donor or to remove T-lymphocytes from allogeneic BM or PBSC to decrease the risk of GVHD. Techniques for RBC depletion are described in Section 4.

It is theorized that GVHD occurs when CD4 antigen-positive effector T-lymphocytes in the graft recruit host CD8 antigen-positive cytotoxic/suppressor cells to the recipient's skin, liver, and gastrointestinal tract, inducing an immunologic response *(59)*. This reaction is especially severe in the mismatched related and matched unrelated settings, in which administration of immunosuppressive drugs alone may not be sufficient to prevent this often fatal complication. Various pharmacologic, immunologic, and mechanical procedures have been devised for inactivation and removal of T-cells and T-cell subsets to prevent or reduce the severity of GVHD *(60)*. Unfortunately, because some of these subsets seem to be necessary for hematopoietic reconstitution and antitumor responses, graft failure and disease recurrence may be higher than with unmanipulated allogeneic grafts *(61,62)*. In addition, increases in the incidence of viral infections and Epstein-Barr virus associated lymphomas that may be secondary to removal of immunocompetent T-cells have also been noted *(63)*. A number of centers are attempting to reverse the negative effects of T-cell depletion by infusing donor leukocytes, including T-lymphocytes to the recipient, in the posttransplant period. Reversal of lymphoma and relapsed CML has been observed using this technique. However, this type of adoptive immunotherapy has been complicated by chronic GVHD, predominantly involving the liver *(64)*.

5.2.1. Pharmacologic T-Depletion

Because T-lymphocytes are sensitive to the immunosuppressive effects of corticosteroids, drugs such as methylprednisolone have been used to reduce T-cell activity in allogeneic grafts. Other agents including L-leucyl-L-leucine methyl ester and vincristine have also been used as modulators of the alloreactive response *(65,66)*.

5.2.2. Immunologic T-Depletion

The first form of immunologic T-cell depletion was developed by Reisner et al. *(67)* and depended on the phenomenon whereby T-cells incubated with soybean lectin will form rosettes around sheep red blood cells. These rosettes can then be removed by density gradient centrifugation.

5.2.3. Mechanical T-Depletion

Counterflow centrifugal elutriation actually removes most of the lymphocytes in the graft by taking advantage of the significant difference in size between HSC and lymphocytes. Smaller cells such as RBC and lymphocytes are removed first, with the media flow rate increasing as each progressively larger cell type is harvested. The final fraction collected contains the majority of the progenitor cells *(68,69)*.

6. STORAGE OF HSC

Once the cells have been concentrated and manipulated using the techniques previously described, the HSC must be stored until the time of transplantation. This storage period can range from a few hours to many years, depending on the purpose of the collection. Allogeneic BM and PBSC are usually infused directly after collection or processing, although they are occasionally frozen for short periods prior to transplantation. Fresh cells can be stored and transported at room or refrigerator temperatures, with care being taken not to expose them to extremes of either heat or cold.

6.1. Cryopreservation

For cryopreservation, the cell suspension is divided among a number of freezing bags and an equal amount of freezing solution mixed with the cells. The usual cryoprotectant is dimethyl sulfoxide (DMSO) which is added at a final concentration of 5–10%, depending on the other ingredients in the freezing mixture *(70)*. An isotonic saline or electrolyte solution and a source of protein, usually autologous plasma or human serum albumin (HSA), are also used *(71)*. A modification of the conventional 10% DMSO procedure was published by Stiff et al. *(72)* in which they supplemented the freezing solution with Pentastarch, a low molecular weight fraction of hydroxyethyl starch (HES) (McGaw, Irvine, CA), as an additional cryoprotectant. This extracellular freezing agent makes it possible to use less DMSO (final concentration 5%), with cell recovery and viability comparable to the standard method. Since there may be unpleasant side effects experienced during or following DMSO infusion, a lower concentration of this agent may be desirable *(73–75)*.

6.1.1. Freezing Rate

Viable HSC recovery appears to be related to a slow freezing rate (1–5°/min) followed by rapid thawing *(71)*. The cells are placed in a programmable chamber into which liquid nitrogen is periodically injected to maintain the chosen freezing rate. When the program is complete, the cells are transferred to a storage freezer.

It is also possible to attain a comparable freezing rate by placing the cells into a mechanical freezer (− 70 to − 80°C) and allowing them to remain undisturbed until frozen. Stiff et al. *(72)* demonstrated no difference in recovery when cells in a HES/DMSO solution were frozen in a mechanical or a controlled rate liquid nitrogen freezer. The cells can then either remain in the mechanical freezer until transplantation or be transferred to a liquid nitrogen freezer.

6.2. Storage

6.2.1. Nitrogen Storage: Liquid and Vapor

Cryopreserved HSC can be maintained under a variety of conditions, but are most commonly stored in a liquid nitrogen freezer. The cells may be stored in either the liquid or vapor phase of liquid nitrogen, with definite advantages and disadvantages to each method. Although liquid storage permits all components to be stored at a uniform temperature (− 196°C), there is some risk of cross-contamination by microorganisms transmitted through the liquid *(76)*. On the other hand, with vapor phase storage, there is a gradual increase in temperature from the bottom to the top of the freezer, so that bags stored at different levels are stored at different temperatures. One report described engraftment failure in a number of dogs transplanted with marrow stored in the vapor phase *(77)*. Furthermore, the small amount of liquid nitrogen in the bottom of a vapor phase freezer does not provide extended protection if the nitrogen source becomes depleted.

6.2.2. Mechanical Freezer Storage

Some centers store HSC in a mechanical freezer (− 80°C) until the time of transplantation, with no obvious damage to the graft over short periods of time *(72)*. However, there is some evidence that cessation of enzymatic and metabolic activity does not occur until the temperature of the cell suspension has dropped to − 135°C or below *(71)*. The continuation of metabolic processes, even at an exceedingly slow rate, might be of concern when cells are to be stored for long periods, as might occur with remission marrow storage for leukemia patients or with banked UCB. A number of centers have reported storage of autologous HSC for 1–5 d at refrigerator temperatures, with no delay in engraftment after infusion *(78,79)*.

7. QUALITY ASSURANCE

Quality assurance of HSC components is necessary to evaluate their engraftment potential, the efficiency of any processing and purging, recovery of HSC after processing, and sterility of the infused component. As the number and types of manipulation increase, the opportunities for cell damage and loss increase as well.

7.1. Graft Evaluation

7.1.1. Quantitation of Cells

Nucleated cells must be quantitated before and after every processing step to determine which, if any, processes may be responsible for losses of progenitor cells. This quantitation is done by performing a standard WBC count using either manual or automated techniques. The total number of nucleated cells in the component is calculated by multiplying the volume of the product by the WBC count. In addition to enumerating the nucleated cells, a differential is performed on a Wright–Giemsa-stained smear to determine the percentage of MNCs in the graft. Because the stem cell is found in the MNC fraction, the recovery of MNC after processing is more important for engraftment potential than the recovery of other nucleated cells. Adequate cells must remain after processing to anticipate complete engraftment in a reasonable amount of time. The criteria for adequate engraftment potential must be determined by the individual transplant center. There is an essential need to correlate clinical outcomes with processing data obtained from the cellular processing laboratory.

7.1.2. Viability

Although the quantitation of nucleated and MNC is critical, it is also important to evaluate the viability of the graft. The most common technique for measuring cell viability is the dye exclusion technique, usually can performed using Trypan Blue dye. The test is based on the ability of the viable cell membrane to exclude the dye, whereas the nonviable cell will stain and appear blue under the microscope (80). Viability can also be determined by using fluorescent dyes and analyzing the cells by flow cytometry or with a fluorescent microscope.

7.1.3. Progenitor Cell Function

In addition to cell recovery and viability, the clonogenic potential of the HSC can also be measured. The colony-forming unit assay (CFU) is a semisolid culture system that generates colonies from committed myeloid and erythroid hematopoietic progenitors. Four colony types can be detected and identified in this system. The most common are the colony-forming unit-granulocyte macrophage (CFU-GM) and, the burst-forming unit-erythroid (BFU-E); whereas the colony-forming unit-granulocyte, erythrocyte, macrophage, megakaryocyte (CFU-MIX or CFU-GEMM) and colony-forming unit-megakaryocyte (CFU-MK) are found less frequently. Although some investigators have claimed to observe a correlation between number of colonies and days to engraftment, this assay is generally used as a qualitative assessment of the graft (81–83). Furthermore, this assay is not standardized, with different laboratories using different culture components, cell concentrations, and scoring criteria. Also, because this culture requires a 14-d incubation period, immediate evaluation of graft function is not possible.

7.1.4. Phenotypic Analysis

A more rapid evaluation of the HSC in the graft can be performed using flow cytometry and fluorescent-tagged MAbs to myeloid antigens such as CD34, expressed on early hematopoietic progenitor cells (84). However, because this antigen can be found on both uncommitted and committed HSC, it is only a surrogate marker for the pluripotent hematopoietic stem cell. This assay is especially useful for evaluating PBSC collections because results can be available in a few hours for use in determining the need for continued PBSC harvests *(85)*. Because this marker also appears on some acute and chronic leukemia cells, results of this assay must be carefully interpreted in patients with hematologic malignancies.

7.1.5. Sterility Testing

Bacterial and fungal contamination of BM, PBSC, and UCB are always a possibility, especially when multiple manipulations are performed. The contamination can come from the patient's or donor's skin or blood, from improperly sterilized equipment and materials, or from poor handling of the graft *(86,87)*. Bacterial and fungal cultures should be performed at collection and at various stages of processing to determine whether the processing techniques and materials are compromising the purity of the graft.

7.2. Evaluation of Purging

Until recently, it was not possible to detect or identify minimal residual tumor cells in vivo or in vitro. Although flow cytometric analysis may be used to identify tumor cells when the tumor burden is large and the necessary antibodies are available, it is not a sensitive enough technique to detect the few, but possibly clonogenic, occult tumor cells in remission BM or PBSC grafts. In addition, cells that have been damaged by purging agents usually cannot be morphologically or phenotypically distinguished from undamaged cells.

The limiting dilution assay, which measures T-cell expansion in response to IL-2 and phytohemagglutinin, is the most sensitive technique for determining the number of functional T-cells remaining after depletion *(88)*. However, because this culture system requires a 2-wk incubation period, it is not useful in situations requiring immediate quantitation of T-cells. Flow cytometry, although a less sensitive technique, is the most practical and rapid method for enumerating T-cells and T-cell subsets, because of the easy availability of monoclonal antibodies to T-cell antigens and receptors.

Although a number of sophisticated cell culture and molecular techniques have been developed for detection of rare tumor cells in BM and PBSC *(89)*, these are not practical for clinical laboratory use. Even in cases where there is a genetic marker that can be used to detect residual tumor cells *(90)*, these molecular methods are difficult and expensive to perform. Some of the immunocytochemical assays currently under development may ultimately result in accurate and reproducible assays for identifying infrequently occurring tumor cells in BM and PBSC, but at this time none of them are standardized or commercially available *(91)*.

7.3. Standards and Regulations

Professional societies such as the Foundation for Accreditation of Hematopoietic Cell Therapy (FAHCT) and the American Association of Blood Banks (AABB) have issued standards for collection and processing of HSC. In addition, the Food and Drug Administration (FDA) has recently published draft regulations for this lished draft regulations for this field *(92)*. Compliance with these standards and field *(92)*. Compliance with these standards and regulations should ensure the collection and preparation of the safest and most efficacious HSC components.

8. HSC INFUSION

Once the patient has completed myeloablative chemo- and/or radiotherapy, the HSC can be infused. Although allogeneic BM and PBSC are usually infused in the fresh state, with or without processing, they are occasionally collected and cryopreserved before the patient is treated, as are autologous BM and PBSC. The cryopreserved HSCs are then thawed and infused following conditioning therapy. Because cryopreserved cells seem to be less prone to injury when thawed quickly, the container of frozen cells is immersed in a 37 °C water bath. Thawing of a 50-mL bag of frozen cells occurs in a matter of minutes. The cells are usually transported to the patient's room, thawed at the bedside and infused through a central venous catheter. Alternatively, the bags of HSC may be thawed, diluted, and pooled in the laboratory, a more controlled environment out of sight of the patient *(93)*. Some centers also wash the cell suspension in order to remove DMSO, which, when infused in large amounts, has been implicated in infusion-related toxicity *(94)*. Because some cells in the HSC product may lyse with freezing and thawing, DNase should probably be added to those components that will be manipulated after thawing *(95)*. This enzyme reduces clumping caused by single-stranded DNA released from cells that did not survive the freeze–thaw process. A recombinant human DNase is now commercially available (Pulmozyme®, Genentech, San Francisco, CA).

9. SUMMARY

The HCS, collected from BM, PBSC, or UCB can be used to replace diseased BM in a variety of genetic disorders and hematological malignancies or to restore marrow function after myeloablative therapy. Procedures for the collection, processing, and storage of these cells are developing rapidly. The laboratories called on to perform these services must be prepared to develop and evolve to accommodate the needs of the HSC transplantation field.

REFERENCES

1. Bortin MM, Horwitz MM, Rowlings PA, et al. 1993 Progress report from the International Bone Marrow Transplant Registry. *Bone Marrow Trans* 1993;12:97–104.
2. Moreb J, Johnson T, Kubilis P, et al. Improved survival of patients with chronic myelogenous leukemia undergoing allogeneic bone marrow transplantation. *Am J Hematol* 1995;50:304–306.
3. Wagner JL, Deeg HJ, Seidel K, et al. Bone marrow transplantation for severe aplastic anemia from genotypically HLA-nonidentical relatives. An update of the Seattle experience. *Transplantation* 1996;61:54–61.
4. Klingemann HG. When should marrow transplantation be considered? In: Deeg HG, Lingeman HG, Phillips GL, eds. *A Guide to Bone Marrow Transplantation*. Berlin: Springer-Verlag, 1988, p. 18.
5. Advisory committee for the International Autologous Bone Marrow Transplant Registry. Bone marrow autotransplantation in man: report of an international cooperative study. *Lancet* 1986;2:960–962.

6. Haas R, Ho A, Bredthauer U, et al. Successful autologous bone marrow transplantation of blood stem cells mobilized with recombinant human granulocyte-macrophage colony-stimulating factor. *Exp Haematol* 1990;18:94.

7. Bensinger W, Singer J, Appelbaum F, et al. Autologous transplantation with peripheral blood mononuclear cells collected after administration of recombinant granulocyte stimulating factor. *Blood* 1993;81:3158–3163.

8. Peters WP, Rosner G, Ross M, et al. Comparative effects of granulocyte macrophage colony stimulating factor (G-CSF) on priming peripheral blood stem cells for use with autologous bone marrow after high dose chemotherapy. *Blood* 1993;81:1709–1719.

9. Charak BS, Areman EM, Dickerson SA, et al. A novel approach to immunomodulation of frozen human bone marrow with interleukin 2 for clinical application. *Bone Marrow Transplant* 1993;11:147–154.

10. Verma UN, Areman EM, Sacher RA, Mazumder A. *In vitro* activation of PBSCs with interleukin 2. In: Gee AP, Gross S, Worthington-White DA, eds. *Advances in Bone Marrow Purging and Processing, Fourth International Symposium.* New York: Wiley Liss,1994, pp. 245–255.

11. Anderson WF. Human gene therapy. *Science* 1992;256:808–813.

12. Sykes M, Khan A, Sachs DH, Tomita Y. Bone marrow transplantation for the induction of tolerance (abstract). *Exp Hematol* 1944;22:1.

13. Anasetti C, Etzioni R, Petersdorf EW, Martin PJ, Hansen JA. Marrow transplantation from unrelated volunteer donors. *Ann Rev Med* 1995;46,169–179

14. Dicke K, Hood D, Hanks S, Vaughn M. The efficiency of outpatient marrow harvesting under local anesthesia (abstract). *Exp Hematol* 1994;22:373.

15. Spitzer TR, Areman EM, Cirenza E, et al. The impact of harvest center on quality of marrows collected from unrelated donors. *J Hematother* 1994;3:65–70.

16. Thomas ED, Storb R. Technique for human marrow grafting. *Blood* 1970;36:507–515.

17. Schwartzberg LS, Birch R, Hazelton B, et al. Peripheral blood stem cell mobilization by chemotherapy with and without recombinant human granulocyte colony stimulating factor. *J Hematother* 1992;1:317–327.

18. Stiff PJ, Murgo AJ, Wittes RE, DeRisi MF, Clarkson BD. Quantification of the peripheral blood colony forming unit culture rise following chemotherapy. *Transfusion* 1983;23:500–503.

19. Juttner CA, To LB. Collection and processing of peripheral blood stem cells. In: Areman E, Deeg HJ, Sacher RA, eds. *Bone Marrow and Stem Cell Processing: a Manual of Current Techniques.* Philadelphia: FA Davis, 1992, pp. 68–73.

20. Passos-Coelho JL, Braine HG, Davis JM, et al. Predictive factors for peripheral-blood progenitor-cell collections using a single large-volume leukopheresis after cyclophosphamide and granulocyte-macrophage colony-stimulating factor mobilization. *J Clin Onc* 1995;1:705–714.

21. Davis JM, Rowley SD, Braine HG, et al. Clinical toxicity of cryopreserved bone marrow graft infusion. *Blood* 1990;75:781–786.

22. Hillyer CD, Tiegerman KO, Berkman EM. Increase in circulating colony forming units granulocyte macrophage during large volume leukapheresis; evaluation of a new cell separator. *Transfusion* 1991;14:187–196.

23. Varadi G, Elchalal U, Shushan A, Schenker JG, Nagler A. Umbilical cord blood for use in transplantation. *Obstet Gynecol Surv* 1995;50;611–617.

24. Apperly JF, Meeting report: umbilical cord blood progenitor cell transplantation. *Bone Marrow Transplant* 1994;14:187–196.

25. English D, Cooper S, Douglas G, Broxmeyer HE. Collection and processing of cord blood for preservation and hematopoietic transplantation. In: Areman E, Deeg HJ, Sacher RA, eds. *Bone Marrow and Stem Cell Processing: A Manual of Current Techniques.* Philadelphia: FA Davis, 1992, pp. 383–385.

26. Gale RP, Feig S, Ho W, et al. ABO blood group system and bone marrow transplantation. *Blood* 1977;50:185–194.
27. Buckner CD, Clift RA, Sanders JE, et al. ABO-incompatible marrow transplants. *Transplantation* 1978;26:233–238.
28. Areman EM. Mononuclear cell concentration and processing techniques. In: Sacher RA, AuBuchon JP, eds. *Marrow Transplantation: Practical and Technical Aspects of Stem Cell Reconstitution.* Bethesda: American Association of Blood Banks, 1992, pp. 131–150.
29. Jansen J. Processing of bone marrow for allogeneic transplantation. In: Sacher RA, McCarthy LJ, Smit Sibinga CT, eds. *Processing of Bone Marrow for Transplantation.* Arlington, VA: American Association of Blood Banks, 1990, pp. 19–39.
30. Dinsmore RE, Reich LM, Kapoor N, et al. ABH incompatible bone marrow transplantation: removal of erythrocytes by starch sedimentation. *Br J Haematol* 1983;54:441–449.
31. Ho WG, Champlin RE, Feig SA, et al. Transplantation of ABO incompatible bone marrow: gravity sedimentation of donor marrow. *Br J Haematol* 1984;57:155–162.
32. Warkentin PI, Hilden JM, Kersey JH, et al. Transplantation of major ABO incompatible bone marrow depleted of red cells by hydroxyethyl starch. *Vox Sanguinis* 1985;48:89–105.
33. Gilmore MJ, Prentice HG, Corringham RE, et al. Separation of mononuclear bone marrow cells using the COBE 2991 blood cell separator. *Vox Sanguinis* 1985;45:294–302.
34. Jin N, Hill R, Segal G, et al. Preparation of red blood cell depleted marrow for ABO incompatible marrow transplantation by density gradient separation using the IBM 2991 Blood cell processor. *Exp. Hematol* 1987;15:93–98.
35. Areman EM, Cullis H, Spitzer T, Sacher RA. Automated processing of human bone marrow can result in a population of mononuclear cells capable of achieving engraftment following transplantation. *Transfusion* 1991;31:724–730.
36. Faradji A, Andreau G, Pillier Loriette C, et al. Separation of mononuclear bone marrow cells using the Cobe 2991 blood cell separator. *Vox Sanguinis* 1988;55:133–138.
37. Carter CS, Goetzman H, Read EJ. Automated bone marrow processing and density gradient separation using the Fenwal CS3000. In: Areman E, Deeg HJ, Sacher RA, eds. *Bone Marrow and Stem Cell Processing: A Manual of Current Techniques.* Philadelphia: FA Davis, 1992, pp. 158–162.
38. Brenner MK, Rill DR, Moen RC, et al. Gene marking to trace origin of relapse after autologous bone marrow transplantation. *Lancet* 1993;341:85–86.
39. Kaiser H, Stuart RK, Brookmeyer R, et al. Autologous bone marrow transplantation in acute leukemia: a phase I study of *in vitro* treatment of marrow with 4 hydroperoxycyclophosphamide to purge tumor cells. *Blood* 1985;65:1504–1510.
40. Yeager AM, Kaiser H, Santos GW, et al. Autologous bone marrow transplantation in patients with 4 hydroperoxycyclophosphamide. *N Engl J Med* 1986;315:141–147.
41. Gorin NC, Douay 1, Laporte JP, et al. Autologous bone marrow transplantation using marrow incubated with ASTA Z 7557 in adult acute leukemia. *Blood* 1986;67:1367–1376.
42. Ciobanu N, Paietta E, Andreeff M, et al. Etoposide as an *in vitro* purging agent for the treatment of acute leukemias and lymphomas in conjunction with autologous bone marrow transplantation. *Exp Hematol* 1986;14:626–635.
43. Rizzoli V, Mangoni L. Pharmacological mediated purging with mafosfamide in acute and chronic myeloid leukemias. In: Gross SR, Gee AP, Worthington-White DA, eds. *Bone Marrow Purging and Processing.* New York: Liss, 1990, pp. 21–38.
44. Rowley SD, Piantadosi S, Marcellus DC, et al. Analysis of factors predicting speed of hematologic recovery after transplantation with 4 hydroperoxycyclophosphamide purged autologous bone marrow grafts. *Bone Marrow Transplant* 1991;7:183–191.

45. Ball ED, Mills LE, Cornwall III GG, et al. Autologous bone marrow transplantation for acute myeloid leukemia using monoclonal antibody-purged bone marrow. *Blood* 1990;75:1199–1206.
46. Howell AL, Fogg Leach M, Davis BH, et al. Continuous infusion of complement by an automated cell processor enhances cytotoxicity of monoclonal antibody sensitized leukemia cells. *Bone Marrow Transplant* 1989;4:317–322.
47. Ucken FM, Gajl Peczalska K, Meyers DE, et al. Marrow purging in autologous bone marrow transplantation for T lineage acute lymphoblastic leukemia; efficacy of ex vivo treatment with immunotoxins and 4-hydroperoxycyclophosphamide against fresh leukemia marrow progenitor cells. *Blood* 1987;69:361–366.
48. Gee AP, Lee C, Bruce KM, et al. Immunomagnetic purging and autologous transplantation in stage D neuroblastoma. *Bone Marrow Transplant* 1987;2(suppl 2):89–98.
49. Kvalheim G, Sorensen O, Fodstad O, et al. Immunomagnetic removal of B-lymphoma cells from human bone marrow: a procedure for clinical use. *Bone Marrow Transplant* 1988;3:31–41.
50. Shimazaki C, Wisniewski D, Scheinberg DA, et al. Elimination of myeloma cells from bone marrow using monoclonal antibodies and magnetic immunobeads. *Blood* 1988;72:1248–1254.
51. Civin CI, Strauss LC, Brovall C, et al. Antigen analysis of hematopoiesis. III. A hematopoietic progenitor cell surface antigen defined by a monoclonal antibody raised against KG-la cells. *J Immunol* 1984;133:157–161.
52. Stray KM, Corpuz S, Kalamasz D, Colter M, Berenson R, Heimfeld S. Purging tumor cells form bone marrow or peripheral blood using avidin biotin immunoadsorption. In: Gee AP, Gross S, Worthington-White DA, eds. *Advances in Bone Marrow Purging and Processing, Fourth International Symposium*. New York: Wiley Liss, 1994, pp. 97–103.
53. Thomas L, Mansour V, Jain R, et al. Use of the CS-3000 Plus to prepare apheresed blood cells for immunomagnetic positive cell selection. *J Hematother* 1995;4:315–321.
54. Verma UN, Bagg A, Brown E, Mazumder A. Interleukin-2 activation of human bone marrow in long-term cultures: an effective strategy for purging and generation of anti-tumor cytotoxic effectors. *Bone Marrow Transplant* 1994;13:115–123.
55. Allieri MA, Lopez M, Douay L, et al. Clonogenic leukemia progenitor cells in acute myelocytic leukemia are highly sensitive to cryopreservation: possible purging effect for autologous bone marrow transplantation. *Bone Marrow Transplant* 1991;7:101–105.
56. Herrman RP, O'Reilly J, Meyer BF, Lazzaro G. Prompt haemopoietic reconstitution following hypothermia purging autologous marrow and peripheral blood stem cell transplantation in acute myeloid leukemia. *Bone Marrow Transplant* 1992;10:293–295.
57. Barnett MJ, Eaves CJ, Phillips GL, et al. Successful autografting in chronic myeloid leukemia after maintenance of marrow in culture. *Bone Marrow Transplant* 1989;4:345–351.
58. Sharp JG, Mann SL, Murphy B, Weeks C. Culture methods for the detection of minimal tumor contamination of hematopoietic harvest: a review. *J Hematother* 1995;4:141–148.
59. Deeg HJ, Acute graft-versus-host disease. In: Deeg HJ, Klingemann HG, Phillips GL, eds. *A Guide to Bone Marrow Transplantation*. Berlin: Springer Verlag, 1988, pp. 86–87.
60. Champlin R, Lee K. T cell depletion to prevent graft versus host disease following allogeneic bone marrow transplantation. In: Areman E, Deeg HJ, Sacher RA, eds. *Bone Marrow and Stem Cell Processing: A Manual of Current Techniques*. Philadelphia: Davis, 1992, pp. 163–170.
61. Goldman JM, Gale RP, Horowitz MM, et al. Bone marrow transplantation of chronic myelogenous leukemia in chronic phase. Increased risk of relapse associated with T cell depletion. *Ann Intern Med* 1988;108:806–814.

62. Martin PJ, Hansen JA, Torok Storb B, et al. Graft failure in patients receiving T cell depleted HLA identical allogeneic marrow transplants. *Bone Marrow Transplant* 1988;3:445–456.

63. Zutter MM, Martin PJ, Sale GE, Shulman HM, Fisher L, Thomas ED, Durman DM. Epstein-Barr virus lymphoproliferation after bone marrow transplantation. *Blood* 1988;72:520.

64. Van Rhee F, Lin F, Cullis JO, et al. Relapse of chronic myeloid leukemia after allogeneic bone marrow transplant: the case for giving donor leukocyte transfusions before the onset of hematologic relapse. *Blood* 1994;83:3377–3383.

65. Kapoor N, Beck EX, Lanfranchi A. Methylprednisolone and vincristine treatment of bone marrow in HLA mismatched bone marrow transplants. In: Areman E, Deeg HJ, Sacher RA, eds. *Bone Marrow and Stem Cell Processing; A Manual of Current Techniques.* Philadelphia: Davis, 1992, pp. 201–204.

66. Tutschka PJ, Korbling M, Hess AS, Beschorner WG, Santos GW. Prevention of GVHD by chemoseparation of marrow cells. *Transplant Proc* 1981;13:1202–1206.

67. Reisner Y, Kapoor N, Kirkpatrick D, et al. Transplantation for acute leukemia with HLA-A and- B nonidentical parental marrow cells fractionated with soybean agglutinin andsheep red blood cells. *Lancet* 1981;2:327–336.

68. DeWitt T, Raymakers R, Plas A. Bone marrow repopulation capacity after transplantation of lymphocyte depleted allogeneic bone marrow using counterflow centrifugation. *Transplantation* 1984;37:151–155.

69. Noga SJ, Schwartz CL, Civin CL, et al. Rapid separation of whole human bone marrow aspirates by counterflow centrifugal elutriation. *Transplantation* 1986;43:438–440.

70. Lovelock JE, Bishop MWH. Prevention of freezing damage to living cells by dimethylsulfoxide. *Nature* 1959;183:1394.

71. Gorin NC. Cryopreservation and storage of stem cells. In: Areman E, Deeg HJ, Sacher RA, eds. *Bone Marrow and Stem Cell Processing; A Manual of Current Techniques.* Philadelphia: Davis, 1992, pp. 292–308.

72. Stiff PJ, Koester AR, Weidner MK, et al. Autologous bone marrow transplantation using fractionated cells cryopreserved in dimethylsulfoxide and hydroxyethyl starch without controlled rate freezing. *Blood* 1987;70:974–978.

73. Smith DM, Weisenburger DD, Bierman P, et al. Acute renal failure associated with autologous bone marrow transplantation. *Bone Marrow Transplant* 1994;2:196–201.

74. Keung YK, Lau S, Elkayam U, Chen SC, Douer D. Cardiac arrhythmia after infusion of cryopreserved stem cells. *Bone Marrow Transplant* 1994;14:363–367.

75. Stroncek DF, Fautsch SK, Lasky LC, et al. Adverse reactions in patients transfused with cryopreserved marrow. *Transfusion* 1991;31:521–526.

76. Tedder RS, Zuckerman MA, Goldstone AH, et al. Hepatitis B transmission from contaminated cryopreservation tank. *Lancet* 1995;346:137–140.

77. Appelbaum FR, Herzig GP, Graw RG, et al. Study of cell dose and storage time on engraftment of cryopreserved autologous bone marrow in a canine model. *Transplantation* 1978;26:245–248.

78. Burnett AK, Tansey P, Hill C, et al. Hematological reconstitution following high dose and supralethal chemoradiotherapy using stored noncryopreserved autologous bone marrow. *Br J Haematol* 1983;54:309–316.

79. Koppler H, Pfluger KH, Havemann K. Hematopoietic reconstitution after high dose chemotherapy and autologous nonfrozen bone marrow rescue. *Ann Hematol* 1991; 63:253–258.

80. Wilson AP. Cytotoxicity and viability assays. In: Freshney RI, ed. *Animal Cell Culture: A Practical Approach.* Washington DC: IRL Press 1986, pp. 183–216.

81. Spitzer G, Verma DS, Fisher R, et al. The myeloid progenitor cell—its value in predicting hematopoietic recovery after autologous bone marrow transplantation. *Blood* 1980;55:317–323.

82. Rowley SD, Zuehlsdorf M, Braine HG, et al. CFU-GM content of bone marrow graft correlates with time to hematologic reconstitution following autologous bone marrow transplantation with 4-hydroperoxycyclophosphamide-purged bone marrow. *Blood* 1987;70:271–275.

83. Messner HA, Curtis JE, Minden MD, et al. Clonogenic hemopoietic precursors in bone marrow transplantation. *Blood* 1987;70:1425–1432.

84. Chen CH, Lin W, Shye S, et al. Automated enumeration of CD34 cells in peripheral blood and bone marrow. *J Hematother* 1994;3:3–13.

85. Siena S, Bregni M, Brando B, et al. Flow cytometry for clinical estimation of circulating hematopoietic progenitors for autologous transplantation in cancer patients. *Blood* 1991;77:400–409.

86. Rowley SD, Davis J, Dick J, et al. Bacterial contamination of bone marrow grafts intended for autologous and allogeneic bone marrow transplantation. *Transfusion* 1988;28:109–112.

87. Centers for Disease Control. Reported contamination of sodium heparin with Pseudomonas putida. *MMWR* 1986;35:123–124.

88. Marciniak E, Romond EH, Thompson JS, et al. Laboratory control in predicting clinical efficacy of T cell-depletion procedures used for prevention of graft-versus-host disease: importance of limiting dilution analysis. *Bone Marrow Transplant* 1988; 3:589–598.

89. Joshi SS, Kessinger A, Mann SL, et al. Detection of malignant cells in histologically normal bone marrow using culture techniques. *Bone Marrow Transplant* 1987;303–310.

90. Huang W, Sun G-L, Li XS. Acute promyelocytic leukemia: clinical relevance of two major PNL-RARα isoforms and detection of minimal residual disease by retrotranscriptase/polymerase chain reaction to predict relapse. *Blood* 1993;82:1264–1269.

91. Moss TJ. Sensitive detection of metastatic tumor cells in bone marrow. In: Gee AP, Gross S, Worthington-White, DA, eds. *Advances in Bone Marrow Purging and Processing, Fourth International Symposium.* New York: Wiley Liss, 1994, pp. 567–577.

92. Draft document concerning the regulation of peripheral blood hematopoietic stem cell products intended for transplantation or further manufacture into injectable products. Food and Drug Administration, February 1996.

93. Kotula P, Areman E, Hancock S, Sacher R. An alternative to bedside thawing of peripheral blood stem cells. (abstract) *J Hematother* 1995;4:222.

94. Beaujean F, Hartmann O, Kuentz M, et al. A simple, efficient washing procedure for cryopreserved human hematopoietic stem cells prior to reinfusion. *Bone Marrow Transplant* 1991;8:291–294.

95. Rowley SD. Recombinant human deoxyribonuclease for hematopoietic stem cell processing. *J Hematother* 1995;4:99–104.

9

Massive Transfusion

Richard K. Spence

1. INTRODUCTION

Massive transfusion is commonly defined as transfusion approximating or exceeding the patient's blood volume within a 24-h period *(1)*. In the adult male who weighs 70 kg, this translates to an estimated replacement of 4–5 L of blood, or transfusion of 16–20 U of packed red blood cells (RBCs). These estimates are generally helpful only after the fact in classifying or defining the situation, because both blood loss and volume replacement occur in a short time period and are dynamic processes.

A second definition that is suitable for most patients is loss of between 30 and 50% of total blood volume *(2)*. This definition is more useful in the clinical setting because amounts of blood loss can be tied to clinical signs and symptoms and the development of shock. Trunkey *(3)* added further clarification by expressing hemorrhage in terms of rate of blood loss. He defined severe hemorrhage as a rate of blood loss >150 mL/min, which could lead to the loss of one half of the victim's blood volume within 20 min. Although these patients are relatively easy to recognize from their obvious signs of shock, patients with less severe hemorrhage are more difficult to define on clinical grounds. Blood loss and hemorrhagic shock may be classified as follows:

1.1. Class I Hemorrhage

Blood loss is < 15% of total blood volume (approx 750 mL or 3 units of packed RBCs). Clinical manifestations include normal or slightly increased pulse rate, normal blood pressure and pulse pressure, and no changes in signs of tissue perfusion. Volume losses are typically restored from extracellular fluid resources *(4)*.

1.2. Class II Hemorrhage

Blood loss is 15–30% of total blood volume (750–1500 mL or 3–6 units of packed RBCs). Heart rate is increased and systolic blood pressure is typically normal, but pulse pressure decreases in response to vasoconstriction and tachycardia. A drop in blood pressure will be seen with change in posture from supine to seated (positive tilt test). Capillary refill may be delayed, respiratory rate may be increased, and patients may demonstrate some signs of anxiety as a result of decreased cerebral perfusion *(5)*.

From: *Red Cell Transfusion: A Practical Guide*
Edited by: M. E. Reid and S. J. Nance Humana Press Inc., Totowa, NJ

1.3. Class III Hemorrhage

Blood loss is 30–40% of total blood volume (1500–2000 mL or 6–8 units of blood). Symptoms include tachycardia, decreased systolic blood pressure and pulse pressure, delayed capillary refill, and a progressively increasing respiratory rate. Urine output may become decreased and the patient may become confused at this level.

1.4. Class IV Hemorrhage

Blood loss is >40% of total blood volume (>2000 mL or 8 units of blood). Clinical signs are those of shock: tachycardia, hypotension, oliguria, and lethargy or coma. Patients with Class IV hemorrhage are those considered to fall into the massive transfusion category.

2. ASSESSMENT OF PATIENTS

Clinical assessment should be coupled with laboratory specimens for assessment. Initial laboratory studies should be drawn when iv lines are placed and should include blood for both a type and crossmatch, and hemoglobin and hematocrit to assess blood loss. An initial low hemoglobin in patients with a history of trauma or obvious blood loss (e.g., from a gastrointestinal source) should be considered evidence of ongoing blood loss. Such low hemoglobin levels may be a result of initial massive losses or continuous bleeding. Those patients whose presenting hemoglobin is consistent with a 40–50% loss of blood volume (6–8 g/dL) should be treated as having massive blood loss *(6)*.

Massive transfusion is needed most commonly in trauma victims, patients with gastrointestinal hemorrhage *(7)*, or ruptured aortic aneurysms *(8,9)*. Massive transfusion may also follow elective surgical procedures such as liver resections, aortic repairs, and coronary artery bypass, especially in those patients with a congenital or acquired bleeding diathesis *(10,11)*. Surprisingly, the majority of trauma patients are managed without blood transfusion. Wudell et al. *(12)* at Vanderbilt University found only 27% of patients admitted to the hospital for trauma over a 5-yr period required transfusion. Of these, only 9.6% of the blunt trauma patients required 20 or more units of blood. However, this small percentage contributes a disproportionate share to total deaths following motor vehicle accidents. Frey et al. *(13)* reported that 41% of such deaths are related to uncontrolled hemorrhage.

Certain injury patterns in combination with hypotension will prompt the clinician to institute early transfusion. Penetrating injuries of the chest, neck, abdomen, or proximal extremities frequently lead to ongoing blood loss. Approximately 2% of patients with abdominal injury will present with "exsanguinating hemorrhage" *(14)*. Pelvic fracture associated with severe abdominal injury characteristically causes high blood loss and leads to transfusion *(15)*.

Overall survival among patients with massive transfusion is 40–60%, and correlates with several factors including the duration and magnitude of shock, age, severe head injury, abdominal trauma as a source of hemorrhage, pelvic fracture, underlying medical conditions particularly of hepatic origin, and nontraumatic surgical emergencies as well as the number of transfusions given *(16–22)*. Morbid complications, including multisystem organ failure, increases following massive transfusion in trauma patients *(23)*.

Two approaches to red cell transfusion may be used in the trauma patient with massive or ongoing hemorrhage—transfusion on the scene or transfusion in the hospital. Transfusion on the scene is rarely done. Proponents of this approach believe that early transfusion offers the theoretical advantage of providing earlier oxygen-carrying capacity through the provision of RBCs as volume replacement *(24,25)*. This must be weighed against the risks and potential disadvantages, which include:

1. Blood is not the ideal resuscitation fluid. It cannot be infused as rapidly through small-bore iv lines as crystalloid solutions.
2. No type and crossmatch can be done, therefore type-specific blood cannot be used.
3. Because of logistics, Group O D-positive cells will be used in most circumstances. This could cause D-negative, premenopausal females future problems.
4. Acute hemolysis may occur in the patients with RBC alloantibodies. This may be confusing and/or misdiagnosed in the trauma setting.

In addition, blood transfused on the scene may be lost again before the source of bleeding is identified and controlled. Infusions of large volumes of crystalloid fluids or blood transfusion at the scene may lead to increased blood pressure, which perpetuates or increases bleeding from open vessels. Some major trauma centers now advocate the use of a ''scoop-and-run'' approach that attempts to minimize blood loss *(26)*. Trauma victims are moved rapidly from the scene to the trauma center where the source of bleeding is identified and controlled. Transfusion is given as needed to replace RBC losses.

Most transfusions are given on arrival in the hospital emergency department or trauma unit. Transfusion in the hospital can be done in life-threatening situations when blood type is unknown. A rapid crossmatch can be done to provide type-specific blood in 5–10 min. Delays may occur in transport and specimen processing, extending the time from blood sampling to transfusion to 30–40 min. In these cases, uncrossmatched Group O packed RBCs can be used as initial therapy *(27–29)*. During their preparation, red blood cells are usually centrifuged and resuspended in an additive solution to extend cell viability and improve flow rates. Packed red cells may need to be transfused along with a saline solution to attain rates of flow needed for adequate resuscitation. The transfusion of packed type O cells containing anti-A and anti-B is usually not a significant problem, since only small quantities of residual plasma (approx 20–30 mL) remain in the red cell concentrates resuspended in additive solutions. When the patient's blood type is determined, the patient can safely be switched to his or her own type or a compatible blood type without concern for hemolysis resulting from passive transmission of these naturally occurring antibodies.

Care must be taken to follow transfusion protocols in the trauma setting because of the risk of human error that can lead to ABO incompatibility reactions, especially when multiple trauma victims are being treated together. Errors in patient identification, sample labeling, multiple simultaneous typing procedures, STAT testing, and the urgent nature of the clinical setting all may increase the risk of clerical errors. ABO reactions may be misdiagnosed as coagulopathy due to hypothermia or hemodilution.

The use of D-positive and D-negative RBCs for transfusion in emergency room/ trauma situations varies in different parts of this country. As a general rule, Group

O D-positive red cells should be used in males with penetrating or blunt trauma with no history of prior transfusion. Group O D-negative blood is reserved for premenopausal females who have the potential of becoming pregnant and for individuals with known or suspected sensitization to the D antigen. Because only 6% of the population is Group O D-negative, the universal use of this product for all emergency room/trauma center patients can not be justified. Hemoglobin-derived blood substitutes are on the horizon, and may provide an answer in the future *(30,31)*.

3. COAGULOPATHIES

Coagulopathy is a frequent finding in the trauma patient and may be caused by a combination of events including dilution of clotting factors and platelets following transfusion, hypothermia, and disseminated intravascular coagulation. Dilutional coagulopathy may occur, depending upon the amount of blood lost and transfused. Nearly 37% of the original blood elements remain in circulation following the controlled exchange of a single blood volume (10 U in a 70 kg adult) *(35)*. Remaining levels of coagulation factors and platelets (>100,000) are usually adequate to maintain hemostasis. With progressive exchanges of two volumes (equivalent to a 20 U transfusion), blood elements drop to levels of approx 5%, and coagulopathy follows *(32–34)*. These levels serve only as basic estimates in the clinical setting, since both platelet counts and amounts of circulating clotting factors will vary depending on both rate of blood loss and rate of transfusion.

Dilutional thrombocytopenia occurs following the equivalent of more than one exchange transfusion of blood and is compounded by large-volume fluid replacement *(35–38)*. Clinical evidence of thrombocytopenia includes diffuse microvascular bleeding and oozing from mucosa, raw wounds and puncture sites. Platelet activity decreases in the presence of hypothermia, a condition that is common in the trauma patient *(39–41)*, and may also be affected by the type and volume of resuscitation fluid *(23)*. If available, whole blood can be used to restore coagulation factors and platelets *(33–35)*.

Prothrombin (PT) and activated partial thromboplastin (aPTT) times may be prolonged when coagulation factors decrease below 30% of normal. The exact activity levels of clotting factors needed for hemostasis when multiple factor deficiencies coexist are not well defined *(2,18,22)*. Hiippala and associates *(38)* found that critical levels of platelets and clotting factors were not reached with blood loss and replacement until more than 2 estimated blood volumes had been replaced. However, fibrinogen deficits appeared much earlier.

It may be difficult to directly correlate the clinical observation of bleeding with prolongation of the PT and aPTT, which are reagent and temperature dependent *(42)*. Because coagulation testing is routinely performed at 37 °C, rather than at the patient's actual in vivo temperature, normal coagulation tests can be obtained even in the presence of clinical evidence of a coagulopathy *(43)*. Normal test results in this setting suggest that sufficient clotting factors are available for coagulation if normothermia is restored *(44)*.

Dilutional coagulopathy may be mistaken for or aggravated by the development of disseminated intravascular coagulation (DIC) *(10,21,45,46)*. DIC in the setting of massive transfusion is reported to occur in 5–30% of trauma patients *(33,37)*, and is associated with high morbidity and mortality rates of nearly 70% *(10,11,47)*. Tissue injury and hemolysis with release of cytokines and tissue thromboplastin into the circulation may cause immediate activation of both the coagulation and the fibrinolytic systems, resulting in severe DIC *(42)*. At the present time, no single laboratory test can be used to confirm or exclude the diagnosis of DIC. However the combination of a low platelet count, a low fibrinogen, an elevated D-dimer, and the presence of soluble fibrin monomers in the context of the patient's underlying condition are the most helpful indicators of DIC.

Coagulation factors and platelets can be replaced as needed by infusing fresh frozen plasma or platelets. The following guidelines for specific component therapy during massive transfusion in patients with clinical evidence of microvascular bleeding may be used:

1. Platelets should be given if the platelet count drops below 80–100 × 10⁹/L.
2. Fresh frozen plasma (FFP) should be given when the PT and/or aPTT are >1.5 times normal.
3. Cryoprecipitate and FFP should be given when fibrinogen drops below 10 g/L.

Although specific guidelines can be helpful in deciding when to use component therapy, they may also lead to undertransfusion if the decision to transfuse is based only on laboratory values. Bleeding in trauma patients is often multifactorial and may not correlate directly to laboratory measurements. The location and extent of injury, the duration of shock, the response to resuscitation and the risk of complicating factors such as intracranial bleeding are important clinical considerations. With prompt management of bleeding, debridement of devitalized tissue, and the skilled use of component therapy, the coagulopathy can usually be controlled. In the end, clinical judgement must prevail, even if this results in what appears to be overuse of components, based on laboratory measurements. Conversely, prophylactic or empiric transfusion of components using a "cookbook" approach without clinical evidence of bleeding should be avoided, since this depletes precious supplies and leads to increased risk of transfusion-related complications.

4. COMPLICATIONS OF MASSIVE TRANSFUSION

Massive transfusion may lead to complications in up to 10% of patients *(2,7,9,10)*. Antibody-mediated hemolysis and transfusion-related acute lung injury (TRALI) may appear, masquerading as dilutional coagulopathy and acute respiratory distress syndrome (ARDS). Metabolic problems including citrate toxicity, hyperkalemia, acidosis, and a shift in the oxygen-dissociation curve may develop. The impact of delayed problems such as transfusion-transmitted disease, and possibly immunosuppression, is difficult to quantify.

Plasma-containing blood products (FFP, platelets) are the major source of citrate during massive transfusion. Amounts of citrate vary, depending on the storage additive. CPDA-1 and Adsol red cell concentrates contain only 5 and 2 mg/mL of citrate, respectively, compared to the plasma from an Adsol unit, which contains nearly 30 mg/mL of citrate. Citrate is excreted in the urine and metabolized rapidly to bicarbonate by the normal liver. Citrate infusions cause a transient decrease in ionized calcium that is restored under normal circumstances by mobilization of skeletal calcium stores. The ability to metabolize and to excrete citrate may be limited in trauma patients with severe hypotension, hypothermia, hepatic injury or pre-existing hepatic disease. In these patients, citrate toxicity can cause muscle tremors, increased myocardial irritability including irreversible ventricular fibrillation, and decreased cardiac output *(48)*. Irreversible ventricular fibrillation may occur at citrate levels of 60 mg/mL. The infusion of calcium salts should be reserved for selected massively transfused patients with clinical manifestations of citrate toxicity.

Potassium leaks from red cells during storage and may accumulate, reaching levels of 7.5 mmol/U *(2)*. Massive transfusion of units containing increased potassium may lead to hyperkalemia, adding to the elevated potassium levels caused by severe shock, renal dysfunction, and muscle necrosis. In most patients, this amount causes little harm, since potassium re-enters red cells within a few hours after transfusion. Some patients may experience a paradoxical hypokalemia resulting from the metabolism of citrate to bicarbonate and increased urinary excretion of potassium *(45)*. In recent years, the ability to infuse large volumes of stored blood rapidly using high-capacity blood warmers has increased the risk of hyperkalemia in trauma patients. Potassium levels must be monitored closely if cardiac dysfunction is to be avoided.

Red blood cells lose 2,3-DPG after 10 d of storage, which causes the oxygen-dissociation curve to shift to the left. These decreases in 2,3-DPG lead to increased oxygen affinity and decreased oxygen offloading of the red cell *(49)*. The cell's deformability may also be limited, restricting it's ability to pass through the microcirculation. This capability is dependent on cellular adenosine triphosphate (ATP) levels. Whole blood in CPDA-1 at 35 d of storage retains only 45% of initial ATP levels. Special additive solutions (Adsol) used in the preparation of red cell concentrates have effectively reduced ATP loss (60–65% of initial levels are retained) and increased red cell storage to 42 d *(50)*.

ABO-incompatible hemolytic transfusion reactions are the most common cause of acute fatalities from blood transfusion and are related to human error *(51,52)*. Acute hemolytic reactions caused by naturally occurring isoagglutinins (anti-A or anti-B) lead to complement activation, red cell lysis, and liberation of free hemoglobin within the vascular system *(53)*. This combination of events may lead to acute renal failure, DIC, and death. A hemolytic reaction in a critically injured or massively transfused patient may be overlooked. Clinical findings of hemoglobinuria, hypotension, fever, and microvascular hemorrhage may be attributed to traumatic injury. Prevention of clerical error is essential.

Kroll et al. *(54)* reported posttransfusion purpura caused by incompatible platelet transfusions, emphasizing that care must be taken with all components *(54)*. First episodes of incompatibility can only be detected clinically or by random screening.

Both animal and human data have demonstrated the immunosuppressive effect of allogeneic blood transfusion *(55,56)*. Although the impact of this effect on the clinical condition is still controversial, evidence points to an increased incidence of infection. This may be devastating in the trauma patient, who is already immunologically compromised from the injury and may have been exposed to a wide variety of both community and nosocomial pathogens. The use of leuko-reduced blood components may hold an answer in the future treatment of patients who are massively transfused *(57)*.

REFERENCES

1. Adverse effects of blood transfusion. In: *Technical Manual,* 11th ed. Bethesda, MD: American Association of Blood Banks, 1993.
2. Jeter E, Ross S. Massive transfusion. In: Petz L, ed. *Clinical Practice of Transfusion Medicine,* 3rd ed. New York: Churchill-Livingstone, 1995, pp. 563–579.
3. Trunkey D. Trauma. *Sci Am* 1983;249:28–30.
4. American College of Surgeons. *Advanced Trauma Life Support Manual,* 1993, American College of Surgeons, Chicago, IL.
5. Schriger D, Baraff L, Capillary Refill—Is it a Useful Predictor of Hypovolemic States. *Ann Emerg Med* 1991;20:601–605.
6. Knottenbelt J. Low initial hemoglobin levels in trauma patients: an important indicator of ongoing hemorrhage. *J Trauma* 1991;31:1396–1399.
7. Yavorski R, Wong R, Maydonovitch C, Battin L, Furnia A, Amundson D. Analysis of 3,294 cases of upper gastrointestional bleeding in military medical facilities. *Am J Gastroenterol* 1995;90:568–573.
8. Harrigan C, Lucas C, Ledgerwood A, Mannen E. Primary hemostasis after massive transfusion for injury. *Surgery* 1985;98:836–840.
9. Phillips T, Soulier G, Wilson R. Outcome of massive transfusion exceeding two blood volumes in trauma and emergency surgery. *J Trauma* 1987;27:903–908.
10. Wilson R, Mammen E, Walt E. Eight years of experience with massive blood transfusion. *J Trauma* 1971;11:275–278.
11. Rutledge R, Sheldon G, Collins M. Massive transfusion. *Crit Care Clinics* 1986;2: 791–783.
12. Wudel J, Morris J, Yates K, Wilson A, Bass S. Massive transfusion: outcome in blunt trauma patients. *J Trauma* 1991;31:1–7.
13. Frey C, Huelke D, Gikas P. Resuscitation and survival in motor vehicle accidents. *J Trauma* 1969;9:292–298.
14. Olsen W. Quantitative peritoneal lavage in blunt abdominal trauma. *Arch Surg* 1972; 104:536–539.
15. Mucha P, Welch T. Hemorrhage in major pelvic fractures. *Surg Clin North Am* 1988; 68:757–780.
16. Sawyer P, Harrison C. Massive transfusion in adults. *Vox Sanguinis* 1990;58:199–202.
17. Kivioja A, Myllynen P, Rokkanen P. Survival after massive transfusions exceeding four blood volumes in patients with blunt injuries. *Am Surg* 1991;57:398–402.
18. Harvey M, Greenfield T, Sugrue M, Rosenfeld D. Massive blood transfusion in a tertiary referral hospital. Clinical outcomes and hemostatic complications. *Med J Aust* 1995;163:356–359.
19. Harrigan C, Lucas C, Ledgerwood A. The effect of hemorrhagic shock on the clotting cascade in injured patients. *J Trauma* 1989;29:1416–1420.
20. Mitchell KJ, Moncure KE, Onyeije C, Rao MS, Siram S. Evaluation of massive volume replacement in the penetrating trauma patient. *J Natl Med Assoc* 1994;86(12):926–929.
21. Canizaro P, Possa M. Management of massive hemorrhage associated with abdominal trauma. *Surg Clin North Am* 1990;70:621–625.
22. Faringer P, Mullins R, Johnson R, Trunkey D. Blood component supplementation during massive transfusion of AS-1 red cells in trauma patients. *J Trauma* 1993;34: 481–486.
23. Samama CM. Traumatic emergencies and hemostasis. *Can J Anesthesiol* 1995;43(5): 479–482.
24. Schmidt P. Use of Rh positive blood in emergency situations. *Surg Gyn Ob* 1988;167: 229–233.
25. Schwab C, Shayne J, Turner J. Immediate trauma resuscitation with type O uncrossmatched blood: a two-year prospective experience. *J Trauma* 1986;26:897–401.

26. Bickell WH, Wall MJ, Jr., Pepe PE, et al. Immediate versus delayed fluid resuscitation for hypotensive patients with penetrating torso injuries. *N Engl J Med* 1994;331: 1105–1109.
27. Janvier G, Fialon P, Guinier MC, Sztark F, Lassie P, Roger I. Strategy of erythrocyte transfusion and plasma use in traumatic emergencies. *Can J Anesthesiol* 1994;42: 643–649.
28. Audibert G. Indications of blood components and outcome of transfusion practices in hemorrhage of multiple trauma. *Can J Anesthesiol* 1994;42:391–394.
29. Gervin A, Fischer R. Resuscitation of trauma patients with type-specific uncrossmatched blood. *J Trauma* 1984;24:327–331.
30. Gervin A. Transfusion, autotransfusion, and blood substitutes. In: Moore E, Mattox K, Feliciano D, eds. *Trauma,* 2nd ed. Norwalk, CT: Appleton and Lange, 1991, pp. 165–173.
31. Bowersox JC, Hess JR. Trauma and military applications of blood substitutes. *Artif Cells Blood Substit Immobil Biotechnol* 1994;22(2):145–157.
32. Humphries JE. Transfusion therapy in acquired coagulopathies. *Hematol Oncol Clin North Am* 1994;8:1181–1201.
33. Counts R, Haisch C, Simon T, Maxwell N, Heimbach D. Hemostasis in massively transfused trauma patients. *Ann Surg* 1979;190:91–96.
34. Murray DJ, Pennell BJ, Weinstein SL, Olsen JD. Packed red cells in acute blood loss: dilutional coagulopathy as a cause of surgical bleeding. *Anesth Analg* 1995;80:336–342.
35. Harke H, Rahman S. Haemostatic disorders in massive transfusion. *Bibliotheca Haemat* 1980;46:179–183.
36. Noe D, Graham S., Luff R, Sohmer P. Platelet counts during rapid massive transfusion. *Transfusion* 1982;22:392–396.
37. Mannucci P, Federici A, Sirchia G. Hemostasis testing during massive blood replacement. *Vox Sanguinis* 1982;42:113–118.
38. Hiippala ST, Myllyla GJ, Vahtera EM. Hemostatic factors and replacement of major blood loss with plasma-poor red cell concentrates. *Anesth Analg* 1995;81:360–365.
39. Schmied H, Kurz A, Sessler DI, Kozek S, Reiter A. Mild hypothermia increases blood loss and transfusion requirements during total hip arthroplasty. *Lancet* 1996;347: 289–292.
40. Nathan HJ, Polis T. The management of temperature during hypothermic cardiopulmonary bypass: II—Effect of prolonged hypothermia. *Can J Anaesth* 1995;42: 672–676.
41. Valeri C, Cassidy G, Khuri S, Feingold H, Ragno G. Hypothermia-induced reversible platelet dysfunction. *Ann Surg* 1987;205:175–180.
42. Bick R. Disseminated intravascular coagulation and related syndromes: a clinical review. *Sem Thromb Hemo* 1988;14:299–305.
43. Rohrer MJ NA. Effect of hypothermia on the coagulation cascade. *Crit Care Med* 1992;20:1402–1408.
44. Nicholls MD, Whyte G. Red cell, plasma and albumin transfusion decision triggers. *Anaesth Intensive Care* 1993;21:156–162.
45. Collins J. Problems associated with the massive transfusion of stored blood. *Surgery* 1974;75:274–278.
46. Lucas C, Ledgerwood A. Clinical significance of altered coagulation test after massive transfusions for trauma. *Am Surg* 1981;47:125–129.
47. Hewson J, Neame P, Kumar N, Ayrton A, Gregor P. Coagulopathy related to dilution and hypotension during massive transfusion. *Crit Care Med* 1985;13:387–392.
48. Bunker J. Metabolic effects of blood transfusions. *Anesthesiology* 1966;27:446–450.
49. Valeri C, Gray A, Cassidy G, Riordan W, Pivacek L. The 24-hour post-transfusion survival, oxygen transport function, and residual hemolysis of human outdated-

rejuvenated red cell concentrate after washing and storage at 4 degrees C for 24 to 72 hours. *Transfusion* 1984;24:323–328.

50. Wolfe L. The membrane and lesions of storage in preserved red cells. *Transfusion* 1985;25:185–189.
51. Sazama K. Reports of 355 transfusion-associated deaths: 1976 through 1985. *Transfusion* 1990;30:583–588.
52. Gloe D. Common reactions to transfusions. *Heart Lung* 1991;20:506–512.
53. Seyfried H, Walewska I. Immune hemolytic transfusion reactions. *World J Surg* 1987;11:25–29.
54. Kroll H, Kiefel V, Mueller-Eckhardt C. Post-transfusion purpura: clinical and immunologic studies in 38 patients. *Infusionsther Transfusionsmed* 1993;20:198–204.
55. Blumberg N, Hea IJ. Transfusion-induced immunomodulation and its possible role in cancer recurrence and perioperative bacterial infection. *Yale J Biol Med* 1990;63:429–433.
56. Crosby ET. Perioperative haemotherapy: II. Risks and complications of blood transfusion. *Can J Anaesth* 1992;39:822–837.
57. Rieger A, Saefkow M, Hass I, Spies C, Eyrich K. Feasibility and rate of leucocyte depletion with a single leucocyte depletion filter during massive transfusion. *Infusionsther Transfusionsmed* 1995;22:355–359.

10

Autogeneic and Directed Blood Transfusions

Pearl T. C. Y. Toy

1. INTRODUCTION

Transfusion with autogeneic or autologous blood (the patient's own blood) remains safer than allogeneic blood transfusion (someone else's blood), because of the reduction of the risk of transmitting viruses *(1,2)*. If transfusion is likely for a planned surgical procedure, several types of autogeneic transfusion can be used either alone or in combination: preoperative autogeneic blood donation/collection (PABD), intraoperative blood salvage, postoperative blood salvage, and acute normovolemic hemodilution *(2)*. In contrast, there is no evidence that directed donor blood (blood from friends and relatives) is safer than volunteer allogeneic blood *(3)*.

The awareness of transfusion-associated AIDS has increased the demand for both autogeneic and directed-donor blood. Autogeneic blood donations increased by 70% and directed donations by almost 25% between 1989 and 1992. In 1992, autogeneic units were 4.1% and directed units were 1% of all red cell transfusions *(4)*.

The American Association of Blood Banks (AABB) has established standards, guidelines, and regulations for autogeneic and directed-donor blood *(5)*. These should be used by each hospital in establishing and monitoring autogeneic and directed-donor programs.

2. AUTOGENEIC TRANSFUSION

2.1. Preoperative Donation

Although PABD was underused in the past *(6)*, its use has grown substantially in the last decade *(4)*.

2.1.1. Surgical Procedures for Which PABD May Be Indicated

Autogeneic donation is appropriate for elective procedures in which expected blood loss is large, e.g., coronary artery bypass graft, major vascular surgery, hip replacement, major spine surgery, hepatectomy, and radical prostatectomy. Tables for the amount of blood to be crossmatched for specific procedures are available in hospitals *(7)*. The transfusion experience of patients who have undergone similar procedures at a hospital can serve as a guide. Tables can be established for the amount of autogeneic blood that should be collected *(2,8)*.

From: *Red Cell Transfusion: A Practical Guide*
Edited by: M. E. Reid and S. J. Nance Humana Press Inc., Totowa, NJ

Whether PABD should be combined with other autogeneic techniques depends, in part, on the surgical procedure planned. For example, PABD and postoperative salvage are often appropriate for patients undergoing revisions of total hip arthroplasty. However, PABD but not intraoperative blood salvage would be effective for total knee replacement because tourniquets are used and intraoperative blood loss is minimal.

Autogeneic techniques are considered inappropriate for many surgical procedures because the expected blood loss is small and it is unlikely the patient will receive a transfusion. These procedures, (e.g., cervical spine fusion, discectomy, mastectomy, hysterectomy, reduction mammoplasty, cholecystectomy, tonsillectomy, vaginal and cesarean deliveries, and transurethral resection of the prostate) usually require a type and screen or no blood order. Patients should not be encouraged to donate autogeneic blood for surgery unless there is a realistic possibility of transfusion *(2)*.

2.1.2. Medical Considerations in Candidates for PABD

Among patients who are having elective surgery for which blood is usually transfused, requirements for PABD are: a hemoglobin of no less than 11 g/dL (Hct 33%), and no bacteremia.

2.1.2.1. COEXISTING MEDICAL CONDITIONS

Autogeneic donations have been safely obtained from patients with stable coronary artery disease, stable valvular disease, and congenital heart disease *(9–12)*. One report using normal healthy controls suggested that donation may be associated with increased risks in patients with cerebral cardiovascular disease *(13)*.

2.1.2.2. AGE

The patient's condition, rather than age alone, should determine whether a patient should donate. Elderly patients—even those who have never donated blood—can safely donate autogeneic blood *(14)*. For patients under 110 pounds, including children, the volume drawn at each donation is reduced in proportion to the body weight. Other factors, such as venous access and emotional tolerance of venipuncture, may limit collection of autogeneic blood from children *(15)*.

2.1.2.3. OBSTETRIC PATIENTS

Among obstetric patients, several studies have not detected complications for either mother or baby from autogeneic blood donations *(16–18)*. However, since so few mothers need transfusions during or after delivery, autogeneic donations should not be encouraged for pregnant women in general. An exception may be placenta previa because of the greater likelihood of transfusion *(19)*.

2.1.3. PABD Strategy

In general, patients should begin blood donation 4–6 wk before surgery to allow for liquid storage of a sufficient number of units and to enable more red cell regeneration. Some patients can give blood as frequently as every 3 d, although once a week is more common. Patients should also take oral iron. Patients donating autogeneic blood should take oral supplementation; for example, $FeSO_4$ 325 mg po tid or ferrous gluconate 325 mg po five times a day. The last blood donation should not be collected later than 72 h before surgery to allow for restoration of intravascular volume *(3)*. In addition, increasing the time between the last donation and surgery should allow greater red cell regeneration.

2.1.4. PABD Risks

2.1.4.1. REACTIONS

Vasovagal reactions occur in about 2–5% of donors—either autogeneic or allogeneic *(20)*. Most vasovagal reactions consist of lightheadedness owing to transient hypotension and bradycardia and are self-limited. More severe reactions with loss of consciousness, seizures, or local vascular access problems are uncommon *(21)*.

2.1.4.2. ERRORS AND ACCIDENTS

Despite the use of special systems to avoid administering the wrong unit of blood to patients, errors occur. Autogeneic units have been transfused to unintended recipients and allogeneic units have been transfused prior to transfusion of autogeneic units. The likelihood that autogeneic blood is given to the wrong patient is not zero but can be estimated to be 1:30,000 to 1:50,000 *(23,24)*. In addition, autogeneic units may not be available when needed because they were lost in transit, broke during processing or shipping, or were improperly identified *(22)*. Systems should be developed to minimize such events.

2.1.5. Positive Tests for Infectious Diseases

When autogeneic blood will be transfused outside the collecting facility, the following tests must be performed on the first unit from a given donor during a 30-d period: HbsAg, anti-HIV1/2, anti-HCV, anti-HBc, serologic test for syphilis, and any other tests recommended or required by the FDA *(5)*. These tests are not yet required for autogeneic blood that will be used within the collecting facility and only for the autogeneic donor. The patient's physician shall be informed of any abnormal results obtained for the aforementioned tests. The shipping facility must notify the receiving transfusion service if an autogeneic unit shipped is positive for any of these tests. A written permission from the receiving transfusion service and a written request from the patient's physician are required if the units to be shipped are confirmed positive for anti-HIV or HbsAg *(5)*. All personnel should handle all blood as biohazard material, regardless of whether the blood is autogeneic or allogeneic, tested or not tested.

Author's Practice: UCSF does not test autogeneic units collected, processed, and transfused at Moffitt-Long Hospital. However, UCSF does test autogeneic units collected at Mt. Zion Hospital, because they are transported to Moffitt-Long Hospital for processing and transported back to Mt. Zion Hospital for transfusion.

2.1.6. Unused Autogeneic Units

Unused autogeneic blood is stored for the patient's perioperative needs for a variable period of time after the operation, in accordance with local policies and procedures. Typically, this blood is stored until the patient's discharge or the unit's outdate. If a second surgical procedure is anticipated or if the scheduled procedure is delayed, the transfusion service may be able to arrange for extended frozen storage of the autogeneic blood. Between one-third and one-half of collected autogeneic blood components are not used by their donors *(4,25,26)*. Although inappropriate excess collections may occur, some collections in excess of transfusions are inevitable in order to provide sufficient blood to meet the needs of most patients *(8)*, and is an inherent cost of autogeneic blood. Most unused units are not suitable for other patients because autogeneic donors often do not meet the health criteria required for allogeneic blood donors. Furthermore, the suitable unit, when no longer needed by the donor, often has a very short shelf-life. Adding of unused autogeneic blood to the inventory would have little impact on the overall blood supply and should not be considered a justification for requesting autogeneic donations from patients who are not likely to require transfusion. Thus, unused autogeneic blood is usually destroyed rather than being added to the allogeneic blood inventory.

Author's Practice: We do not add autogeneic units to the allogeneic inventory except those from bone marrow or organ transplant donors. If unused by the donor, they may be transfused to the transplant recipient, but not added to the general allogeneic inventory.

2.1.7. Autogeneic Platelet-Rich Plasma

Autogeneic platelet-rich plasma can be collected from patients in the operating room using apheresis equipment. For cardiac surgery patients, this plasma is removed before cardiopulmonary bypass and returned after heparin reversal. Although the procedure has been advocated as a technique to improve hemostasis and limit blood loss *(27–29)*, other data do not support its routine use *(30–32)*.

2.1.8. Recombinant Erythropoietin

Most studies show that recombinant erythropoietin increases capacity for PABD *(33)*. It reduced allogeneic transfusion in anemic *(34)* but not in nonanemic PABD patients who underwent orthopedic surgery *(35)*. Recombinant erythropoietin is not routinely recommended for PABD because of its high cost. It has been licensed by the FDA for autogeneic donation. Lower doses administered subcutaneously, if effective, would lower cost and increase usage.

2.1.9. Indications for Autogeneic vs Allogeneic Blood Transfusion

Whether the indications for autogeneic and allogeneic transfusions should be the same is an interesting and difficult question. The benefits of allogeneic and autogeneic red cell transfusions are similar, but the risks of autogeneic blood are less. Hence, the risk–benefit ratio supports the more liberal use of autogeneic blood. Although some physicians may choose to use autogeneic blood components more liberally than allogeneic components for a given indication, autogeneic blood should not transfused merely because it has been collected. For example, it is inappropriate to transfuse autogeneic red blood cells (RBCs) to the slightly or nonanemic patient, or to transfuse autogeneic fresh frozen plasma in the absence of coagulopathy.

Author's Practice: We usually consider an autogeneic transfusion inappropriate, when given to a nonbleeding patient with a hemoglobin of 10 g/dL or higher. Autogeneic transfusions in patients with a hemoglobin of 7–10 g/dL may or may not be appropriate, depending on the medical circumstances.

2.2. Intraoperative Salvage

Blood shed intraoperatively may be recovered by suction and transfused into the patient.

2.2.1. Indications

Patients who are expected to have large intraoperative blood loss can benefit from intraoperative salvage, especially when preoperative donation is impossible or inadequate. Examples of such procedures are cardiac surgery, intra-abdominal vascular surgery, complex spine surgery, and liver transplantation.

In general, it is not recommended to reinfuse blood contaminated with bacteria, cancer cells, or amniotic fluid *(2)*. Bacteria can contaminate shed blood in procedures that involve spilled intestinal contents, bacterial peritonitis, abscesses, or osteomyelitis. Cancer cells may theoretically metastasize when reinfused, but this has never been demonstrated. Amniotic fluid may contaminate blood salvaged in ruptured ectopic pregnancy.

2.2.2. Risks

2.2.2.1. DILUTIONAL COAGULOPATHY

Because washed, salvaged blood is deficient in platelets and plasma, patients who receive one blood volume or more of salvaged blood may develop dilutional coagulopathy. Patients with pre-existing coagulation deficiency owing to liver disease may develop dilutional coagulopathy with less than one blood volume transfusion. As expected, the abnormalities are hypofibrinogenemia, thrombocytopenia, and prolonged prothrombin and partial thromboplastin time. Fibrin degradation products may be reinfused and have been detected by laboratory testing. These abnormalities may be misinterpreted as disseminated intravascular coagulation. Treatment with fresh frozen plasma and platelets should be guided by laboratory tests and clinical judgment regarding the amount of existing and anticipated further blood loss.

2.2.2.2. OTHER RISKS

Heparin may be reinfused when blood is unwashed or when the cell-washer is not functioning properly. Air embolis may occur with improper technique. Hemolysis can be caused by vigorous suctioning of shed blood.

2.3. Postoperative Salvage

Postoperative blood lost and collected from mediastinal, chest, and joint drains can be transfused without washing. Such blood is deficient in fibrinogen and thus does not require anticoagulation. This technique is not often used because the amount of blood salvaged is small and there are some risks involved.

2.3.1. Indications

When the amount of postoperative bleeding is small, as in first-time knee replacement, salvage may not be worthwhile *(35)*. It can be considered after traumatic hemothorax, cardiac surgery, or orthopedic surgery in which the amount of RBCs lost and collected is larger.

2.3.2. Risks

Small amounts of salvaged blood have been transfused with no apparent side effects *(37)* but, in some cases, fever *(38)*, hypotension *(37)*, and upper airway edema *(39)* have been reported.

2.4. Acute Normovolemic Hemodilution

Acute normovolemic hemodilution is the intentional lowering of the hematocrit while maintaining normal blood volume prior to a surgical procedure. In principle, fewer red cells will be lost if the hematocrit were lowered, for any given volume of whole blood lost during surgery. In theory, significant red cell savings will be achieved only with very low hematocrit levels and large whole blood losses *(40)*.

2.4.1. Indications

The use of hemodilution is controversial and requires considerable vigilance and expertise *(2)*. It may be considered when preoperative donation or intraoperative salvage is impossible. The anticipated intraoperative blood loss should be 50% or more of the patient's blood volume. Initial hematocrit should be close to normal. Since the hematocrit will be lowered to about 0.20, the patient should not have cardiovascular, cerebrovascular, pulmonary, hepatic, or renal disease *(2)*.

2.4.2. Risks

Because of the induced anemia, there is potential for critical organ ischemia. Dilutional coagulopathy may also occur and laboratory tests of hemostasis should be closely monitored.

Author's Practice: We perform hemodilution on a research basis.

3. DIRECTED DONATIONS

Directed donations are made by family or friends and are reserved for transfusion to a recipient. Although demand for directed donations stemmed from lay concern regarding the safety of the allogeneic blood supply, there is no evidence that a directed donor supply is any safer *(3)*. The pros and cons of directed donations have been described in detail *(3)*. Current practices vary. Some centers believe that it is less safe and either do not accept directed donors or do not crossover directed donor blood. At other centers that do accept directed donors, they must meet all donor requirements, but may donate more frequently for individual patients with the approval of both the blood bank and recipient's physicians *(5)*. Directed-donor units from blood relatives are irradiated to prevent graft-vs-host disease associated with transfusion of blood from human leukocyte antigen (HLA)-homozygote persons to HLA-heterozygote persons who share the haplotype *(42)*. Overall, in 1992 in the United States, 31.2% of directed-donor transfused to the intended recipient, whereas 13.1% crossed over, and 55.7% were discarded *(4)*.

Author's Practice: We provide a directed-donor service to patients and their families. They are very grateful for the opportunity to contribute to the care of the patient. Most of our directed donors are first-time donors, and after donation, most sign up to become accessible as volunteer donors to their local community blood center.

4. QUALITY PROGRAM: AUTOGENEIC AND DIRECTED DONATIONS

A quality program on autogeneic and directed donor (AU/DD) should select patients most likely to benefit and provide the safest donation experience. In addition, a quality program should help prevent accidents, errors, and miscommunication that result in a unit not being available when needed or a unit transfused to the wrong patient. Such accidents or errors include units that are lost in transit, broken, damaged, misfiled, mislabeled, or inadvertently outdated, crossed over or discarded *(22,23)*. Miscommunication can occur over whether a unit was actually donated, compatible with the recipient, and actually in the transfusion service ready to be transfused. Prevention of such AU/DD mishaps requires a system different from the traditional random, volunteer donor blood system. Special procedures must be developed and preferably, a special coordinator assigned to the program. Redundant and consistent clerical checks are important to such a system. In addition, physicians and patients should be correctly informed of the currently available AU/DD units and updated on that information in a timely manner.

The transfusion service must have a good tracking system. As soon as it is determined that AU/DD blood will be required, the patient should be assigned a medical record number that will be entered into the computer and recorded on the unit tag. AU/DD patients who do not yet have an inpatient medical record number should be identifed and checked daily until a medical record number is obtained. Upon receipt, AU/DD units must be entered computer and/or manual card system. After verification of information, it is desirable to notify physicians via facsimile about blood availability. If patients are seen in presurgical clinic, they usually know what AU/DD units should be available for their upcoming surgery. Their expectations should be verified with the blood bank so that the blood bank can track AU/DD units not yet received and clear up any misunderstandings with the patient. All AU/DD units should be arranged in an orderly manner in the refrigerator and freezer to prevent units from unnecessarily outdating, and to ensure that all expired units are removed. Autogeneic units about to expire should be identified in order to determine whether these units should be discarded or frozen for subsequent surgery. Directed-donor units that are incompatible with the patient must be discarded or crossed over, depending on the institution's policy. Directed-donor units that are compatible with the patient but are about to expire should be identified and the physician informed. Discrepancies in patient identification information on the unit, physician order, or computer record must be resolved. A dedicated phone line in the blood bank is desirable for incoming calls from hospital staff, patients, families, and outside blood centers.

Author's Practice: On a quarterly basis, the hospital-wide quality improvement committee meets to discuss any AU/DD incidents and problems. The committee is represented by blood bank personnel, administration, operating room nurses, clinical ward nurses, and presurgical clinic staff. Depending on the need, education material is developed and procedures are revised.

On a daily basis, transfusion service staff review inventory and discard, freeze, or cross-over appropriate AU/DD units; maintain AU/DD units in refrigerators and freezers in alphabetical order and by order of outdate for each patient; and make new cards for new orders or new units received.

The special AU/DD coordinator in the transfusion service must on a daily basis, answer calls regarding AU/DD units, verify AU/DD unit availability and inform the attending physician, review all autogeneic units that will expire in 7 d and ask the attending physicians whether to freeze the units, obtain physician consent for transfusion of HbsAg and anti-HIV positive units, resolve discrepancies in patient identification such as discrepant names and date of births, determine AU/DD unit availability for patients coming to presurgical clinic and inform the clinic, obtain any missing medical record numbers for patients, and maintain AU/DD patient records, e.g., update records if units are transfused or if the patient is discharged, call physician on units about to expire, pull units to be returned to general inventory, pull units that have expired, and pull and file inactive records.

On a weekly basis, the special AU/DD coordinator checks the AU/DD refrigerator for correct order and outdates, and checks the card file to remove inactive cards, clarify surgery dates, and correct discrepancies.

5. COSTS

5.1. Cost of PABD

Autogeneic blood components require special handling and segregated processing and storage compared with allogeneic units. In addition, increased personnel time is associated with collecting blood from patients with complex medical histories as opposed to healthy donors. Therefore, autogeneic blood often costs more than regular volunteer blood and may result in billing surcharges.

Autogeneic transfusions cost more because the donation process is more labor-intensive and not all donated units are transfused. The cost-effectiveness values ranged from $235,000 to over $23 million per quality-adjusted year of life saved, when the only benefit considered is avoidance of the major known transfusion-transmitted infectious diseases (41). Benefits of PABD not included in this estimate include peace of mind for the patient, avoidance of most acute transfusion reactions, delayed hemolytic reactions, alloimmunization, immunosuppression, and other transfusion-transmitted diseases for which donors are not yet tested (43).

Decrease in the cost of PABD can be achieved by streamlining the donation process and by judicious selection of appropriate candidates. Nurses can assist in streamlining the process by guiding patients through their institutions' procedures and by helping to reduce costly clerical errors in donation, storage, and transfusion. Unnecessary donations may be avoided by informed discussions between patients and physicians. Through such judicious use, PABD will likely remain a valuable service to elective surgery patients.

5.2. Other

Similar to PABD, other autogeneic techniques are costly for procedures associated with little blood loss. A preliminary study (40) found that the cell-saver is costly and should not be used if two or more PABD units exist and the preoperative hemoglobin is above 11 g/dL for total hip replacement. Another study found postoperative salvage costly and not worthwhile when the amount of postoperative bleeding is small (44). With regard to acute normovolemic hemodilution, one study found the procedure a cost-effective alternative to PABD by patients undergoing radical retropubic prostatectomy (45). Directed donations also involve more complex logistics and thus higher cost.

Cost is a major issue to hospitals and blood centers in the era of managed care. Without a doubt, autogeneic and directed-donor blood is more costly than volunteer allogeneic blood. In some situations, the use of this blood does not meet the general expectations for cost-effective medical therapies. These extra costs will be carefully scrutinized in the next decade.

ACKNOWLEDGMENTS

I thank Helen Oless and Daniel Tatum for help in the preparation of the manuscript. This work was supported in part by Public Service Awards R03 HL50282 and R01 HL36715 from the National Heart, Lung and Blood Institute, National Institutes of Health.

REFERENCES

1. Sloand EM, Pitt E, Klein HG. Safety of the blood supply. *JAMA* 1995;274:1368–1373.
2. Transfusion alert: Use of autologous blood. NIH Expert Autologous Transfusion. *Transfusion* 1995;35:703–711.
3. Silvergleid NJ. Autologous and designated donor programs. In: Petz LD, Swisher SN, Kleinman S, Spence RK, Strauss RG, eds. *Clinical Practice of Transfusion Medicine,* 3rd ed. New York: Churchill Livingstone, 1996, p. 287.
4. Wallace EL, Churchill WH, Surgenor DM, et al. Collection and transfusion of blood and blood components in the United States, 1992. *Transfusion* 1995;35:802–812.
5. American Association of Blood Banks. *Standards for Blood Banks and Transfusion Services,* 17th ed. Bethesda, MD: 1996.
6. Toy PT, Strauss RG, Stehling LC, et al. Predeposited autologous blood for elective surgery. *N Engl J Med* 1987;316:517–520.
7. Friedman BA. An analysis of surgical blood use in United States hospitals with application to the maximum surgical blood order schedule. *Transfusion* 1979;19:268–278.
8. Axelrod FB, Pepkowitz SH, Goldfinger D. Establishment of schedule of optimal preoperative collection of autologous blood. *Transfusion* 1989;29:677–680.
9. Britton LW, Eastlund DT, Dziuban SW, et al. Predonated autologous blood use in elective cardiac surgery. *Ann Thorac Surg* 1989;47:529–532.
10. Dzik WH, Fleisher AG, Ciavarella D, Karlson KJ, Reed GE, Berger RL. Safety and efficacy of autologous blood donation before elective aortic valve operation. *Ann Thorac Surg* 1992;54:1177–1180.
11. Love TR, Hendren WG, O'Keefe DD, Daggett WM. Transfusion of predonated autologous blood in elective cardiac surgery. *Ann Thorac Surg* 1987;43:508–512.
12. Owings DV, Kruskall MS, Thurer RL, Donovan LM. Autologous donations prior to elective cardiac surgery. Safety and effect on subsequent blood use. *JAMA* 1989;262: 1963–1968.
13. Spiess BD, Sassetti R, McCarthy RJ, Narbone RF, Tuman KJ, Ivankovich AD. Autologous blood donation: hemodynamics in a high-risk patient population. *Transfusion* 1992;32:17–22.
14. Pindyck J, Avorn J, Kuriyan M, Reed M, Iqbal MJ, Levine SJ. donation by the elderly. Clinical and policy considerations. *JAMA* 1987;257:1186–1188.
15. Tasaki T. Ohto H, Noguchi M, Abe R, Kikuchi S. Hoshino S. Autologous blood donation elective surgery in children. *Vox Sanguinis* 1994;66:188–193.
16. Droste S, Sorensen T, Price T, et al. Maternal and fetal hemodynamic effects of autologous blood donation during pregnancy. *Am J Obstet Gynecol* 1992;167:89–93.
17. Kruskall MS, Leonard SS, Klapholz H. Autologous blood donation during pregnancy. Analysis of safety and blood use. *Obstet Gynecol* 1987;70:939–941.
18. McVay PA, Hoag RW, Hoag MS, Toy PT. Safety and use of autologous blood donation during the third trimester of pregnancy. *Am J Obstet Gynecol* 1989;160:1479–1486.

19. Combs CA, Murphy EL, Laros RK, Jr. Cost-benefit analysis of autologous blood donation in obstetrics. *Obstet Gynecol* 1992;80:621–625.

20. McVay PA, Andrews A, Hoag MS, et al. Moderate and severe reactions during autologous blood donations are no more frequent than during homologous blood donations. *Vox Sanguinis* 1990;59:70–72.

21. Popovsky MA, Whitaker B, Arnold NL. Severe outcomes of allogeneic and autologous blood donation: frequency and characterization. *Transfusion* 1995;35:734–737.

22. Anonymous Autologous Survey Report. American Association of Banks. Associated Bulletin 95-4. AABB Newsbriefs, May 1995, p. 8.

23. Shulman IA. 1992. CAP Surveys, Set J-C. Comprehensive Transfusion Medicine Survey, College of American Pathologists.

24. Linden JV, Paul B, Dressler KP. A report of 104 transfusion errors in New York State. *Transfusion* 1992;32:601–606.

25. Kruskall MS, Glazer EE, Leonard SS, et al. Utilization and effectiveness of a hospital autologous preoperative blood donor program. *Transfusion* 1986;26:335–340.

26. Renner SW, Howanitz PJ, Bachner P. Preoperative autologous donation in 612 hospitals: a College of American Pathologists' Q-probes study of quality issues in transfusion practice. *Arch Pathol Lab Med* 1992;116:613–619.

27. DelRossi AJ, Cernaianu AC, Vertrees RA, et al. Platelet-plasma reduces postoperative blood loss after cardiopulmonary bypass. *J Thorac Cardiovasc Surg* 1990; 100:281–286.

28. Ferraris VA, Berry WR, Klingman RR. Comparison of blood reinfusion techniques used during coronary artery bypass grafting. *Ann Thorac Surg* 1993;56:433–439.

29. Jones JW, McCoy TA, Rawitscher RE, Lindsley DA. Effects of intraoperative plasmapheresis on blood loss in cardiac surgery. *Ann Thorac Surg* 1990;49:585–590.

30. Ereth MH, Oliver WC Jr, Beynen FM, et al. Autologous platelet-rich plasma does not reduce transfusion of homologous blood products in patients undergoing repeat valvular surgery. *Anesthesiology* 1993;79:540–547.

31. Tobe CE, Vocelka C, Sepulvada R, et al. Infusion of autologous platelet-rich plasma does not reduce blood loss and product use after coronary artery bypass. *J Thorac Cardiovasc Surg* 1993;105:1007–1013.

32. Wong CA, Franklin ML, Wade LD. Coagulation tests, blood transfusion requirements in platelet-rich plasmapheresed versus nonpheresed cardiac surgery patients. *Anesth Analg* 1994;78:29–36.

33. Markham A, Bryson HM. Epoetin Alfa. A review of its pharmacodynamic and pharmacokinetic properties and therapeutic use in nonrenal applications. *Drugs* 1995;49: 232–254.

34. Mercuriali F, Zanella A, Barosi G, et al. Use of erythropoietin to increase the volume of autologous blood donated by orthopedic patients. *Transfusion* 1993;33:55–60.

35. Goodnough LT, Price TH, Friedman KD, et al. A phase III recombinant human erythropoietin therapy in nonanemic orthopedic patients subjected to aggressive removal of blood for autologous use: dose, response, toxicity, and efficacy. *Transfusion* 1994;34:66.

36. Umlas J, Foster RR, Dalal SA, O'Leary SM, Garcia L, Kruskall MS. Red cell loss following orthopedic surgery: the case against postoperative blood salvage. *Transfusion* 994;34:402–406.

37. Clements DH, Sculco TP, Burke SW, Mayer K, Levine DB. Salvage and reinfusion of postoperative sanguineous wound drainage. *J Bone Joint Surg* 1992;74:646–651.

38. Heddle NM, Brox WT, Klama LN, Dickson LL, Levine MN. randomised trial on the efficacy of an autologous blood draininage and tranfusion device in patients undergoing elective knee arthroplasty. *Transfusion* 1992;32:742–746.

39. Woda R, Tetzlaff JE. Upper airway oedema following autologous blood transfusion from a wound drainage system. *Can J Anaesth* 1992;39:290–292.

40. Weiskopf RB. Mathematical analysis of isovolemic hemodilution indicates that it can decrease the need for allogeneic blood transfusion. *Transfusion* 1995;35:37–41.

41. Etchason J, Petz L, Keeler E, et al. The cost effectiveness preoperative autologous blood donations. *N Engl J Med* 1995;332:719–723.

42. Wagner FF, Flegel WA. Transfusion-associated graft-versus disease: risk due to homozygous HLA haplotypes. *Transfusion* 1995;35:284–291.

43. Rutherford CJ, Kaplan HS. Autologous blood donation—Can we bank on it? *N Engl J Med* 1995;332:740–742.

44. Sizemore JC, Sammons TD. Criteria for use of intra-operative cell salvage on orthopaedic cases. *Transfusion* 1995;355:A31.

45. Monk TG, Goodnough LT, Birkmeyer JD, Brecher ME, Catalona WJ. Acute normovolemic hemodilution is a cost-effective alternative to preoperative autologous blood donation by patients undergoing radical retropubic prostatectomy. *Transfusion* 1995;35:559–565.

11

Triggers for the Transfusion of Red Cells

William C. Sherwood

1. INTRODUCTION

Although the transfusion of human blood dates back at least 200 years, our current understanding of indications for the transfusion of blood products have been been shaped only during the past decade. Curiously, a driving force in the molding of these practices has been the perceived risks of transfusion transmissible diseases, most particularly the transmission of HIV *(1)*. The concern for these risks has imposed a conservatism in the transfusion of red cells that has probed the bottom limits of true physiologic need for red cell mass in a number of clinical circumstances *(2–6)*.

In 1980, before concerns about HIV, Friedman *(7)*, in analyzing transfusion practice in surgical patients coined the term "transfusion trigger." He questioned the indications for red cell transfusion, as determined by hemoglobin concentrations that were the same for women as for men, although women normally maintain lower hemoglobin levels than men.

Friedman is not the first to raise such questions. Rawstron *(8)*, in an exhaustive search of the literature, chronicled the practice of evaluating hemoglobin concentrations prior to surgery. He noted that in 1890 Miculicz first made a recommendation that hemoglobin content should be at least 30% of normal (4.5 g/dL) before undertaking general surgery. With regard to the risks of blood transfusion, this low level was, perhaps, a harbinger to the current conservative practice since the ABO blood groups would not be described for another 10 years!

Following 1900, the recommendations by experts of the day for minimum presurgical hemoglobin concentration gradually increased. By 1960, Davis *(9)*, in a popular surgical text, recommended a minimum preanesthetic hemoglobin of 70% of normal (10 g/dL). This advice was followed until the current wave of conservatism emerged in the mid 1980s. Usually these recommendations were made arbitrarily or with only anecdotal experience. However, even in earlier years, such recommendations were often accompanied with the caution that the decision for red cell transfusion should not be based on hemoglobin levels alone, but should consider the clinical circumstances of the patient.

To some, the term "transfusion trigger" connotes an exactness that calls for precise formulas to be used in the decision to tranfuse red cells. However, this is not

From: *Red Cell Transfusion: A Practical Guide*
Edited by: M. E. Reid and S. J. Nance Humana Press Inc., Totowa, NJ

the case when observing the similarities between the "triggers" associated with the decision to transfuse blood and the trigger in hunting or marksmanship. When comparing the two:

1. Triggers and their fingers are different.
2. The weapons and ammunition vary.
3. The targets are diverse and frequently moving.

Even with today's knowledge and techniques there is no uniform formula to be used in the decision to transfuse red cells. There are, however, an array of clinical and laboratory guidelines that assist the physician in the decision to pull, or not pull, the transfusion trigger. In addition, there is a growing wealth of clinical and surgical experience on this subject.

As a fundamental rule, the maintenance of adequate oxygen delivery is the goal of red cell transfusions. Before proceeding, it is useful to review briefly the physiology of oxygen transport, tissue oxygenation, and the compensatory mechanisms that come into play during disease states in order to provide a greater understanding of the various indications for red cell transfusions.

2. OXYGEN DYNAMICS

Although there a number of important functions for the red cell, such as the transport of CO_2 or acid–base buffering, oxygen transport from the lungs to the tissues is the primary function. In this capacity, the red cell is a critical player in the chain of events of oxygen delivery. When there is a deficiency of red cells, a deficiency in oxygen delivery may occur.

2.1. Oxygen Delivery

Oxygen delivery (Do_2, mL/kg/min) is a term that describes the end result of a series of functions and overlapping circumstances that transport oxygen to the tissues. In simple organisms in which the ambient air or water is nearby the tissue cells, oxygen transport systems may be simple or unnecessary. However, the process becomes more complex as the complexity of the organism increases. In the human, these functions begin with the ventilation process of the lungs and end with the dissociation of oxygen from hemoglobin at the capillary endothelium and presentation to the cell wall by the interstitial fluid (*see* Fig. 1).

During stress and disease states, in order to maintain the status quo, there is the ability for considerable compensation by one function of the oxygen delivery chain to overcome deficiencies of another. Overall, the process is dynamic and compensatory adaptations are the rule. As an example, in order to maintain adequate oxygen delivery a fall in hemoglobin level may be accompanied by:

1. Increased ventilation.
   a. Rate and depth of respirations.
2. Increased blood flow.
   a. Increased cardiac output.
      i. Increased stroke volume.
      ii. Increased heart rate.
   b. Decreased peripheral vascular resistance.

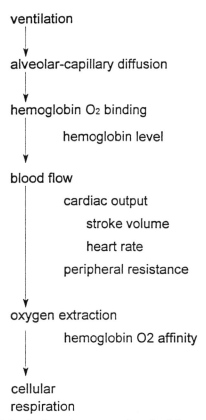

ventilation

alveolar-capillary diffusion

hemoglobin O₂ binding

    hemoglobin level

blood flow

    cardiac output

       stroke volume

       heart rate

    peripheral resistance

oxygen extraction

    hemoglobin O2 affinity

cellular
respiration

Fig. 1. Physiologic functions associated with oxygen delivery.

3. Increased oxygen extraction.
   a. Decreased hemoglobin oxygen affinity.

Many of the compensatory mechanisms take time to develop to their full efficiency. If the hemoglobin concentration falls slowly, over days or weeks, these compensatory mechanisms are allowed time to completely develop. The patient may not recognize a developing anemia until it becomes severe. However, an acute fall in hemoglobin does not allow time for compensatory mechanisms to become fully effective. Under these circumstances, oxygen delivery is less and tissue anoxia may occur at hemoglobin levels that would not invoke such effects if compensatory mechanisms were fully developed.

2.2. Oxygen Extraction and Consumption

Oxygen consumption (Vo_2, mL/kg/min) is the processes of utilization of oxygen by the cell in its aerobic glycolytic process. The end result is the production of high-energy phosphate bonds, CO_2 and water. Oxygen consumption is greatest for highly active cells such as muscle cells and the brain. With oxygen deprivation, some active cells may continue energy production temporarily using an anaerobic glycolytic pathway. However, an oxygen "debt" develops. Energy production is less efficient and glycolysis is not complete. There is a build up of lactic acid leading toward acidosis. This worsening condition can only be corrected by the restoration of adequate oxygen delivery.

The oxygen extraction ratio (ER = Vo_2/Do_2) is that fraction of the oxygen delivered that becomes consumed by tissue cells. Under normal and resting circumstances, more than ample oxygen is supplied. The tissues will extract only 20–25% of the oxygen delivered. If oxygen consumption increases without a compensatory increase in oxygen delivery, the oxygen extraction ratio increases. As a corollary, the ratio also increases if oxygen delivery falls without a proportionate fall in oxygen consumption. Any weakness in the oxygen delivery sequence, without adequate compensatory changes, can cause a fall in oxygen delivery. Low hemoglobin concentration is a convenient example.

When available, the oxygen extraction ratio is used as a guide to the adequacy of tissue oxygenation since it takes into account both oxygen delivery and consumption. An extraction ratio >50% indicates there is a sufficient imbalance between oxygen delivery and consumption to signify tissue anoxia. At such levels, oxygen consumption becomes linearly dependent on oxygen delivery. Lactic acidosis has occurred or is not far behind. Falling oxygen extraction ratios often indicate improved oxygen delivery and pay back of oxygen debt.

Of importance, in the otherwise normal and resting subject, with full compensatory mechanisms employed, the hemoglobin level must fall to very low levels (<5.0 g/dL) before oxygen delivery and the oxygen extraction ratio will signal serious concern *(2,10–12)*. As is discussed, this phenomenon appears to be an important clinical finding as well.

2.3. Drawbacks of the Measurements of Oxygen Dynamics

These measurements of oxygen dynamics have certain disadvantages and weaknesses.

1. A simple and readily available clinical tool for the measurement of oxygen delivery and consumption does not exist. The most informative techniques are invasive and may require the use of the balloon-tipped, flow-directed, pulmonary arterial (PA) catheter. Using oxygen dynamics and cardiac index results from PA techniques, Shoemaker et al. *(13)*, developed effective therapeutic goals to monitor the high-risk patient. However, most patients that require red cell transfusions are not sufficiently high-risk to warrant such invasive supervision, and there are no practical methods to assess oxygen delivery in these patients.

   An exception are the techniques in use for measuring oxygen consumption in the newborn. The small size allows biocontainment of the infant using sealed hoods, in-line ventilators, and flow-through circuit pumps. Oxygen consumption can be continually monitored.

2. These techniques measure oxygen dynamics at a "global" level. The results depict an average of all body tissues and only indirect information about specific organs such as the heart, brain, or kidneys. There is some evidence in animal studies that the oxygen extraction ratio is a valid indicator of myocardial metabolism, but information in humans is lacking *(12,14)*. With global information, the status of organs or tissues that experience isolated blood flow restrictions will not be known. In the young patient in whom the absence of vascular disease is assumed, global data is useful. In the older patient in whom the presence of vascular disease is evident or likely, such data may be misleading.

   Some have attempted to overcome the drawbacks of global measurements by using techniques to monitor the oxygen delivery and consumption of specific organs. Lindahl

(15) suggested "on-line vector cardiography" to monitor myocardial oxygenation in the critically ill patient.

A novel and noninvasive technique, is the use of near-infrared spectrophotometry (NIRS) described by Jobsis in 1977 *(16)*, to measure cerebral oxygenation. The technique was reintroduced recently by Nollert *(17)* to monitor cerebral oxygenation during cardiac bypass surgery. Small devices that transmit and receive light (optodes) are placed on the scalp or other tissue. An emitted laser wave of 770–910 nm is able to penetrate and become dispersed in tissue such as the brain. Light of specific wavelengths is absorbed by the chromophores of the tissue: oxygenated and deoxygenated hemoglobin and oxygenated cytochrome a,a,3, the final enzyme in the cell respiratory pathway. By measuring the reflected light, these chromophores can be quantitated.

3. As a final drawback, the available measurements of oxygen dynamics do not reflect reserve capacity for oxygen delivery. They indicate the current status of the patient, but do not measure reserves or project subsequent events. As a result, attempts to correct or improve the oxygen delivery pathway such as red cell transfusion often take the safest approach and assume that capacity is running out.

Despite the drawbacks of these measurements of oxygen delivery, the aforementioned methods are useful under varied circumstances. However, even these are not used for many patients that receive red cell transfusions. As stated earlier, no single method of arterial oxygen tension or saturation can describe the complex oxygenation system in terms that are most useful to the clinician *(17)*. The desirable transfusion trigger of the future will be associated with simple and practical methods that will provide information on oxygen delivery, consumption, and reserve, for critical organs as well as globally.

3. THE HEMOGLOBIN OR HEMATOCRIT AS INDICATORS OF OXYGEN DELIVERY

A number of investigators have noted that hemoglobin or hematocrit measurements are less than satisfactory determinants of oxygen delivery *(6,10,14,15, 18–22)*. The hemoglobin concentration must fall to very low levels before global oxygen dynamics are affected. With falling hemoglobin levels, the status of critical organs usually remains unknown, and some compensatory changes cannot be predicted or easily measured. These features appear to be particularly true in the critically ill patient with unstable cardiovascular dynamics, when fluid shifts are rapidly occurring, and during metabolic derangements such as renal failure and sepsis. However, active blood loss is directly reflected by the hemoglobin or hematocrit when time allows for volume reconstitution *(23,24)*.

For most patients requiring red cell transfusions, the hemoglobin or hematocrit is one of the simple and readily available objective measures of the oxygen delivery system. But such measurements must be coupled with the clinical circumstances of each patient when used in the decision to transfuse red cells. The physician formulates the hemoglobin or hematocrit measurement with cardiovascular status, fluid balance, pulmonary factors, medications, age, and other associated diseases *(18)*. He or she then balances the benefits against the risks in order to decide whether or not to transfuse red cells *(25)*.

The clinical circumstances among patients are highly variable and rigid criteria for the use of hemoglobin or hematocrit values as indicators for the transfusion of red cells is not appropriate. One reason for the variation of the use of red cells among institutions *(26,27)* is the differing clinical requirements of patients. Attempts have been made to assess the appropriateness of red cell transfusions by matching against preset criteria, which include hemoglobin or hematocrit and clinical circumstances. During such an evaluation, Renner *(28)* found only 2% of red cell transfusions unjustified. However, using more strict criteria, Mozes *(29)* found 40% inappropriate. Although there appears to be considerable room for improvement, these variations in red cell usage are likely to continue until simple, noninvasive methods are available to measureuseful oxygen dynamics.

4. PROBES FOR THE MINIMUM ACCEPTABLE HEMOGLOBIN AND OXYGEN DELIVERY IN HUMANS

There are a number of animal studies intended to determine the physiologic parameters of oxygen dynamics and outcomes at low hemoglobin levels. This information, coupled with a wide array of studies in humans, have pushed the minimum acceptable levels of hemoglobin and of oxygen delivery continually downward for many patients. These explorations have been patient driven, such as those that refuse blood transfusion for religious reasons, at the risk of death; as well as physician driven, when considering risk:benefit ratios. These clinical probes that test the lower limits of oxygen delivery are made possible by newer measurement techniques that, as noted in Section 2., are able to continually monitor oxygen delivery and consumption in the critically ill patients *(2,3,6,11,13,17,30,31)*.

4.1. Patients Who Refuse Blood Transfusions

There are both anecdotal reports and well-designed analyses of the clinical course and outcome of critically ill patients who refuse blood transfusions, usually for religious reasons. These reports cover a wide variety of circumstances and include: organ transplants, cardiac bypass surgery, extensive trauma, neurosurgery, gynecologic and obstetric surgery, vascular surgery, joint replacement, sickle cell anemia, and leukemia. As expected from anecdotal reports, outcomes were usually favorable although hemoglobin levels and, presumably, oxygen delivery dipped to extremely low levels.

The analyses of a small number of patient series provide more meaningful information. Spence *(6,32)* and Carson *(18)* reported on a series of patients who refused blood transfusion and underwent a variety of surgical procedures, both elective and emergency. Oxygen dynamics were measured for many of these patients during critical phases. From this series, Spence *(6)* applied a statistical approach to determine predictors of survival of the event. He noted that hemoglobin concentration alone was a poor predictor of survival until the level dipped to 3.0 g/dL and below. However, prediction of survival was much improved if the nadir of hemoglobin concentration was coupled with the oxygen extraction ratio. The mortality rate for patients with hemoglobin values in this range was doubled if the oxygen extraction ratios were > 50%. For these patients, the probability of survival was < 1%.

From this series, Spence also noted that an isolated predictor of survival was sepsis *(32)*. Although the presence of sepsis would be expected to be an important predictor of survival in most patients, the occurrence of sepsis in the anemic patient offers particular concern, as is discussed later in this chapter. A surprising result of this analysis is that no other associated diseases or parameters had a significant effect on outcome. This includes age and cardiovascular status.

4.2. Circumstances in Which Blood is not Available

There are many reports of outcomes of severe anemic and/or bleeding circumstances in which transfusions would have been given had reasonably safe red cells been available. Many of these are evaluations conducted in developing countries and measurements of oxygen dynamic are not available *(5,33,34)*.

An informative study by Lackritz et al. *(4)* evaluated anemia and the results of transfusion in children under the age of 12 admitted to a Kenyan hospital in 1989. In this setting, red cells for transfusion were either scarce or carried an unacceptable risk for HIV transmission except for desperate circumstances. Twenty-nine percent of children admitted had hemoglobin concentrations <5.0 .0 g/dL. Generally, children did not receive transfusions at hemoglobin values above this level. Lackritz observed that transfusions administered to children with hemoglobin concentrations from 5.0–3.9 g/dL did not serve to improve survival unless the patients also exhibited respiratory distress (intercostal retractions, forced expiration, or nasal flaring). However, when hemoglobin concentrations were 3.9 g/dL and below, transfusions improved the probability of survival even in the absence of respiratory symptoms.

The above study in children, as well as the analyses of Spence and Carson, compared their measurements with survival. Unfortunately, there are no such analyses comparing the results of transfusion in such patients with other morbid features and complications or long-term growth and development. In children and infants, the effects of chronic anemia and associated impairment on growth and development are well known *(35)*. However, except for the premature infant, the long-term results of transitory anemia and correction by transfusion have not been well studied.

4.3. Physician-Induced Hemodilution

An additional probe at the nadir of hemoglobin levels and of oxygen delivery is the experience with preoperative hemodilution *(2,3,31,36,37)*. Such procedures are intended to reduce or eliminate the need for allogeneic red cell transfusions by making maximum economy of the patient's own red cell mass. Blood is removed from the patient during the early anesthetic period and replaced with crystalline and colloid solutions, allowing hemoglobin concentrations to reduce to low levels. Any blood lost during surgery is of a reduced hemoglobin concentration and is replaced with the previously collected autogeneic blood. The great advantage of this process is that the patient can be monitored and well controlled. Impending problems in oxygen delivery may be interrupted by the return of autogeneic red cells.

Fontana et al. *(2)* provided the deepest probe by performing preoperative hemodilution on eight children undergoing surgery for scoliosis. During hemodilution hemoglobin, concentrations fell to an average 3.0 ± 0.8 g/dL! Throughout the procedure, the patients received controlled ventilation with 100% oxygen. Although the average oxygen delivery fell to one-half the starting value, the average oxygen extraction ratio rose only to 44% and plasma lactate did not increase. There were no adverse clinical outcomes. Of interest, the majority of oxygen delivered during these procedures was dissolved in plasma rather than carried by hemoglobin.

Table 1
Sample Guideline for the Transfusion of Red Blood Cells [a]

Symptomatic anemia in a normovolemic patient, regardless of hemoglobin level.
Acute blood loss equal to, or greater than, 15% of estimated blood volume.
Acute blood loss with evidence of inadequate oxygen delivery.
Preoperative hemoglobin equal to, or less than, 8.0 g/dL and operative procedure
    associated with major blood loss.
Hemoglobin equal to, or less than, 9.0 g/dL in a patient on a chronic transfusion
    regimen.
Additional considerations:
Criteria for symptomatic anemia may be defined locally and can include categories of
    patients considered at greater risk on the basis of age and/or cardiac or
    pulmonary disease.
The guidelines for the use of autogeneic and allogeneic blood may be the same, or
    those for autogeneic blood may be more lenient.
Transfusion of a single unit may be appropriate.

---

[a] From ref. *43* with permission.

Such profound degree of hemodilution is not without controversy. Lindahl *(15)* criticized this approach, noting that suitable monitoring techniques for vital organs are not yet available and that current monitoring methods provide only late warning signs. He advised that the remaining reserve is too thin to perform such procedures with consistent safety.

5. INDICATIONS FOR RED CELL TRANSFUSIONS

5.1. General Practices

Since the beginning of our century *(8)*, the transfusion of red cells in preparation for surgery has received considerable attention. The recommendations of an NIH consensus conference *(38)* published in 1988 provide a basic guideline for surgical blood use. This consensus panel noted there is no single criterion, such as hemoglobin concentration, that should serve as the basis for transfusion decisions and that clinical judgement should play the major role. However, the panel "bracketed the target" by declaring that uncomplicated patients with hemoglobin concentrations of 10.0 g/dL or more rarely require preoperative transfusions, whereas those with 7.0 g/dL or less frequently will require red cell transfusions. These recommendations, along with others in the literature *(28,29,39,40)* that are more comprehensive, are used by hospitals to establish criteria for transfusion practice. These, in turn, are used in the transfusion utilization review process required by the Joint Commission on Accreditation of Healthcare Organizations *(41,42)*.

There is the general belief that the utilization review process has had an educational effect in transfusion medicine. Often, the utilization review guidelines have become standards of transfusion practice within an institution. Table 1 provides broad recommendations for utilization review of red cell transfusions that were developed by the American Association of Blood Banks (AABB) Transfusion Practices Quality Assurance Committee *(43)*. Although these guidelines seem "hemoglobin-based," clinical circumstances and physician judgement are over-riding requirements. The AABB

Table 2
Audit Criteria for Pediatric Red Cell Transfusions[a]

Whole blood
    Massive or acute blood loss (>1 blood volume in <24 h).
    Exchange transfusion.
    Cardiovascular bypass surgery.
    Extracorporeal membrane oxygenation (ECMO).
Red cells
    Neonatal infants <4 mo old:
        Venous hemoglobin level <130 g/L in neonatal infants <24 h old.
        Hemoglobin level <130 gIL and *severe pulmonary disease,* cyanotic heart disease,
            or heart failure.
        Acute blood loss >10% of the total blood volume.
        Phlebotomy losses >5–10% of the total blood volume.
        Hemoglobin level <80 g/L in stable newborn infants *with clinical manifestations*
            of anemia.
    Patients 4 mo of age or older:
        Significant preoperative anemia; intraoperative blood loss >15% of total blood
            volume; postoperative hemoglobin level <80 g/L, *and symptoms or signs*
            of anemia.
        Acute blood loss with hypovolemia unresponsive to crystalloid or colloid.
        Hemoglobin level <130 g/L in patients with *severe pulmonary disease* requiring
            assisted ventilation.
        Chronic congenital or acquired anemia without an expected satisfactory response
            to medical therapy and a hemoglobin level <80 g/L, or a hemoglobin level
            <100 g/L *with symptoms anchor signs of anemia.*
        Chronic transfusions to suppress endogenous hemoglobin production in *selected*
            patients with sickle cell or thalassemia syndromes.
        Induction of immune tolerance before renal transplantation.

[a]From ref. *39* with permission.

Pediatric Hemotherapy Committee has developed similar guidelines for transfusion utilization review for infants and children *(39)*. The red cell transfusion portion of these guidelines is reproduced in Table 2.

    Although the current wave of conservatism in transfusion practice was motivated by transfusion safety concerns, an additional thrust to this momentum is now "cost" *(44)*. With continued improvement in blood transfusion safety, cost control pressure is likely to continue the push for conservative transfusion practices well into the future.

5.2. Special Circumstances

5.2.1. Autogeneic Red Cells

    There is a sharp controversy on the indications for the transfusion of autogeneic red cells after they are collected and made available to the patient *(24,25)*. The central question is: "Should the utilization review criteria be more liberal for the transfusion of autogeneic red cells (i.e., higher hematocrit or hemoglobin level) than for allogeneic red cells?" The proponents of this practice indicate that since there is greater transfusion safety from autogeneic red cell units, as compared to allogenic units, the risk:benefit ratio is changed *(24)*. Miller *(24)* noted that, in the patient with coronary artery disease, myocardial ischemia, and myocardial infarction are less likely to occur intraoperatively than on the third hospital day *(45)*. He maintained the autogeneic donor-patient should have the benefit of the higher oxygen delivery reserve with which to respond to intra- and postoperative complications.

Those against this practice *(25)* contend that the scientific evidence is not available to justify such differences in transfusion criteria. Gould *(25)* maintained that, currently, there is no documentation of increased patient benefits in terms of mortality, length of hospital stay, rehabilitation, return to work, or cost. Two independent studies, evaluating transfusion practices for total knee and hip arthroplasties, determined that length of hospital stay was independent of patient hemoglobin *(46,47)*. They conclude that, as a result, the transfusion of autogeneic or allogeneic red cells to achieve an increase in hemoglobin level, solely for shortening hospital stay, is unwarranted.

5.2.2. Pregnancy

There appears to be little support for variation in utilization review guidelines for the woman during pregnancy. The infant *in utero* has an anormous capacity to "parasitize" oxygen from the mother. In addition, there are two somewhat independent compensatory systems at hand. The mother's system can increase placental blood flow during anemia. The fetus, in addition to the ability to increase placental blood flow, can produce very high hemoglobin levels even though the mother may be severely anemic *(48)*. The oxygen dissociation curve for fetal hemoglobin is left-shifted indicating a greater tenacity for oxygen than maternal adult hemoglobin. However, the gradient across the placenta resulting from the difference in oxygen affinity between hemoglobins does not appear essential for oxygen transport to the fetus *(49)*.

Although the fetus can withstand maternal anemia quite well, as evidenced by the usual favorable outcome of pregnancies in woman who experience chronic anemia *(50)*, fetal distress creates a circumstance that falls outside of transfusion utilization review guidelines. In such patients some correction of maternal anemia is often recommended *(48,51)*.

Additionally, there are exceptions to transfusion utilization review guidelines for patients with sickle disease under selected circumstances. Such patients may be managed by red cell transfusion or exchange programs intended to reduce the concentration of hemoglobin S. During pregnancy the threat of acute vascular accidents are a serious concern for women with sickle cell disease. Often, such patients are managed aggressively with red cell transfusions during the second and third trimesters in order to surpress their own red cell production *(50–52)*. This practice may require sustained hemoglobin concentrations as high as 10 g/dL. When transfusing the woman with infant *in utero,* consider that the fetus is exposed to the same transfusion transmissible disease risks as the mother.

5.2.3. Radiation Therapy

Reduced oxygen delivery to tumor cells can impair radiation-induced tumor regression by as much as one-third *(53)*. Tumors may have large areas of poor blood supply and reduced gas diffusion. Under these conditions, relative hypoxia of tumor cells is common. Efforts to overcome this restriction include such maneuvers as: breathing high oxygen concentrations, hyperbaric oxygen chambers, and radio-sensitizing drugs such as nitroimiidazoles that are electron affinity sensitizers of DNA, similar to oxygen.

The radiation-induced cure rate for carcinoma of the cervix is significantly impaired by anemia, an affect which is improved if the anemia is corrected by red cell transfusion *(54)*. Some have proposed aggressive correction of anemia in the radiation therapy patient, using red cell transfusions if necessary *(55)*. However, Hunt *(56)* suggested caution with this approach, noting that tumor hypoxia is usually a result of poor perfusion, an effect which usually cannot be improved by increasing the hematocrit.

5.2.4. Bacterial Sepsis

During the course of bacterial sepsis, oxygen consumption may be severely decreased. Usually, efforts are made to improve oxygen delivery and aggressively correct any anemia that exists. However, the causes of tissue hypoxia are frequently at tissue and cellular levels rather than a failure of oxygen delivery *(21)*. In addition to direct injuries to the cellular respiratory process, sepsis can result in endothelial damage, loss of microvascular regulation, edema, and impaired oxygen diffusion to the cell. Because of these effects, lactic acidosis, a common feature of bacterial sepsis, may not be relieved by improving oxygen delivery with red cell transfusion *(21,57)*.

Importantly, these effects at a tissue level are inconsistent phenomena and there are no clear methods to determine which patients will exhibit improvement of tissue oxygenation with improvement of oxygen delivery. But, sepsis submits the patient to a serious threat *(6)* and aggressive treatment is the rule.

5.2.5. End-Stage Renal Disease

Patients with end-stage renal disease present a particular paradox for improving oxygen delivery by raising the hemoglobin concentration. Metra et al. *(58)* has showed that the at-rest cardiac index in such patients is significantly enhanced by raising the average hemoglobin concentration with erythropoietin from 6.0–9.9 g/dL. The sense of well-being and quality of life in such patients is much improved. However, Raine *(59)* cautioned against such success reminding us that such elevations in hemoglobin concentration increase blood viscosity and diastolic blood pressure in patients with renal disease *(60)*. These authors noted that one half the deaths of patients with end-stage renal disease are from myocardial infarction, congestive heart failure, or stroke; sequelae associated with hypertension.

So far these cautions by Raine and the similar initial concerns of raising the hemoglobin concentration with erythropoietin in the end-stage renal disease patient have not materialized. In practice, erythropoietin is used to its maximum benefit. In patients refractory to erythropoietin, particularly while being supported by hemodialysis, transfusions are used to maintain hemoglobin levels in the 8.0–9.0 g/dL range.

6. SUMMARY

The maintenance of adequate oxygen delivery is the goal of red cell transfusions. For most patients that may require transfusions, the need for oxygen delivery, the reserve capacity, and the results of improvements cannot be easily measured. As a result, the decision to transfuse red cells is a formulation by the treating physician using the hemoglobin or hematocrit coupled with an array of clinical circumstances. The benefits are then balanced against the risks and a decision is made. When considering this process, it should not be surprising that there are no firmly established guidelines for transfusing red cells. The wide variation in clinical circumstances cannot be incorporated into useful guidelines.

Even when more informative data about oxygen delivery are available, they may not reflect the status of the critical organs if cardiovascular disease is present. The potential presence of coronary or cerebral vascular disease in the many patients that may need transfusions has a decided effect on the decision process.

In the absence of cardiovascular disease, the human body maintains a robust system of compensatory mechanisms that will provide for adequate oxygen delivery to the tissues with hemoglobin concentrations that may fall as low as 4.0 g/dL. However, patients frequently have many other complicating factors and red cell volumes in this low range provide no reserve.

The risk of transfusing transmissible diseases, along with other risks of transfusion therapy, have fueled a wave of conservatism in transfusion practices. These practices have come under a hospital committee review process, requiring that transfusion guidelines be established. Appropriate, or not, these guidelines are often referred to as transfusion triggers. However, they should be regarded only as guidelines. Until our technology improves, the need to pull the transfusion trigger remains a decision for the physician who must use his or her best clinical judgment.

REFERENCES

1. Dodd RY. The risk of transfusion-transfusion infection (editorial). *N Engl J Med* 1992;327:419–421.
2. Fontana JL, Welborn L, Mongan PD, Sturm P, Martin G, Bunger R. Oxygen consumption and cardiovascular function in children during profound intraoperative normovolemic hemodilution. *Anesth Anal* 1995;80:219–225
3. van Woerkens E, Trouborst A, van Lanschot J. Profound hemodilution: what is the critical level of oxygen delivery-dependent oxygen consumption in humans. *Anesth Anal* 1992;75:818–821.
4. Lackritz EM, Campbell CC, Ruebush TK, Hightower AW, Wakube A, Steketee RW, Were JBO. Effect of blood transfusion on survival among children in a Kenyan hospital. *Lancet* 1992,340:524–528.
5. Dorward JA, Knowles JK, Dorward JM. Treatment of severe anemia in children in a rural hospital. *Trop Doct* 1989;19:155–158.
6. Spence RK, Costabile JP, Young JS, Norcross ED, Alexander JB, Pello MJ, Atabek UM, Camishon RC. Is hemoglobin level alone a reliable predictor of outcome in the severely anemic surgical patient? *Am Surg* 1992;58:92–95.
7. Friedman BA, Burns TL, Schork MA. The analysis of blood transfusion of surgical patients by sex: A quest for a transfusion trigger. *Transfusion* 1980;20:179–188.
8. Rawstron RE. Preoperative hemoglobin levels. *Anaes Intens Care* 1976;4:175–185
9. Davis HS. In: *Complications in Surgery and Their Management.* Philadelphia: Saunders. 1960, pp. 314.
10. Shoemaker WC, Ayers S, Holbrook P, Thompson W. *Textbook of Critical Care.* Philadelphia: Saunders, 1989.

11. Bland RD, Shoemaker WC, Shabot MM. Physiologic monitoring goals for the critically ill patient. *Surg Gyn Obst* 1978;1407:833–841.
12. Levy PS, Chavez RP, Crystal GJ. Oxygen extraction ratio: a valid indicator of transfusion need in limited coronary vascular reserve. *J Trauma* 1992;32;769–773.
13. Shoemaker WC, Appel PL, Kram HB, Waxman K, Lee T-S. Prospective trial of supranormal values of survivors as therapeutic goals in high-risk surgical patients. *Chest* 1988;94:1176–1186.
14. Wilkerson DK, Rosen AL, Gould MD, Sehgal LR, Sehgal HL, Moss GS. Oxygen extraction ratio: a valid indicator of myocardial metabolism in anemia. *J Surg Res* 1987;42:629–634
15. Lindahl SGE. Thinner than blood (editorial). *Anesth Anal* 1995;80:217–218
16. Jobsis FF. Non-invasive infrared monitoring of cerebral and myocardial oxygen sufficiency and circulatory parameters. *Science* 1977;198:1264–1267.
17. Nollert G, Mohnle P, Tassani-Prell P, Reichart B. Determinants of cerebral oxygenation during cardiac surgery. *Circulation* 1995;92(9 Suppl):327–333.
18. Carson JL, Willett LR. Is a hemoglobin of 10 g/dL required for surgery? *Med Clin N Amer* 1993;77:335–347.
19. Bland RD, Shoemaker WC, Shabot MM. Physiologic monitoring goals for the critically ill patient. *Surg Gynecol Obstet* 1978;147:833–841.
20. Baxter BT, Minion DJ, McChance CL, Eskildsen JM, Heffele JJ, Lynch TG. Rational approach to postoperative transfusion in high risk patients. *Am J of Surg* 1993;166:720–725.
21. Steffes CP, Bender JS, Levison MA. Blood transfusion and oxygen consumption in surgical sepsis. *Crit Care Med* 1991;19:512–517.
22. Carson JL, Poses RM, Spence RK. Anemia and surgery: the relationship between the severity of anemia and surgical mortality and morbidity. *Lancet* 1988;1:727–729.
23. Czer LS, Shoemaker WC. Optimal hematocrit values in critically ill postoperative patients. *Surg Gynecol Obstet* 1978;14:363–368.
24. Miller RD, von Ehrenburg W. Controversies in transfusion medicine: indications for autologous and allogeneic transfusion should be the same: con. *Transfusion* 1995;35:450–452.
25. Gould SA, Forbes SM. Controversies in transfusion medicine: indications for autologous and alloganeic transfusion should be the same: pro. *Transfusion* 1995;35:446–449
26. Surgenor DM, Wallace EL, Churchill WH, Hao SHS, Chapman RH, Poss R. Red cell transfusions in total knee and total hip replacement surgery. *Transfusion* 1991;31:531–537.
27. Goodnough LT, Johnston MFM, Toy PTCY and the Transfusion Medicine Academic Award Group. The variability of transfusion practice in coronary artery bypass surgery. *JAMA* 1991;265:86–90.
28. Renner SW, Howanitz JH, Fishkin BG. Towards meaningful blood usage review: comprehensive monitoring of physician practice. *QRB* 1987;13:76–80.
29. Mozes B, Epstein M, Ben-Bassat I, Modan B, Halkin H. Evaluation of the appropriateness of blood and blood product transfusion using pre-set criteria. *Transfusion* 1989;29:473–546.
30. Swain JA. Cardiac surgery and the brain. *N Engl J Med* 1993;329:1119–1120.
31. Komatsu T, Shinbutani K, Okamoto K. Critical level of oxygen delivery after cardiopulmonary bypass. *Crit Care Med* 1987;15:194–197.
32. Spence RK, Carson JA, Poses R, McCoy S, Pello M, Alexander J, Popovich J, Norcross E, Camishon R. Elective surgery without transfusion: influence of preoperative hemoglobin loss on mortality. *Am J Surg* 1990;1S9:320–324.

33. Global Blood Safety Initiative. *Guidelines for the Appropriate Use of Blood:* World Health Organization, 1989.
34. Greenberg AK, Nguyen-Dinh P, Mann JM. The association between malaria, blood transfusion and HIV seropositivity in a pediatric population in Kinshasa, Zaire. *JAMA* 1988;259:545–549.
35. Skuse D, Pickles A, Wolke D, Reilly S. Postnatal growth and mental development: evidence for a sensitive period. *J Child Psychol Psychiat* 1994;35:521–545.
36. Sunder-Plassmann L, Klovekorn W, Messner K. Preoperative hemodilution. Basic adaptation mechanism and limitations of clinical application. *Anaesthetist* 1976;25: 124–130.
37. Messmer K, Kreimeier U, Intaglietta M. Present state of intentional hemodilution. *Eur Surg Res* 1986;18:254–263.
38. Perioperative red blood cell transfusion. NIH Consensus Conference. *JAMA* 1988; 260:2700–2703.
39. Strauss RG, Blanchette VS, Hume H. Levy GJ, Schloz JF, Blazina AL, Werner C, Sotelo-Avila C, Barrass C, Hines D. National acceptability of American Association of Blood Banks Pediatric Hemotherapy Committee guidelines for auditing pediatric transfusion practices. *Transfusion* 1993;33:168–171.
40. Coffin C, Matz K, Rich E. Algorithms for evaluating the appropriateness of blood transfusion. *Transfusion* 1989;29:298–303.
41. Grindon AJ, Tomasulo PS, Bergin JJ. The hospital transfusion committee. *JAMA* 1985;253:540–543.
42. Silberstein LE, Kruskall MS, Stehling LC. Strategies for the review of transfusion practices. *JAMA* 1989;262:1993–1997.
43. Stehling L, Luban NLC, Anderson KC, Sayers MH, Long A, Attar S, Leitman SF, Gould SA, Kruskall LT, Goodnough LT, Hines DM. Guidelines for blood utilization review. *Transfusion* 1994;34:438–471.
44. Etchason J. Petz L, Keeler E. The cost-effectiveness of preoperative autologous blood donations. *N Engl J Med* 1995;332:719–724.
45. Mangano DT, Browner WS, Hollenberg M. Association of perioperative myocardial ischemia with cardiac morbidity and mortality in men undergoing non-cardiac surgery. *N Engl J Med* 1990;323:1781–1788.
46. Kim DM, Brecher ME, Estes TJ, Morrey BF. Relationship of hemoglobin level and duration of hospitalization after total hip arthroplasty: implications for the transfusion target. *Mayo Clin Proc* 1993;68:37–41.
47. Goodnough LT, Verbrugge D, Vizmeg K, Riddell J. Identifying elective orthopedic surgical patients transfused with amounts of blood in excess of need: the transfusion trigger revisited. *Transfusion* 1992;32:648–653.
48. Meschia G. Supply of oxygen to the fetus. *J Reprod Med* 1979;23:160–165.
49. Carache S, Catalano P. Burns S. Jones RT, Koler RD, Rutstein R, Williams RR, Hathaway PJ. Pregnancy in carriers of high-affinity hemoglobins. *Blood* 1985;65: 713–718.
50. Milner PF, Jones BR, Dobler J. Outcome of pregnancy in sickle cell anemia: hemoglobin C disease. *Am J Obst Gynecol* 1980;138:239–243.
51. Morrison JC, Blake PG, Reed CD. Therapy for the pregnant patient with sickle cell hemoglobinopathies: A natural focus. *Am J Obgt Gynecol* 1982;144:268–269.
52. Carache S, Scott J, Niebyl J. Managament of sickle cell disease in pregnant patients. *Obstet Gynecol* 1980;55:407–111.
53. Gray LH, Conger AD, Ebert M, Hornsey S, Scott OCA. The concentration of oxygen in the tissues at the time of irradiation as a factor in radiotherapy. *Br J Radiol* 1953; 26:638–648.

54. Brown JM. Sensitizers and protectors in radiotherapy. *Cancer* 1985;55:2222–2228.

55. Mullins JD, Glatstein E. Hemoglobin, tissue hypoxia and radiation therapy. *JAMA* 1988;260:3580.

56. Hunt TK. Blood transfusion before radiation for malignancy. *JAMA* 1989;262:2234.

57. Mink RB, Murray M, Pollack M. Effect of blood transfusion on oxygen consumption in pediatric septic shock. *Crit Care Med* 1990;18:1087–1091.

58. Metra M, Cannella G, La Canna G. lmprovement in exercise capacity after anemia correction with recombinant erythropoietin in end-stage renal failure. *Am J Cardiol* 1991;68:1060–1066.

59. Raine AEG. Hypertension blood viscosity and cardiovascular morbidity in renal failure: implications of erythropoietin therapy. *Lancet* 1988;1 :97–99.

60. Neff MS, Kim KE, Persoff M, Onesti G, Swartz C. Hemodynamics of uremic uremia. *Circulation* 1971;43:876–883.

12

Chronic Transfusion Support

Karen E. King and Paul M. Ness

1. INTRODUCTION

The purpose of this chapter is to describe the underlying principles of chronic red cell transfusion therapy and its complications. In addition, specific diseases are addressed in which a chronic transfusion protocol may be a reasonable option; current recommendations and potential alternatives to transfusion are also considered for patients affected by these diseases. With the development of new therapies, some diseases that previously required chronic transfusion support are no longer initially treated with transfusions. Although many diseases are addressed specifically, this discussion is not intended to be comprehensive. The featured diseases were chosen as representative examples; many of the diseases not specifically addressed bear similarities to those that are included.

2. GENERAL PRINCIPLES OF CHRONIC TRANSFUSION THERAPY

The specific protocol of chronic transfusion support must be individualized for the patient depending on the underlying disease. The exact transfusion trigger will vary from patient to patient and depends in large part on the physiologic impact of the anemia, the patient's ability to compensate and the activity level of the patient. Physiologic compensation occurs at several levels during chronic anemia. As the hemoglobin concentration decreases, red cell 2,3-diphosphoglycerate (2,3-DPG) increases and shifts the oxygen dissociation curve to the right, reducing oxygen affinity and enhancing oxygen delivery to the tissues (1). Cardiac compensation occurs with increased cardiac output by increasing stroke volume (2,3). Respiratory compensation also occurs with increased respiratory rate and depth (3).

When a patient is initially placed on a chronic transfusion protocol, it may take some time to determine the optimal transfusion schedule for the patient. Both the amount of blood required and the interval of transfusions must be determined. It is ideal to avoid large fluctuations in hematocrit over time and better to maintain a relatively stable level. Most adult patients can tolerate the transfusion of 2 U of red cells in 1 d. We have found that an average adult with no red cell production will require 2 U of red cells every 2 wk, unless there is an increased hemolytic component. Thus, most of our chronic transfusion patients receive 2 U of red cells every 2–4 wk.

From: *Red Cell Transfusion: A Practical Guide*
Edited by: M. E. Reid and S. J. Nance Humana Press Inc., Totowa, NJ

3. HEMOGLOBINOPATHIES

3.1. Sickle Cell Disease

Transfusion therapy has been a mainstay of treatment for many complications of sickle cell disease. The best indication for the use of chronic transfusion therapy for patients with sickle cell disease is for the prevention of recurrent cerebrovascular accidents *(4)*. Acute transfusions are indicated for patients with acute splenic sequestration *(5)*. Acute chest syndrome is an indication for exchange transfusion, especially in children *(6,7)*.

Exchange transfusions were routinely performed as a part of preoperative preparation for patients with sickle cell disease. A recent study evaluating preoperative transfusion protocols, however, found that a conservative preoperative protocol, in which the hemoglobin was raised to 10 g/dL, was as effective in preventing perioperative complications as an aggressive approach, designed to suppress the hemoglobin S level below 30% *(8)*.

When transfusing patients with sickle cell disease, one must be aware of the relationship of viscosity to both hematocrit and percent hemoglobin S red cells. At a fixed percent of hemoglobin S red cells, viscosity increases with the hematocrit. At a fixed hematocrit, viscosity increases with increased percent hemoglobin S red cells *(9,10)*. Raising the hematocrit above 35% without a significant reduction in percent sickle cells could result in increased viscosity, which could negate the beneficial effects of the transfusion *(11)*. We have seen this complication in patients with elevated hematocrits associated with hydroxyurea therapy.

We recommend the use of leukocyte-reduced red cell products for these complicated patients to avoid febrile, nonhemolytic transfusion reactions that may confound an already complicated clinical situation.

3.2. Thalassemia Major

Patients with thalassemia major require chronic transfusion therapy from a very young age. Those patients with milder forms of the disease may not require chronic transfusions until the age of 4 yr. Allogeneic bone marrow transplantation is being used in some centers as a cure for this disease. However, not all centers are advocating bone marrow transplantation, since this procedure has high morbidity and mortality with potential graft-vs-host disease (GVHD), and engraftment failure *(12)*. Long-term evaluation of patients who are conservatively treated with chronic transfusions and chelation therapy shows prolonged survival when there is good compliance with iron chelation therapy (serum ferritin levels below 2500 ng/mL) *(13)*. Some have advocated the use of neocytes to extend the transfusion interval and reduce transfused iron; however, the neocyte preparations are more costly, lead to increased donor exposures, and are not of clearcut benefit *(14)*. We recommend the use of leukocyte-reduced red cell products to avoid febrile, nonhemolytic transfusion reactions in these chronically transfused patients.

4. HEMATOLOGIC MALIGNANCIES

4.1. Myelodysplastic Syndromes (MDS)

The MDS comprise a group of clonal stem cell disorders with abnormal bone marrow differentiation, peripheral cytopenias, and a high risk of transformation to acute leukemia. Much of the morbidity associated with MDS is related to the cytopenias leading to symptomatic anemia, bleeding, and infection *(15)*. Currently, there is no effective therapy for MDS. Bone marrow transplantation is considered in younger patients; however, for most patients, only supportive therapy is available. These patients usually develop increasing red-cell transfusion requirements over time, with ultimate transfusion dependence.

The possible role of erythropoietin (EPO) therapy for patients with MDS has been extensively investigated. Studies have shown a variability in serum EPO levels and a variability in therapeutic response to exogenous EPO treatment among patients with MDS *(16)*. Some patients have an unexpectedly low EPO level for their degree of anemia. It has been shown that a low pretreatment EPO level is the best predictor of response to exogenous EPO therapy *(17)*. Overall, only 20–30% of patients with MDS respond to exogenous EPO therapy. A trial of EPO is only recommended for transfusion-dependent patients with MDS who have a low serum EPO level (< 500 mU/mL) *(18)*.

4.2. Leukemia

Patients with acute leukemia do not usually require chronic transfusion support, although they will need short-term transfusion therapy during induction chemotherapy. At initial presentation, one must be aware of possible hyperleukocytic leukostasis in the acute leukemic patient, with a markedly elevated white cell count, frequently owing to acute myelocytic leukemia. Although white cells do not usually contribute significantly to whole blood viscosity, hyperleukocytosis with malignant white cells can have associated hyperviscosity because of abnormal flow characteristics of the malignant white cells. These patients frequently present with hyperleukocytosis, anemia, and evidence of poor perfusion, which may be caused by leukostasis or infiltration of blood vessels by leukemic cells. In these patients, the white cell count should be reduced by leukopheresis before the patient is given red cell transfusions. If leukopheresis technology is not available, the patient's white cell count can be reduced by manual whole blood exchange or chemotherapy *(19,20)*.

5. OTHER HEMATOLOGIC DISORDERS

5.1. Aplastic Anemia

Patients with severe aplastic anemia should undergo bone marrow transplantation as quickly as possible. While an appropriate donor is being identified, these patients may require transfusion support. The number of transfusions should be kept at a minimum, and family donors should be avoided. Patients with aplastic anemia who undergo bone marrow transplantation are more likely to have engraftment failure if they have been multiply transfused or have received blood products from family members. If an appropriate donor can not be identified, patients can be treated with immunosuppressive therapy. Although immunosuppressive therapy rarely results in normal marrow function, the goal of this therapy is to achieve independence from transfusion support *(21)*.

We recommend the use of leuko-reduced blood products for patients with aplastic anemia in order to reduce the risk of alloimmunization against human leukocyte (HLA) antigens. Alloimmunization in these patients can be devastating; it can complicate bone marrow transplantation and also lead to platelet refractoriness.

5.2. Paroxysmal Nocturnal Hemoglobinuria (PNH)

PNH is an acquired clonal disorder of the bone marrow that affects red cells, platelets, granulocytes, and possibly lymphocytes. Several membrane protein deficiencies have been observed in PNH involving proteins that are attached to the glycosylphosphatidylinositol (GPI) anchor. The defect is found in the X-linked PIG-A (phosphatidylinositol glycan class A) gene that has a role in an early step in the synthesis of the GPI anchor *(22,23)*.

Patients with PNH will have intermittent episodes of hemolysis owing to the increased sensitivity of their red cells to complement-mediated lysis. Patients with severe PNH require chronic transfusion support, since they essentially have a chronic hemolytic anemia. Because these patients have intravascular hemolysis with hemoglobinuria, they lose iron in their urine and may not require chelation therapy despite chronic transfusions.

Many hematologists suggest that patients requiring red cell transfusions should receive washed red cells to avoid the transfusion of complement, which is present in plasma *(24)*. Studies have shown that unwashed red cells are safely transfused to patients with PNH *(25)*. In vitro studies have shown that PNH red cells undergo hemolysis in the presence of white cell antigen–antibody reactions *(26)*. Theoretically, any reaction which generates C5b-7 complexes can potentially lead to hemolysis in these patients *(27)*. Since PNH patients are multiply transfused, many have white cell antibodies. It has been recommended that patients with PNH receive leuko-reduced red cells *(28)*.

5.3. Bone Marrow Transplantation

Patients who undergo bone marrow transplantation may require red cell transfusions at various points in their clinical course, especially during ablative therapy and before engraftment occurs. Some patients with partial/incomplete engraftment will need indefinite transfusion support.

Patients undergoing bone marrow transplantation should receive irradiated cellular blood products to prevent transfusion-associated (TA) GVHD. In addition, recipients who are cytomegalovirus (CMV)-seronegative and are transplanted with CMV-seronegative donor marrow should receive CMV-seronegative blood products. If CMV-seronegative products are not available, leuko-reduced blood products should be given. Leuko-depleted red cells may also have a role in reducing the risk of alloimmunization.

The possible role of EPO in reducing the red cell transfusion needs of bone marrow transplant patients is controversial. Studies have shown that inappropriately low endogenous erythropoietin levels are seen in patients following bone marrow transplantation, especially allogeneic transplantation *(29,30)*. Two randomized studies have shown a beneficial effect of EPO treatment in allogeneic transplant patients, with decreased transfusion requirements *(31,32)*.

6. ANEMIA OF CHRONIC DISEASE

The anemia of chronic disease occurs in patients with chronic infections, chronic inflammatory conditions, such as rheumatoid arthritis, or in patients with neoplasms in the absence of marrow replacement. The anemia of chronic disease is usually mild to moderate and features a lower than expected reticulocyte count for the degree of anemia. The pathogenesis of this anemia is unclear. Many have speculated that EPO plays a central role. More recent studies have implicated the role of various cytokines that can inhibit erythropoiesis, by affecting EPO and/or iron metabolism *(33)*.

6.1. Rheumatoid Arthritis

Patients with rheumatoid arthritis often have a moderate anemia, usually not requiring transfusion therapy. These patients have a blunted EPO response and their EPO levels are lower than expected for the degree of anemia *(34)*. Patients with rheumatoid arthritis respond to therapeutic EPO treatment with no significant change in the status of their rheumatologic disease *(35)*. Recombinant human EPO will stimulate erythropoiesis in surgical candidates with rheumatoid arthritis to enable them to donate autologous blood *(36)*.

6.2. Malignancies Without Bone Marrow Involvement

Patients with solid tumors may have anemia despite a lack of bone marrow involvement even before the initiation of chemotherapy. The etiology of the anemia of cancer is unclear. A blunted EPO response has been seen in these patients in whom EPO levels are lower than expected for the degree of anemia *(37)*. This blunted EPO response was corrected with hypoxemia and EPO production increased. These studies suggest that EPO therapy may be helpful in the treatment of anemia associated with cancer. If EPO therapy is unsuccessful, these patients may require chronic transfusions.

Patients with malignancies also have anemia associated with combination chemotherapy. The blunted endogenous EPO response is exacerbated with chemotherapy, but therapeutic EPO has been successfully used in the treatment of these patients. In one prospective study of patients undergoing myelosuppressive chemotherapy, EPO treatment resulted in a significant increase in hematocrit; however, transfusion requirements did not decrease until the second and third months of treatment. The EPO-treated patients did have a significant improvement in their energy level and ability to perform daily activities *(38)*.

6.3. Chronic Infections

Many infections that previously required chronic transfusion therapy are currently treatable and are no longer appropriate indications for red cell replacement. Some parasitic infections may still require acute transfusions. In cases of heavy infection by malaria or babesia organisms, there may be massive hemolysis. In these situations, an exchange transfusion may be considered to reduce the parasitic load acutely and to prevent further acute intravascular hemolysis that can lead to renal damage.

Currently, the most common infectious agent requiring chronic transfusion therapy is the human immunodeficiency virus (HIV) and resultant acquired immunodeficiency syndrome (AIDS). Patients with AIDS have numerous hematologic disorders including anemia, leukopenia, and thrombocytopenia *(39)*. The etiology of the anemia in these patients is multifactorial. Most patients with AIDS are treated with the antiviral drug zidovudine (azidothymidine, AZT) which is associated with myelosuppression, anemia, and neutropenia *(40)*. In a study evaluating the underlying reason for transfusion in patients with AIDS and AIDS-related complex, transfusion was associated with numerous factors including drugs and other infections (mycobacterium avium complex). The most frequent association producing severe anemia requiring transfusion was AZT *(41)*. All treatable causes of anemia must be excluded in these patients. Frequently, patients with advanced disease will become transfusion dependent. It is prudent to provide CMV-seronegative blood products to AIDS patients who are seronegative for CMV, since primary infection with CMV can cause devastating ophthalmalogic and respiratory complications. This clinical setting arises most commonly in the pediatric AIDS population.

EPO therapy has been used in anemic patients with AIDS treated with AZT. EPO may be effective in treating the anemia of HIV and AZT in selected patients. In one randomized study, reduced transfusion requirements were seen in the EPO treated patients who had low endogenous EPO levels (< 500 IU/L) before treatment *(42)*.

There is concern about the immunomodulatory effects of transfusion in patients with AIDS. A retrospective study revealed that transfused patients with AIDS had a higher incidence of opportunistic infections, especially clinically significant CMV infection. These transfused patients also had an increased death rate *(43)*. In addition, a carefully performed in vitro study has shown that allogeneic donor leukocytes in cellular blood products can upregulate HIV-1 expression and dissemination *(44)*. These studies imply that leukocyte reduction of blood products for patients with AIDS may have therapeutic benefit. The NIH has sponsored the Virus Activation and Transfusion Study to evaluate the possible immunomodulatory effects of transfusion and methods to circumvent these adverse effects, if they exist.

Parvovirus B19 infection has a pathologic effect on hematopoiesis, especially erythroid progenitors. Parvovirus infection has been associated with aplastic crises that occur in patients with chronic hemolytic anemia. Chronic infection can occur in immunocompromised patients, including patients with HIV infection or AIDS, immunosuppressed states such as transplantation, and congenital immunodeficiency. Persistent infection can result in pure red cell aplasia and require chronic transfusion support *(45,46)*.

6.4. Renal Insufficiency

Although frequently considered in this category, the anemia associated with renal insufficiency is not truly an anemia of chronic disease, since the etiology of the anemia is clearly associated with decreased erythropoietin production by the impaired kidneys. At one time, virtually all patients with end-stage renal disease became transfusion dependent. Since the development of recombinant human EPO, only a minority of these patients require transfusions. It is estimated that over 95% of hemodialysis patients will successfully respond to EPO therapy with a hematocrit of 35% within 12 wk of initiating treatment *(47)*. This therapy has had numerous beneficial effects, including the elimination of transfusion dependence and the potential adverse effects of transfusion, improvement in quality of life, and improvement in uremic pruritus *(48)*.

The use of EPO in predialysis renal failure was initially questioned since EPO was suspected to accelerate the progression to end-stage renal disease. Theoretically,

EPO therapy could lead to deleterious systemic and renal hemodynamic changes, including increased blood viscosity and increased systemic blood pressure. It has now been shown that EPO is safe and efficacious to treat patients with predialysis renal failure *(49)*; patients have improvement in hematocrit and quality of life, without the feared consequences. A large multicenter study of EPO in predialysis patients showed no significant acceleration in progression of renal disease *(50)*. An increase in systemic blood pressure may require adjustment of hypertensive medications *(51)*.

7. ADVERSE EFFECTS OF CHRONIC RED CELL TRANSFUSIONS

7.1. Transfusion Reactions

Transfusion reactions are potential adverse sequelae in any transfusion and are not unique to chronic red cell transfusions. These reactions are thoroughly discussed in Chapter 13.

7.2. Transfusion-Associated Graft-vs-Host Disease

TAGVHD is a risk for some chronically transfused patients who are severely immunocompromised, such as patients undergoing bone marrow transplantation. This transfusion-related complication occurs when immunocompetent lymphocytes are transfused that are capable of engrafting and reacting against host tissues *(52)*. γ-Irradiation inactivates immunocompetent lymphocytes and is used to prevent TAGVHD. Thus, it is recommended that γ-irradiation be performed on cellular products given to immunocompromised patients, and recipients of bone marrow or progenitor cell transplantation. Since situations of partial HLA identity between the donor and recipient are also associated with TAGVHD, blood products donated by a relative should be γ-irradiated *(53,54)*.

7.3. Transfusion-Transmitted Infections

Transfusion-transmitted infections may be a complication of any transfusion episode and are not limited to chronic transfusion recipients. Of course, a chronically transfused patient has an overall higher risk, due to the exposure to multiple donors over an extended period of time.

Currently the risk of transfusion-associated hepatitis B is estimated to be as high as 1 in 25,000 components transfused or as low as 1 in 200,000 *(55,56)*. The incidence of transfusion-associated hepatitis C has been greatly reduced with the development of improved testing. In a multicenter study of cardiac surgery patients from April 1985 through February 1991; patients were divided into three groups representing different donor screening procedures. They found that the risk of post-transfusion hepatitis C declined from 0.55% to 0.36% to 0.06% per unit transfused over each time period with the implementation of new testing procedures *(57,58)*. The hepatitis C risk is now even smaller as a result of improved hepatitis C serologic detection methods. The most recent estimate of the risk of HIV transmission by screened blood in the United States is between 1 in 450,000 to 1 in 660,000 donations as a result of efficacious donor screening and highly sensitive HIV antibody and antigen detection systems *(59)*.

7.4. Alloimmunization

Although alloimmunization is a risk of any transfusion, multiply transfused patients have a higher rate of alloimmunization because of the exposure to a greater number of donors. The development of alloantibodies is multifactorial and involves such variables as the immunogenicity of the antigen, the immunoresponsiveness of the patient, the number of exposures, and possibly the age of initial transfusion.

An increased risk of alloimmunization has been seen in patients with sickle cell disease (18–36%) *(60–63)*, as compared to other multiply transfused patients. It has been suggested that this increased rate of alloimmunization is related to the transfusion of racially discordant red cells, since African Americans are underrepresented in the donor population *(64)*. Differences in red cell antigen frequency between African Americans and Caucasians have been documented.

It is interesting that patients with thalassemia have a lower rate of alloimmunization as compared to patients with sickle cell disease. Thalassemic patients usually have a higher transfusion exposure and began a chronic transfusion protocol at a younger age. Among patients with thalassemia major, the rate of alloimmunization increases for patients who begin transfusion therapy at a later age *(65)*. Thus, it appears that earlier exposure to blood products may induce a tolerance for red cell antigens; however, the issue of racially discordant blood does not usually have as great an impact on thalassemic patients.

Delayed hemolytic transfusion reactions are a well-established risk of multiple transfusions and are seen in alloimmunized patients; these reactions, as well as delayed serologic transfusion reactions are thoroughly discussed in Chapter 13. Of note, in patients with sickle cell disease, delayed hemolytic transfusion reactions may appear clinically like a painful crisis *(66)* or an aplastic crisis *(67)*. Thus, a delayed hemolytic transfusion reaction must be considered as the cause of a variety of complaints in any patient with sickle cell disease who has been recently transfused.

Because of the high rate of alloimmunization and delayed hemolytic transfusion reactions in patients with sickle cell disease, prophylactic antigen matching has been proposed and evaluated by several investigators. A decreased incidence of alloimmunization has been seen with both extensive (17 blood group antigens) *(68)* as well as less extensive (C, E, K, S, and Fy^a or Fy^b) *(69,70)* antigen matching. The best approach to this problem of alloimmunization has been debated and issues of cost effectiveness and the limited number of donors with rare phenotypes remain important concerns. The majority of patients do not become alloimmunized and patients who do develop antibodies usually develop a single antibody first. Thus, we feel that a reasonable approach to this problem is to perform an initial red cell phenotype on all patients with sickle cell disease and then to provide antigen-matched red cells once the patient has made a single alloantibody.

7.5. Iron Overload and Chelation Therapy

An average unit of red cells contains 200–250 mg of iron. Any patient who has received over 100 units of red cells is at risk for iron overload and chelation therapy should be considered. Iron will accumulate within the mitochondria, which will ultimately affect function in the heart, liver, and endocrine glands. Iron accumulation in the heart can be devastating, resulting in cardiac dysfunction and congestive heart failure. At this time, chelation therapy consists of deferoxamine therapy. Although compliance is a problem, deferoxamine is effective in preventing the complications of iron overload in patients with thalassemia major *(72)* and with sickle cell disease *(73)*.

Kim et al. *(74)* recommended a novel approach to managing patients with sickle cell disease who require a chronic transfusion protocol with iron chelation. They utilize automated erythrocytapheresis, which simultaneously achieves the goals of chronic transfusion and chelation. The automated procedure can successfully maintain patients with a low hemoglobin S and a higher total hemoglobin. In addition, this therapy obviates the need for chelation therapy. In fact, their patients with massive iron overload achieve decreased serum ferritin levels over time. Long-term studies will be needed to determine if the improvements in iron balance compensate for the additional donor exposures required with automated erythroctapheresis.

REFERENCES

1. Torrance J, Jacobs P, Restrepo A, et al. Intraerythrocytic adaptation to anemia. *N Engl J Med* 1970;283:165–169.
2. Roy SB, Bhatia ML, Mathur VS, Virmani S. Hemodynamic effects of chronic severe anemia. *Circulation* 1963;28:346–356.
3. Sproule BJ, Mitchell JH, Miller WF. Cardiopulmonary physiological responses to heavy exercise in patients with anemia. *J Clin Invest* 1960;39:378–388.
4. Russell MO, Goldberg HI, Hodson A, et al. Effect of transfusion therapy on arteriographic abnormalities and on recurrence of stroke in sickle cell disease. *Blood* 1984; 63:162–169.
5. Emond AM, Collis R, Darvill D, et al. Acute splenic sequestration in homozygous sickle cell disease: natural history and management. *J Pediatr* 1985;107:201–206.
6. Wayne AS, Kevy SV, Nathan DG. Transfusion management of sickle cell disease. *Blood* 1993;81:1109–1123.
7. Mallouh AA, Asha M. Beneficial effect of blood transfusion in children with sickle cell chest syndrome. *AJDC* 1988;142:178–182.
8. Vichinsky EP, Haberkern CM, Neumayr L, et al. A comparison of conservative and aggressive transfusion regimens in the perioperative management of sickle cell disease. *N Engl J Med* 1995;333:206–213.
9. Charache S, Conley CL. Rate of sickling of red cells during deoxygenation of blood from persons with various sickling disorders. *Blood* 1964;24:25–48.
10. Schmalzer EA, Lee JO, Brown AK, et al. Viscosity of mixtures of sickle and normal red cells at varying hematocrit levels: implications for transfusion. *Transfusion* 1987; 27:228–233.
11. Jan K, Usami S, Smith JA. Effects of transfusion on rheological properties of blood in sickle cell anemia. *Transfusion* 1982;22:17–20.
12. Rund D, Rachmilewitz E. Thalassemia major 1995: older patients, newer therapies. *Blood Rev* 1995;9:25–32.
13. Olivieri NF, Nathan DG, MacMillan JH, et al. Survival in medically treated patients with homozygous B-thalassemia. *N Engl J Med* 1994;331:574–578.
14. Collins AF, Goncalves-Dias C, Haddad S, et al. Comparison of a transfusion preparation of newly formed red cells and standard washed red cell transfusions in patients with homozygous B-thalassemia. *Transfusion* 1994;34:517–520.
15. Greenberg PL. Treatment of myelodysplastic syndromes. *Blood Rev* 1991;5:42–50.

16. Bowen D, Culligan D, Jacobs A. The treatment of anaemia in the myelodysplastic syndromes with recombinant human erythropoietin. *Br J Haematol* 1991;77:419–423.

17. Mittelman M. Recombinant erythropoietin in myelodysplastic syndromes: Whom to treat and how? More questions than answers. *Acta Haematol* 1993;90:53–57.

18. Mittelman M, Lessin LS. Clinical Application of recombinant erythropoietin in myelodysplasia. In: Spivak J, eds. *Erythropoietin: Basic and Clinical Aspects.* Hematology/Oncology Clinics of North America. Philadelphia: Saunders, 1994, pp. 993–1009.

19. Lichtman MA, Rowe JM. Hyperleukocytic leukemias: rheological, clinical, and therapeutic considerations. *Blood* 1982;60:279–283.

20. Harris AL. Leukostasis associated with blood transfusion in acute myeloid leukemia. *Br Med J* 1978;1:1169–1171.

21. Young NS. Aplastic anemia. *Lancet* 1995;346:228–232.

22. Yomtovian R, Prince GM, Medof ME. The molecular basis for paroxysmal nocturnal hemoglobinuria. *Transfusion* 1993;33:852873.

23. Rotoli B, Bessler M, Alfinito F, del Vecchio L. Membrane proteins in paroxysmal nocturnal haemoglobinuria. *Blood Rev* 1993;7:75–86.

24. Dacie JV. Transfusion of saline-washed red cells in nocturnal haemoglobinuria. *Clin Sci* 1948;7:65–75.

25. Brecher ME, Taswell HF. Paroxysmal nocturnal hemoglobinuria and the transfusion of washed red cells: a myth revisited. *Transfusion* 1989;29:681–685.

26. Sirchia G, Ferrone S, Mercuriali F. Leukocyte antigen-antibody reaction and lysis of paroxysmal nocturnal hemoglobinuria erythrocytes. *Blood* 1970;36:334–336.

27. Rosse WF. Transfusion in paroxysmal nocturnal hemoglobinuria: to wash or not to wash? *Transfusion* 1989;29:663–664.

28. Sirchia G, Zanella A. Transfusion of PNH patients. *Transfusion* 1990;30:479.

29. Beguin Y, Clemons GK, Oris R, Fillet G. Circulating erythropoietin levels after bone marrow transplantation: Inappropriate response to anemia in allogeneic transplants. *Blood* 1991;77:868–873.

30. Ireland RM, Atkinson K, Concannon A, et al. Serum erythropoietin changes in autologous and allogeneic bone marrow transplant patients. *Br J Haematol* 1990;76: 128–134.

31. Steegman JL, Lopez J, Otero MJ, et al. Erythropoietin treatment in allogeneic BMT accelerates erythroid reconstitution: results of a prospective controlled randomized trial. *Bone Marrow Transplant* 1992;10:541–546.

32. Klaesson S, Ringden O, Ljungman P, et al. Reduced blood transfusions requirements after allogeneic bone marrow transplantation: results of a randomised, double-blind study with high-dose erythropoietin. *Bone Marrow Transplant* 1994;13:397–402.

33. Means RT, Krantz SB. Progress in understanding the pathogenesis of the anemia of chronic disease. *Blood* 1992;80:1639–1647.

34. Hochberg MC, Arnold CM, Hogans BB, Spivak JL. Serum immunoreactive erythropoietin in rheumatoid arthritis: impaired response to anemia. *Arthritis Rheum* 1988; 31:1318–1321.

35. Pincus T, Olsen JN, Russell IJ, et al. Multicenter study of recombinant human erythropoietin in correction of anemia in rheumatoid arthritis. *Am J Med* 1990;89:161–168.

36. Mercuriali F, Gualtieri G, Sinigaglia L, et al. Use of recombinant human erythropoietin to assist autologous blood donation by anemic rheumatoid arthritis patients undergoing major orthopedic surgery. *Transfusion* 1994;34:501–506.

37. Miller CB, Jones RJ, Piantadosi S, et al. Decreased erythropoietin response in patients with the anemia of cancer. *N Engl J Med* 1990;322:1689–1692.

38. Case DC, Bukowski RM, Carey RW, et al. Recombinant human erythropoietin therapy for anemic cancer patients on combination chemotherapy. *J Natl Cancer Inst* 1993;85:801–806.

39. Spivak JL, Bender BS, Quinn TC. Hematologic abnormalities in the acquired immune deficiency syndrome. *Am J Med* 1984;77:224–228.

40. Richman DD, Fischl MA, Grieco MH, et al. The toxicity of azidothymidine (AZT) in the treatment of patients with AIDS and AIDS-related complex. *N Engl J Med* 1987; 317:192–197.

41. Jacobson MA, Peiperl L, Volberding PA, et al. Red cell transfusion therapy for anemia in patients with AIDS and ARC: incidence, associated factors, and outcome. *Transfusion* 1990;30:133–137.

42. Fischl M, Galpin JE, Levine JD, et al. Recombinant human erythropoietin for patients with AIDS treated with zidovudine. *N Engl J Med* 1990;322:1488–1493.

43. Sloand E, Kumar P, Klein HG, et al. Transfusion of blood components to persons infected with human immunodeficiency virus type 1: relationship to opportunistic infection. *Transfusion* 1994;34:48–53.

44. Busch MP, Lee T-H, Heitman J. Allogeneic leukocytes but not therapeutic blood elements induce reactivation and dissemination of latent human immunodeficiency virus type 1 infection: implications for transfusion support of infected patients. *Blood* 1992;80:2128–2135.

45. Brown KE, Young NS. Parvovirus B19 infection and hematopoiesis. *Blood Rev* 1995;9:176–182.

46. Luban NLC. Human parvoviruses: implications for transfusion medicine. *Transfusion* 1994;34:821–827.

47. Esbach JW, Abdulhadi MH, Browne JK, et al. Recombinant human erythropoietin in anemic patients with end-stage renal disease. *Ann Intern Med* 1989;111:992–1000.

48. De Marchi S, Cecchin E, Villalta D, et al. Relief of pruritus and decreases in plasma histamine concentrations during erythropoietin therapy in patients with uremia. *N Engl J Med* 1992;326:969–974.

49. Watson AJ, Gimenez LF, Cotton S, et al. Treatment of the anemia of chronic renal failure with subcutaneous recombinant human erythropoietin. *Am J Med* 1990;89: 432–435.

50. The US Recombinant Human Erythropoietin Predialysis Study Group. Double-blind, placebo-controlled study of the therapeutic use of recombinant human erythropoietin for anemia associated with chronic renal failure in predialysis patients. *Am J Kidney Dis* 1991;18:50–59.

51. Kleinman KS, Schweitzer SU, Perdue ST, et al. The use of recombinant human erythropoietin in the correction of anemia in predialysis patients and its effect on renal function: a double-blind, placebo-controlled trial. *Am J Kidney Dis* 1989;14: 486–495.

52. Brubaker DB. Transfusion-associated graft-versus-host disease. In: Anderson KC, Ness PM (ed). *Scientific Basis of Transfusion Medicine: Implications for Clinical Practice.* Philadelphia: Saunders, 1994, p. 544.

53. McMilin KD, Johnson RL. HLA homozygosity and the risk of related-donor transfusion-associated graft-versus-host disease. *Transfus Med Rev* 1993;7:37–41.

54. Petz LD, Calhoun L, Yam P, et al. Transfusion-associated graft-versus-host disease in immunocompetent patients: report of a fatal case associated with transfusion of blood from a second-degree relative, and a survey of predisposing factors. *Transfusion* 1993;33:742–750.

55. Foster GR, Carman WF, Thomas HC. Replication of hepatitis B and delta viruses: appearance of viral mutants. *Semin Liver Dis* 1991;11:121–127.

56. Dodd RY. The risk of transfusion-transmitted infection. *N Engl J Med* 1992;327: 419–421.

57. Donahue JG, Munoz A, Ness PM, et al. The declining risk of post-transfusion hepatitis C virus infection. *N Engl J Med* 1992;327:369–373.

58. Nelson KE, Ahmed F, Ness PM, et al. Comparison of first and second generation ELISA screening tests in detecting HCV infections in transfused cardiac surgery patients. In: *Program and Abstracts of the International Symposium on Viral Hepatitis and Liver Disease,* Tokyo, Japan, May 1014, 1993, p. 50.
59. Lackritz EM, Satten GA, Aberle-Grasse J, et al. Estimated risk of transmission of the human immunodeficiency virus by screened blood in the United States. *N Engl J Med* 1995;333:1721–1725.
60. Cox JV, Steane E, Cunningham G, Frenkel EP. Risk of alloimmunization and delayed hemolytic transfusion reactions in patients with sickle cell disease. *Arch Intern Med* 1988;148:2485–2489.
61. Davies SC, McWilliam AC, Hewitt PE, et al. Red cell alloimmunization in sickle cell disease. *Br J Haematol* 1986;63:241–245.
62. Orlina AR, Unger PJ, Koshy M. Post-transfusion alloimmunization in patients with sickle cell disease. *Am J Hematol* 1978;5:101–106.
63. Rosse WF, Gallagher D, Kinney TR, et al. Transfusion and allomimmunization in sickle cell disease. *Blood* 1990;76:1431–1437.
64. Vichinsky EP, Earles A, Johnson RA, et al. Alloimmunization in sickle cell anemia and transfusion of racially unmatched blood. *N Engl J Med* 1990;322:1617–1621.
65. Rebulla P, Modell B. Transfusion requirements and effects in patients with thalassemia major. *Lancet* 1991;337:277–280.
66. Diamond WJ, Brown FL, Bitterman P, et al. Delayed hemolytic transfusion reaction presenting as sickle-cell crisis. *Ann Intern Med* 1980;93:231–234.
67. Milner PF, Squires JE, Larison PJ, et al. Posttransfusion crises in sickle cell anemia: role of delayed hemolytic reactions to transfusion. *S Med J* 1985;78:1462–1469.
68. Ambruso DR, Githens JH, Alcorn R, et al. Experience with donors matched for minor blood group antigens in patients with sickle cell anemia who are receiving chronic transfusion therapy. *Transfusion* 1987;27:94–98.
69. Tahhan HR, Holbrook CT, Braddy LR, et al. Antigen-matched donor blood in the transfusion management of patients with sickle cell disease. *Transfusion* 1994;34:562–569.
70. Tahhan HR, Werner AL, Bergante RA, et al. Antigen-matching in the transfusional management of pediatric patients with sickle cell disease (abstract). *Transfusion* 1995;35:16S.
71. Ness PM. To match or not to match: the question for chronically transfused patients with sickle cell anemia. *Transfusion* 1994;34:558–560.
72. Brittenham GM, Griffith PM, Nienhuis AW, et al. Efficacy of deferoxamine in preventing complications of iron overload in patients with thalassemia major. *N Engl J Med* 1994;331:567–573.
73. Cohen A, Schwartz E. Excretion of iron in response to deferoxamine in sickle cell anemia. *J Pediatr* 1978;92:659–662.
74. Kim HC, Dugan NP, Silber JH, et al. Erythrocytapheresis therapy to reduce iron overload in chronically transfused patients with sickle cell disease. *Blood* 1994; 83: 1136–1142.

Modern Approaches to the Diagnosis and Management of Red Cell Transfusion Reactions

Patricia M. Kopko and Dennis Goldfinger

1. INTRODUCTION

The transfusion of red blood cells (RBCs) can usually be accomplished in a safe and effective manner. However, transfusion reactions are not an uncommon event and can range in severity from mild urticaria to severe, life-threatening hemolytic episodes. Therefore it is important for clinicians, as well as pathologists and blood bankers, to understand how to diagnose and manage various transfusion reactions.

This chapter is divided into two major sections which cover the various types of hemolytic and nonhemolytic transfusion reactions. In each of the sections we emphasize etiology, diagnosis, and our recommendations for patient management.

2. HEMOLYTIC TRANSFUSION REACTIONS

Hemolytic transfusion reactions can be divided into acute reactions, which generally begin during or shortly after the administration of RBCs, and delayed reactions, which usually do not start until a few days or more after the transfusion.

2.1. Acute Transfusion Reactions

2.1.1. Acute Hemolytic Transfusion Reactions (AHTRs)

AHTRs are usually the result of the transfusion of ABO incompatible RBCs. They are less commonly seen secondary to incompatibility of non-ABO antigens. Only a few non-ABO antigens are likely to cause AHTRs; these include antigens of the Kidd, Kell, Duffy, and Rh systems and the S and s antigens of the MNS system. Kidd antibodies possess the unique characteristic of being able to cause severe hemolysis despite being present only weakly in the patient's serum. They are also well known for disappearing with time only to rapidly reappear with future transfusions of Kidd-positive blood (anamnestic response).

2.1.1.1. Signs and Symptoms

The clinical manifestations of AHTRs can be myriad. Expected signs and symptoms can include fever, chills, severe back pain, tachycardia, respiratory distress, hypotension, and hemoglobinuria. In an anesthetized patient the first sign of a

From: *Red Cell Transfusion: A Practical Guide*
Edited by: M. E. Reid and S. J. Nance Humana Press Inc., Totowa, NJ

Table 1
Steps in Evaluating a Suspected Transfusion Reaction

Clinical
    Stop transfusion
    Maintain venous access
    Monitor vital signs
    Check identification of patient and unit of RBCs
    Obtain blood samples (EDTA and clot)
    Deliver samples to blood bank
Laboratory
    Perform clerical check
    Centrifuge posttransfusion blood sample
    Perform visual exam for free hemoglobin and hyperbilirubinemia
    Check ABO group and DAT on posttransfusion sample
    Recheck ABO group on unit of RBCs.
Additional laboratory studies
      (may be indicated if the above studies are abnormal)
    ABO group and DAT on pretransfusion sample
    Antibody screen on pre- and posttransfusion specimens
    Examine urine for free hemoglobin
    Gram stain and culture of unit of RBCs

hemolytic transfusion reaction may be hemoglobinuria and/or unexplained hypotension or uncontrollable generalized bleeding in the operative field. Symptoms can be seen with the administration of only a few milliliters of incompatible blood and are usually evident within 1–2 h of beginning the transfusion. However, severe complications are typically only seen with the administration of 100 mL or more of RBCs.

2.1.1.2. DIAGNOSIS

Any patient in whom an AHTR is suspected needs to be rapidly evaluated and diagnosed, because the severity of the reaction is usually proportional to the volume of incompatible blood transfused (Table 1). The transfusion should be stopped immediately, the iv should be kept open, vital signs should be monitored, and a clerical check of the unit of blood and the recipient should be performed at the bedside. A blood specimen from the patient should be sent to the blood bank for evaluation, where another clerical check should be done. In addition, a visual examination of the patient's serum for free hemoglobin and a direct antiglobulin (Coomb's) test (DAT) should be performed. We also do a repeat ABO type of both the patient's posttransfusion blood specimen and the unit of blood involved, since the majority of serious reactions are owing to ABO incompatibility. No further testing is usually needed if the initial workup is negative. In fact, ordering excessive laboratory tests at the initiation of the workup, such as urinalysis for hemoglobinuria, Gram stain of the remaining RBCs, and serum haptoglobin may only serve to delay not only the resolution of the event, but also the ability to provide needed transfusions to an anemic patient. Details of additional diagnostic steps, if the initial workup is positive, are given in Table 1.

2.1.1.3. Management

If the patient exhibits signs of a serious hemolytic transfusion reaction large bore venous access should be established and he or she should be transferred to an intensive care unit. Treatment should be started while awaiting definitive laboratory evidence that a reaction has occurred, because early intervention may be life saving. Since hypotension, heart failure, and acute renal failure are often present, the insertion of a Swan–Ganz catheter to monitor the patient's hemodynamic status should be considered to aid in proper treatment. The patient's blood pressure should be maintained with iv fluids and possibly low-dose dopamine. Diuretics may be indicated to facilitate adequate renal perfusion. Pulmonary function should be monitored since oxygen therapy and/or ventilator support may be required *(1)*. The therapeutic implications of an AHTR are reviewed in Fig. 1.

Early use of heparin has been suggested as a means of preventing the development of disseminated intravascular coagulation (DIC), although this therapy is somewhat controversial, particularly in a surgical patient who may be at increased risk of bleeding complications *(2)*.

If the patient has received an incompatible unit of blood, the cause of the error must be determined. The most common causes of AHTRs are system and clerical errors, including patient, specimen, and unit mix-up *(3)*. If a mix-up has occurred, another patient could potentially receive an incompatible unit. Finding the cause of the error and acting upon it may make it possible to avoid another incompatible transfusion.

Patients who have experienced an AHTR are often anemic and will need to be further transfused. In extreme circumstances, transfusion should not await final outcome of the transfusion reaction workup. A patient who needs to be transfused should receive group O, Rh-negative blood until the source of error has been identified. This is usually a good choice, since most cases of AHTR are secondary to ABO incompatibility. This approach obviously will not work in AHTRs because of non-ABO antigens. It is permissible to switch to ABO- and Rh-compatible blood once the source of the error and the patient's true blood type have been established.

It is important that the blood bank physician communicate with the clinicians caring for the patient both during the workup of the transfusion reaction and once the results are known. In addition, the reaction should be clearly documented in the patient's chart.

2.1.1.4. Prevention

One of the most important concerns in any discussion of hemolytic transfusion reactions is their prevention. As has been previously mentioned, the most common sources of error are systemic and clerical. Nursing, physician, and phlebotomy staff should be properly trained to draw specimens for crossmatch. Only properly labeled specimens should be accepted by the blood bank; improperly labeled specimens should be discarded. Strict attention to patient and unit identification protocols should be maintained whenever a unit of blood is administered.

Numerous devices designed to prevent the transfusion of ABO incompatible RBCs are on the market. These systems, for the most part, involve an additional clerical

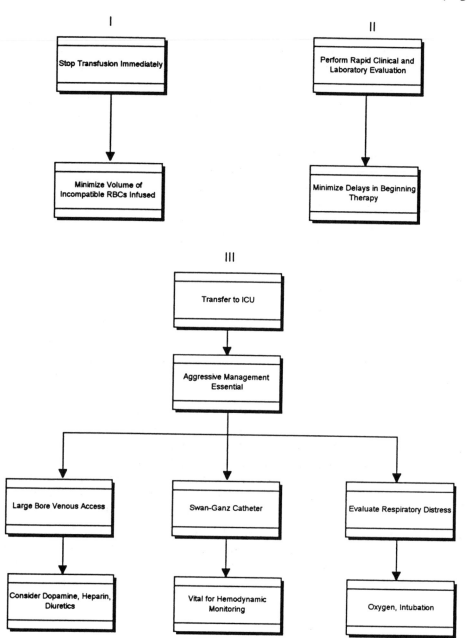

Fig. 1. AHTR: therapeutic implications.

check in the form of a bar-coded bracelet, an additional identification bracelet, or a lock opened with a code or key. We feel that, although these devices may add another barrier to the administration of incompatible blood, none is fail-safe. Also, they can only work if the staff involved in their use is convinced that these devices are needed, because most of these devices can either be ignored or circumvented by staff not committed to their use. These systems can also be quite expensive to use, which is an important consideration in these days of cost containment. To our knowledge, none of these systems includes a method to prevent technical errors in the blood bank, resulting in the assignment of an incorrect ABO type to a patient.

2.1.1.5. PATHOGENESIS

The pathogenesis of the dangerous complications associated with AHTRs has begun to become understood in recent years. The source of renal failure in AHTRs had been thought to be hemoglobin, which was alleged to form hemoglobin casts in the renal tubules, causing tubular obstruction and/or a direct toxic effect on the renal tubular epithelial cells. More recently, the renal failure was explained as a secondary effect of shock and subsequent renal hypoperfusion. However, the physiologic similarities of AHTRs to septic shock and our increased knowledge of the cellular and molecular mechanisms of septic shock have led to new insights into the possible mechanisms involved in the pathogenesis of AHTRs. Cytokines, which have been found to be mediators of inflammation and the immune response, are now thought to play a central role in the pathophysiology of AHTRs. Tumor necrosis factor (TNF) and interleukin-1 are thought to be important in the pathogenesis of shock in both sepsis and AHTRs *(4)*. They are also thought to play a key role in the development of DIC via the induction of changes to the endothelial cell's surface and it's hemostatic properties. Interleukin-8 has chemoattractant and activating effects on neutrophils and has been shown to increase in response to TNF. It may be partially responsible for the respiratory complications seen in AHTRs, via a direct toxic effect of accumulating neutrophils and increased vascular permeability resulting in pulmonary edema. In addition, the renal and pulmonary failure seen in AHTRs have been hypothesized to be in part the result of a decrease in endothelial derived relaxing factor, which is primarily nitric oxide (NO). Free hemoglobin is thought to combine with NO, reducing its bioavailability, resulting in vasoconstriction. The pathophysiology of AHTRs is summarized in Fig. 2. The complexity of cytokines and their various possible actions as biologic mediators of AHTRs is beyond the scope of this chapter. The reader is referred to an excellent review of the topic for further information *(1)*. A better understanding of the pathophysiology of AHTRs may ultimately lead to new therapies for management of these patients.

In summary, we feel that rapid diagnosis and aggressive management are essential in the treatment of AHTRs. We find that these reactions are often not treated in a sufficiently serious manner. We also emphasize that these patients should be treated in a critical care setting and in a similar manner to the treatment of septic shock and by physicians adept in the treatment of critically ill patients.

2.1.2. Hyperhemolysis in Patients with Sickle Cell Disease

Occasional patients with sickle cell disease who are transfused with crossmatch-compatible RBCs develop hemolysis of both the transfused RBCs and their own RBCs *(5)*. Posttransfusion workup may fail to identify any additional antibodies in the patient's serum. Continued transfusion in these patients can result in severe anemia that progresses in an ever-increasing spiral as long as the patient is transfused, and can ultimately end with the patient's demise.

The mechanism of destruction of transfused RBCs is not understood since there often appears to be no laboratory evidence of incompatibility. Furthermore, the means whereby hemolysis of the patient's own RBCs is accelerated cannot currently be explained.

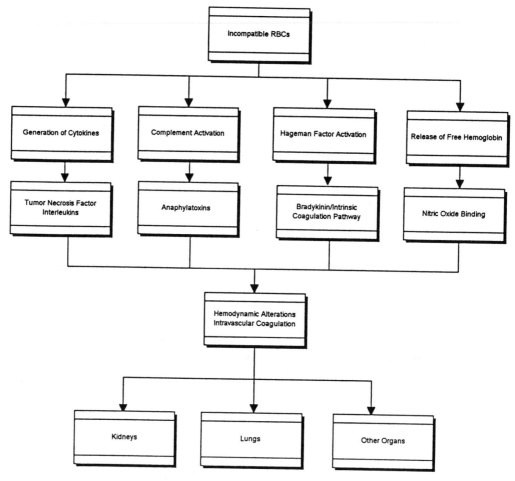

Fig. 2. Pathophysiology of AHTR.

2.1.2.1. MANAGEMENT

In our experience, these reactions are best managed by ceasing transfusion therapy of the patient. If the patient has a hemoglobin concentration (Hgb) of <5 g/dL, we advocate admitting him or her to an intensive care unit where close monitoring will be provided. Oxygen should be administered by mask. We find that the benefits of oxygen therapy in severely anemic patients are not often fully appreciated. Increasing the oxygen content of inspired air raises the oxygen content of the patient's blood, which is useful in someone who cannot be transfused. Its use in severe anemia can not only add to the patient's comfort but has been known to revive comatose patients who had previously steadfastly refused blood transfusion. Hydration by iv should be started and vitamin B12 and folic acid should be given. Patients with sickle cell disease often have minimal reserves of folate which are quickly consumed in crises, thereby impairing adequate hematopoeisis. Both of the authors have seen sickle cell patients with hyperhemolysis and Hgb levels <3.5 g/dL who eventually recovered with the treatment described above.

Transfusion after recovery from an episode of hyperhemolysis should be avoided since the phenomenon could potentially recur. In fact, we recommend adding a note to the patient's blood bank computer record, which states that the blood bank director should be notified if blood is ever requested for this patient.

Although we do not recommend transfusing someone who has previously experienced an episode of hyperhemolysis, there may be no other choice in cases of life-threatening anemia. Cullis et al. *(6)* successfully transfused 6 U of packed RBCs to a woman with hyperhemolysis and a Hgb of 3 g/dL by first administering steroids and iv immunoglobulin.

2.1.3. Transfusion in the Presence of Crossmatch Incompatibility

Occasionally, a patient will need to be transfused with crossmatch incompatible blood. This will usually occur either in the presence of an autoantibody or an allo-antibody to a high incidence antigen when a patient is extremely anemic and antigen-negative blood cannot be found. Complex survival studies using small volumes of radiolabeled RBCs have been described *(7)*, but are typically too complex to be commonly used. The so-called in vivo crossmatch is much simpler to perform. This method involves infusing approx 30 mL of blood over a 20–30 min period. The transfusion is then stopped for 15–30 min. During this time the patient is closely monitored for clinical symptoms of a transfusion reaction. At the end of this period a blood specimen is drawn and then centrifuged to check the plasma for visual evidence of hemolysis. If this test is negative, the remainder of the unit is transfused; however, if it is positive the unit, except under extreme circumstances, is discarded and an in vivo crossmatch is performed on another unit of blood.

Our own experience with the in vivo crossmatch has been less than satisfactory. We have found that the absence of hemolysis, even after as long as a 45 min wait, does not necessarily mean that the patient will not subsequently hemolyze the unit of blood when it is transfused. Conversely, we have seen a patient with cold agglutinin disease, who experienced hemolysis after infusion of a small amount of packed RBCs, who was successfully transfused with the remainder of the unit. In other words, the in vivo crossmatch is subject to both false-negative and false-positive results. To decrease the number of false negatives, we use a 45–60 min waiting period between the initial test dose of RBCs and the visual examination for hemolysis. Although we have found that the in vivo crossmatch is not absolutely predictive of RBC survival, its use is probably considered the standard of care when a unit of crossmatch incompatible blood must be transfused, and should thus probably be utilized.

2.2. Delayed Transfusion Reactions

Ness and associates *(8)* divided delayed transfusion reactions into delayed serologic transfusion reactions (DSTRs), in which there is only serologic evidence of incompatibility following transfusion, and delayed hemolytic transfusion reactions (DHTRs), in which there is both clinical evidence of hemolysis and serologic findings consistent with the administration of an incompatible transfusion.

2.2.1. Delayed Serologic Transfusion Reactions

DSTRs are characterized by the development of a RBC alloantibody following transfusion that was not present prior to transfusion. The presence of a new allo-antibody may result in a positive DAT *(8,9)*. There may be a previous history of pregnancy and/or transfusion. No clinical or laboratory evidence of hemolysis is present in DSTRs.

2.2.1.1. PATHOGENESIS

DSTRs may be the result of primary alloimmunization or may be due to an anamnestic response in a previously exposed patient. The antibodies are usually of the IgG class. The DAT demonstrates IgG, with or without complement, on the surface of the RBCs. Complement can rarely be demonstrated in the absence of IgG. Antibody formation, and hence the development of a positive DAT, usually occurs within 3–7 d following the administration of RBCs in the case of an anamnestic response. Antibody formation may take as long as 2 wk to several months in the case of primary alloimmunization. These reactions are often not initially detected until weeks to months after the original transfusion, when another blood specimen is received in the blood bank for testing prior to additional transfusion of the patient.

Almost any antigen can be involved in the development of DSTR; however, the E antigen is the most common offender. Two, or rarely more, antigens in combination can also cause a DSTR.

2.2.1.2. SIGNS AND SYMPTOMS

Patients undergoing a DSTR are asymptomatic, with the only evidence of a reaction being the development of a new alloantibody and possibly a positive DAT, which can be present for several months.

2.2.1.3. MANAGEMENT

When a DSTR is first suspected, a workup for hemolysis should be initiated. The details of this evaluation are described. The patient's clinical physician should be informed so that he or she can monitor the patient for evidence of hemolysis. It should be emphasized that these patients do not need to be treated. Whenever possible, the patient should be informed that he or she has developed an antibody that may potentially make it more difficult to find compatible blood for future transfusions. Some institutions give the patient an antibody identification card to carry at all times and instruct him or her to present this card whenever admitted to a hospital.

Additional transfusions, if needed, are not contraindicated in patients with DSTRs, as long as blood lacking the offending antigen is given. Any patient who has developed an alloantibody should always receive RBCs that are negative for the corresponding antigen, even if the antibody can no longer be demonstrated in the patient's serum, because a more serious hemolytic transfusion reaction can occur if the patient is given additional incompatible blood. Kidd antibodies, in particular, are notorious for disappearing, only to return rapidly and cause massive hemolysis upon reexposure to the Kidd antigen. Therefore, blood bank records should always be checked for a history of alloantibodies prior to transfusion.

2.2.2. Delayed Hemolytic Transfusion Reactions

DHTRs have all of the characteristics of DSTRs with the exception that they are, by definition, accompanied by clinical and/or laboratory evidence of hemolysis. DHTRs are virtually always the result of an anamnestic response and usually occur within 3–7 d following transfusion. The most common antigens involved are in the Kidd, Duffy, Kell, and Rh systems.

2.2.2.1. SIGNS AND SYMPTOMS

The reactions are almost always of a benign nature and in fact, are usually asymptomatic. The most common signs and symptoms seen are fever, anemia, hyperbilirubinemia, and jaundice. Although there have been rare reports of renal failure, DIC, and even death *(9)* attributed to DHTRs, we feel that severe reactions are so rare that they are probably worthy of a case report.

2.2.2.2. PATHOGENESIS

Why the development of antibody results in hemolysis in some situations but not others is not entirely understood. The fact that the vast majority of these reactions are asymptomatic is probably due to the slow rate of hemolysis as compared to AHTRs. It is known that symptomatic reactions are more likely to occur with antibodies which activate complement. On the other hand, the strength of the positive DAT does not correlate with the presence or degree of hemolysis.

2.2.2.3. MANAGEMENT

As with DSTRs, both the clinician and the patient need to be informed of the reaction. Informing the clinical physician is particularly important, since the knowledge that the patient is hemolyzing will provide an explanation for the falling hematocrit and may prevent an unnecessary workup for occult blood loss. The patient needs to be evaluated for evidence of hemolysis, which includes a positive DAT, decreased Hgb, decreased haptoglobin, and increased indirect bilirubin. Reticulocytosis and microspherocytes on peripheral smear can also be evidence of hemolysis.

The need for additional transfusions to replace hemolyzed RBCs should be evaluated on a case-by-case basis. It is usually safe to transfuse these patients as long as compatible blood can be found. It is important that all future transfusions should be with RBCs that are negative for the antigen that corresponds to the newly developed alloantibody.

3. NONHEMOLYTIC TRANSFUSION REACTIONS

3.1. Allergic Reactions

Allergic reactions are one of the most common complications of transfusion and typically consist of urticaria and itching. More severe anaphylactic reactions are seen only rarely.

3.1.1. Urticarial Reactions

Urticaria during a transfusion is usually caused by an allergic reaction to plasma proteins. These reactions are markedly reduced when plasma proteins are removed by washing RBCs with saline *(10)*. However, administration of an antihistamine 30 min prior to transfusion is a much more economical form of prevention.

If hives are the only sign of a reaction and no fever is present, it is not necessary to perform a laboratory workup for possible hemolysis. The transfusion should be stopped and an antihistamine administered. If the patient responds to treatment, the transfusion can be restarted. We recommend that urticarial reactions are the only type of transfusion reaction in which restarting the unit is permissible.

3.1.2. Anaphylactic Reactions

These reactions are seen in patients with IgA deficiency who form anti-IgA antibodies when transfused with plasma or plasma-containing blood components. Re-exposure to IgA can result in anaphylaxis that can be severe. In fact, fatal reactions have been reported *(11)*. IgA deficiency is present in about 1 in 700 individuals; however, not everyone who is IgA deficient will form anti-IgA antibodies and IgA-mediated anaphylaxis is actually an extremely rare phenomenon.

Vyas et al. *(12)* divided patients with anti-IgA antibodies into two groups. The first group consists of IgA deficient patients who form class specific antibodies and develop anaphylaxis in response to plasma-containing components. The second group has normal IgA levels and forms anti-IgA antibodies of limited specificity. The significance of antibodies with limited specificity is not completely understood.

3.1.2.1. SIGNS AND SYMPTOMS

Patients with class specific anti-IgA antibodies may experience circulatory collapse and respiratory distress associated with wheezing when exposed to plasma. A significant negative finding is that they do not have fever, which is of great help in differentiating anaphylaxis from AHTRs.

3.1.2.2. DIAGNOSIS

The diagnosis is made utilizing a two-step process. First, a sample of the patient's serum is tested for IgA concentration. If the patient has absent IgA he/she should then be tested for antibodies to IgA, which need to be demonstrated for definitive diagnosis of this disorder.

3.1.2.3. MANAGEMENT

Subcutaneous epinephrine is the treatment of choice for most anaphylactic reactions. Severe cases should be treated in an intensive care unit, utilizing more aggressive therapies.

Any IgA deficient patient who has experienced an anaphylactic reaction should not receive blood components containing IgA. These patients can receive any compatible unit of allogeneic packed RBCs as long the unit is either doubled washed or previously frozen and then deglycerolized to remove as much plasma as possible prior to transfusion. For patients requiring plasma transfusions, plasma from IgA-deficient donors can be obtained through rare donor registries. Albumin, plasma protein fraction, and most immunoglobulin preparations contain IgA proteins and should not be used in IgA-deficient patients.

3.2. Fluid Overload

Congestive heart failure (CHF) can potentially occur in any patient who is transfused too rapidly. However, children with small blood volumes and individuals with underlying cardiac disease are more prone to developing CHF secondary to transfusion.

3.2.1. Signs and Symptoms

Patients with fluid overload can experience respiratory distress, particularly while in a supine position. Other signs and symptoms can include low-grade fever, headache, and hypertension. In severe reactions evidence of frank pulmonary edema can develop. This type of reaction typically begins during or shortly after transfusion.

3.2.2. Management

When symptoms occur, the transfusion should be stopped, the patient should be placed in an upright position, and given oxygen by mask. Intravenous diuretics should be administered if there is significant evidence of CHF.

These reactions are not often seen by blood bankers, because they are usually underreported due to the fact that clinicians are quite comfortable with both their diagnosis and management. It should be emphasized, however, that these reactions can be quite severe if pulmonary edema develops, and can ultimately be fatal.

3.2.3. Prevention

We feel that fluid overload can be prevented in most patients if two simple rules of thumb are followed. First, whole blood should not be administered to patients who are not bleeding. Packed RBCs are a much more efficient way to increase Hgb than is whole blood, and their use is much less likely to result in fluid overload. Second, nonbleeding patients should not receive more than 2 U of packed RBCs in a 24-h period. This rule may be somewhat difficult to adhere to in these days of cost containment, particularly with increased pressures to treat patients quickly and release them from the hospital or to treat in an outpatient setting.

Patients with borderline cardiac function can usually tolerate transfusion of a unit of RBCs if it is administered over a 6-h period. Patients with frank CHF who need to be transfused may need to receive RBCs at an even slower rate. This can be accomplished by dividing a unit of RBCs and transfusing each half of the unit over a 6-h period.

3.3. Transfusion-Related Acute Lung Injury (TRALI)

TRALI, which is also known as noncardiogenic pulmonary edema, is thought to occur secondary to accumulation of antibody-coated leukocytes in the pulmonary microvasculature.

3.3.1. Signs and Symptoms

The most common presentation is the development of respiratory distress with difficulty breathing, hypoxia, hypotension, fever, pulmonary edema, and bilateral infiltrates on chest X-ray within a few hours of transfusion. Some patients initially present with a more mild respiratory distress shortly after transfusion, which is followed by clearing of symptoms within a few hours. Marked respiratory distress can then present about 24–48 h posttransfusion. This latter group of patients can be misdiagnosed because they do not display the classic presentation of TRALI. The respiratory distress typically improves within 3–7 d following the transfusion. The infiltrates on chest X-ray generally take a few days longer to resolve.

3.3.2. Pathogenesis

The pathogenesis of TRALI is thought to be related to increased vascular permeability in the lungs as a result of cytokine production secondary to the accumulation of antibody-coated leukocytes in the pulmonary microvasculature. The increased vascular permeability leads to exudation of fluid into the alveoli resulting in pulmonary edema *(13)*. Seeger and associates *(14)* developed an ex vivo model of TRALI using rabbit lung. When the rabbit lungs were perfused with albumin containing neutrophils, antineutrophil antibodies, and rabbit plasma as a source of complement, there was a marked increase in vascular permeability that began approx 3 h after perfusion and became quite marked at 6 h. The time course of the increased vascular permeability seen in this model is similar to that seen in patients experiencing a TRALI reaction.

Literature reports demonstrate two scenarios for the development of TRALI. In the first type the patient has preformed antibodies that react to donor leukocytes. In the second type, donor plasma contains antibodies that react with recipient WBCs. Both antibodies to HLA antigens and neutrophils have been implicated in TRALI reactions.

3.3.3. Diagnosis and Prevention

In our experience, the laboratory diagnosis of TRALI is not always an easy one to make. This is because not all patients with anti-HLA or antineutrophil antibodies develop TRALI. Conversely, these antibodies cannot be demonstrated in all patients with clear-cut clinical evidence of TRALI. For these reasons, we feel the diagnosis is primarily a clinical one and that all patients who develop respiratory compromise without signs of CHF, following a transfusion, should be treated as if they have TRALI. The search for antibodies in the recipient and/or the donor would take place after the fact and should take no part in treatment decisions. We recommend that any patient who has developed TRALI should be restricted to leukocyte-reduced blood components.

3.3.4. Management

Patients with TRALI need to be distinguished clinically from those with pulmonary edema secondary to CHF. The important distinction between the two conditions is that patients with TRALI are normovolemic and will have a normal pulmonary capillary wedge pressure on right heart catheterization. This difference is of great significance because diuretic therapy, which is the mainstay of treatment for fluid overload, can result in severe hypotension in patients with TRALI *(15)*. Therefore, the hemodynamic status of patients with posttransfusion respiratory distress should be carefully monitored. Transfer to an intensive care unit should be strongly considered for patients thought to be suffering a TRALI reaction. The treatment of choice for these patients is aggressive respiratory support, with administration of oxygen and possible intubation with mechanical ventilation.

3.4. Nonhemolytic Febrile Transfusion Reactions (NHFTR)

3.4.1. Signs and Symptoms

NHFTRs are the most common reactions reported to the blood bank and present as fever, associated with transfusion, that cannot be explained by other causes. The fever is often accompanied by other signs and symptoms including: chills, respiratory distress, anxiety, and alterations of blood pressure. These reactions usually occur during or within 2 h following transfusion.

3.4.2. Pathogenesis

Classically NHFTRs have been attributed to the formation of antibodies to donor WBCs in patients who were either multiply transfused or multiparous. These leukocyte antibodies can result in NHFTRs when incompatible WBCs are administered as part of a transfusion. Perkins and colleagues *(16)* demonstrated that at least 0.25×10^9 incompatible WBCs must be present in a transfusion to produce a NHFTR. Therefore, transfusion of components with fewer WBCs can be utilized to decrease the likelihood of a NHFTR. Goldfinger and Lowe *(10)* showed that the incidence of NHFTRs is markedly decreased when saline-washed RBCs that contain both reduced plasma volume and numbers of WBCs, are administered. In addition, leukocyte reduction via filtration has been shown to decrease the incidence of NHFTRs.

More recently, another possible pathogenetic mechanism has been postulated to explain some of these reactions. Cytokines, which are produced by WBCs, can accumulate during storage of RBC units. These cytokines are thought to cause a febrile reaction in the recipient when the RBCs are administered. The accumulation of cytokine in a unit of RBCs can be prevented by leuko-reduction of RBCs following collection and prior to storage. Further clinical studies will be required to clarify the role, if any, of passively administered cytokines in NHFTRs.

3.4.3. Diagnosis

NHFTRs can clinically mimic AHTRs or transfusion of bacterially contaminated RBCs. Thus, the transfusion should always be stopped and a workup for incompatibility should be performed if a patient experiences a febrile reaction during transfusion. Since fever is often present in patients sick enough to require a transfusion, other etiologies such as sepsis must be ruled out as the cause of the temperature elevation. However, a definitive etiology for a febrile episode during administration of RBCs cannot always be established.

3.4.4. Management

Conventional wisdom has mandated that the remainder of the unit of RBCs should never be transfused in a patient who has experienced a NHFTR *(17)*. Recently, some authors have advocated resuming the transfusion if the posttransfusion workup is negative for incompatibility and the patient defervesces with antipyretics *(18)*. The major advantage to restarting the unit of RBCs is that it will potentially decrease donor exposure. The major drawback to resuming transfusion is that the patient will receive more of whatever was causing the febrile reaction. The biggest concern in this regard is that a patient could receive more of a unit of RBCs with bacterial contamination.

We feel that the transfusion should not be restarted in a patient who has suffered a NHFTR, because the logistical problems involved in performing the workup, restarting the transfusion, and administering the remaining RBCs in a timely manner are insurmountable in most hospitals. In addition, the majority of NHFTRs occur after most or all of the component in question has been transfused. This means that the recipient has received most of the therapeutic benefit of the transfusion. Last, additional transfusion of a unit of RBCs that contains bacteria could have disastrous consequences.

3.4.5. Prevention

Leukocyte reduction of RBCs greatly decreases the incidence of NHFTRs. The most efficient means of prevention is with the current, third generation, leukocyte removal filters that decrease the number of WBCs present in a filtered component by 99.9–99.99%, leaving less than 5×10^6 WBCs in a unit of RBCs. Saline washing of RBCs is less effective and only removes approx 90% of the WBCs.

Patients who are chronic transfusion recipients are at great risk of developing NHFTRs. These patients should probably receive leukocyte-reduced blood components as soon as it is evident that they will become transfusion-dependent.

Another use for leukocyte reduction is to prevent alloimmunization to human leukocyte antigen (HLA) or other WBC antigens in patients who will also require platelet transfusions. These patients often become alloimmunized to HLA antigens and thus become refractory to transfusion of random platelets. It can then become very difficult and expensive to find compatible platelets for these patients because they will often only respond to crossmatched or HLA-matched platelets. Some centers routinely leuko-reduce all components, including RBCs, prophylactically to prevent alloimmunization. This practice remains controversial, but if proven effective, could be cost effective.

Patients who have unquestionably experienced a true NHFTR should receive leukocyte-reduced blood components for future transfusions. However, since the diagnosis is not always without question, and the majority of patients who develop a fever associated with transfusion will not experience a NHFTR with subsequent transfusions, we recommend that patients who are not likely to be chronic transfusion recipients should be restricted to leukocyte-reduced components only after they have experienced two suspected febrile reactions.

3.5. Septic Transfusion Reactions

Septic transfusion reactions are a severe complication of transfusion. Strict adherence to protocols designed to maintain sterility have made bacterial contamination of RBC units a rarity. When RBCs are contaminated, it is usually the result of asymptomatic bacteremia in the donor or contamination at the venipuncture site. Gram-negative organisms, particularly *Yersinia enterocolitica,* that are able to grow at storage temperatures of 4°C are usually the offending agents *(19).*

3.5.1. Signs and Symptoms

The signs and symptoms of a septic transfusion reaction can be very similar to those of an AHTR. The reaction usually begins after the administration of only a small amount of RBCs and is often quite severe. The most common associated findings are shock and high fever, although DIC, renal failure, and hemoglobinuria can be seen. The occasional presence of gastrointestinal symptoms, including abdominal cramping and diarrhea can help distinguish these reactions from AHTRs.

3.5.2. Management

The transfusion should be halted as soon as a reaction is suspected and treatment should begin immediately. For all but the mildest reactions, treatment is probably best provided in a critical care setting. Blood pressure should be maintained with iv fluids and pressor support if needed. Empiric therapy with broad spectrum antibiotics should be started before culture results are complete.

3.5.3. Diagnosis

Definitive diagnosis can only be made by culturing the same organism from both the unit of RBCs and the patient's blood stream. The specimen for culture should be taken from the blood remaining in the bag itself, not from a segment, because cultures from segments are likely to give false negative results *(19)*. A Gram stain of the RBC unit can provide a presumptive diagnosis and aid in determining which antibiotics are likely to provide the most effective therapy.

3.5.4. Prevention

Prevention is best accomplished by maintaining sterility during procurement and storage of RBCs, carefully screening donors for potential sources of bacteremia and examining all RBC units for clotting, change in color, and gas bubble formation prior to release from the blood bank.

3.6. Premedication

Febrile and allergic reactions, although often thought of as benign, can be quite uncomfortable and frightening for the transfusion recipient. In addition, the presence of fever can result in an unnecessary workup for infection, which can result in the patient's being cultured and treated with antibiotics. For these reasons, many physicians routinely premedicate transfusion recipients with an antihistamine and an antipyretic. In addition to sparing the patient the symptoms of the reaction, premedication can decrease costs by preventing the loss of blood components due to disposal of the remaining portion of a unit of RBCs after a reaction has developed.

The one drawback to premedication is that antipyretics can potentially mask the febrile component of an AHTR. However, it seems unlikely that an antipyretic would be able to entirely block the febrile response associated with an AHTR. Thus, we feel that premedication of a transfusion recipient poses little risk to most patients. On the other hand, it can result in both increased patient comfort and significant monetary savings both in reduced blood costs and in prevention of unneeded workups for infection.

REFERENCES

1. Capon SM, Goldfinger D. Acute hemolytic transfusion reaction, a paradigm of the systemic inflammatory response: new insights into pathophysiology and treatment. *Transfusion* 1995;35:513–520.
2. Rock RC, Bove JR, Nemerson Y. Heparin treatment of intravascular coagulation accompanying hemolytic transfusion reactions. *Transfusion* 1969;9:57–61.
3. Sazama K. Reports of 355 transfusion-associated deaths: 1976 through 1985. *Transfusion* 1990;30:583–590.
4. Davenport RD, Streiter RM, Kunkel SL. Red cell ABO incompatibility and production of tumour necrosis factor-alpha. *Br J Haematol* 1991;78:540–544.

5. Friedman DF, Kim HC, Manno CS. Hyperhemolysis associated with red cell transfusion in sickle cell disease. *Transfusion* 1993;33:14S.
6. Cullis JO, Win N, Dudley JM, Kaye T. Post-transfusion hyperhaemolysis in a patient with sickle cell disease: use of steroids and intravenous immunoglobulin to prevent further red cell destruction. *Vox Sanguinis* 1995;69:355–357.
7. International Committee for Standardization in Haematology: recommended methods for radioisotope red cell survival studies. *Br J Haematol* 1980;45:659.
8. Ness PM, Shirey RS, Thoman SK, Buck SA. The differentiation of delayed serologic and delayed hemolytic transfusion reactions: incidence, long-term serologic findings, and clinical significance. *Transfusion* 1990;30:688–693.
9. Pineda AA, Taswell HF, Brzica SM. Delayed hemolytic transfusion reaction. An immunologic hazard of blood transfusion. *Transfusion* 1978;18:1–7.
10. Goldfinger D, Lowe C. Prevention of adverse reactions to blood transfusion by the administration of saline-washed red blood cells. *Transfusion* 1981;21:277–280.
11. Pineda AA, Taswell HF. Transfusion reactions associated with Anti-IgA antibodies: report of four cases and review of the literature. *Transfusion* 1975;15:10–15.
12. Vyas GN, Perkins HA, Fudenberg HH. Anaphylactiod transfusion reactions associated with anti-IgA. *Lancet* 1968;1:312–315.
13. Popovsky MA, Moore SB. Diagnostic and pathogenetic considerations in transfusion-related acute lung injury. *Transfusion* 1985;25:573–577.
14. Seeger W, Schneider U, Kreusler B, Witzleben E, Walmrath D, Grimminger F, Neppert J. Reproduction of transfusion-related acute lung injury in an ex vivo lung model. *Blood* 1990;76:1438–1444.
15. Levy GJ, Shabot MM, Hart ME, Mya WW, Goldfinger D. Transfusion-associated noncardiogenic pulmonary edema. Report of a case and a warning regarding treatment. *Transfusion* 1986;26:278–281.
16. Perkins HA, Payne R, Ferguson J. Non-hemolytic febrile transfusion reactions. *Vox Sanguinis* 1966;11:578–600.
17. Widmann FK. Controversies in transfusion medicine: Should a febrile transfusion response occasion the return of the blood component to the blood bank? Pro. *Transfusion* 1994;34:356–358.
18. Oberman HA. Controversies in transfusion medicine: should a febrile transfusion response occasion the return of the blood component to the blood bank? Con. *Transfusion* 1994;34:353–355.
19. Yersinia enterocolitica bacteremia and endotoxin shock associated with red blood cell transfusions—United States, 1991. *MMWR* 1991;40:176–178.

14

Clinical and Laboratory Impact
of Blood Group Antigens and Antibodies

Beat M. Frey and Marion E. Reid

1. INTRODUCTION

The purpose of this chapter is to consider the impact of blood group antigens and antibodies on the practice of transfusion medicine. We describe erythrocyte blood group antigens, explain how antibodies that react with these antigens are detected and identified and describe how suitable blood is selected for transfusion. We summarize cases in which blood group antigens are associated with changes in red blood cell (RBC) morphology, disease susceptibility, and differential diagnosis. We conclude with an overview of how recent advances in biosciences impact on modern transfusion practice.

2. BLOOD GROUP ANTIGENS

Erythrocyte blood group antigens are polymorphic, inherited, structural characteristics on proteins, glycoproteins, or glycolipids on the RBC membrane exofacial surface. The polymorphism of blood group antigens has been used to monitor in vivo survival of transfused RBCs, and in genetic, forensic, and anthropological investigations. More recently, blood group antigens have contributed to our current understanding of cell membrane structure (Fig. 1).

A working party on terminology for red cell surface antigens, sanctioned by the International Society for Blood Transfusion (ISBT) has placed blood group antigens into four categories: systems, collections, low-incidence antigen series, and high-incidence antigen series (*see* Table 1) *(1)*. A blood group system consists of one or more antigens controlled by a single gene, or by very closely linked homologous genes. A collection consists of serologically, biochemically, or genetically related antigens that do not fit the criteria for a system status. The low-incidence and high-incidence antigen series contain infrequent and common antigens, respectively, which cannot be included in a system or collection. Of the 254 recognized antigens, 194 have been placed into the 23 blood group systems, 11 into the five collections, 37 in the low series, and 12 in the high series.

From: *Red Cell Transfusion: A Practical Guide*
Edited by: M. E. Reid and S. J. Nance Humana Press Inc., Totowa, NJ

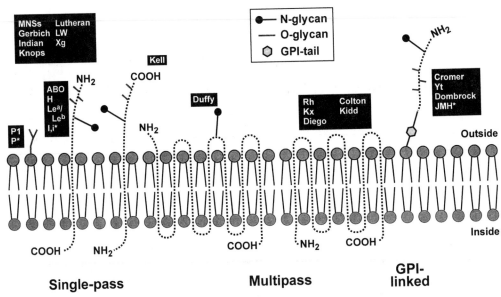

Fig. 1. Model of RBC membrane components carrying antigens.

3. BLOOD GROUP ALLOANTIBODIES

A blood group antigen has no immediate untoward effect on blood transfusion. It is the corresponding antibody that has clinical relevance and dictates the need for pretransfusion testing. The detection and identification of blood group antibodies has contributed significantly to the safe supportive blood transfusion practices used today. Blood group antibodies are clinically important in the immune destruction of RBCs in incompatible allogeneic blood transfusions, maternofetal blood group incompatibility, autoimmune hemolytic anemia, and organ transplantation.

In human blood grouping, most tests involve hemagglutination techniques in which clumping of the RBCs in different test phases serves as the detectable endpoint. The first blood group antigens to be identified were those to which antibodies agglutinated antigen-positive RBCs in a saline medium. These antibodies have since been shown usually to be IgM and to detect carbohydrate antigens, including A, B, P1, Le^a, Le^b, H, and I.

3.1. Clinical Significance of Alloantibodies

By definition, clinically significant antibodies cause an adverse reaction on transfusion of incompatible blood. In contrast, clinically insignificant antibodies manifest themselves during immunohematological testing and can be a confounding factor, but they usually cause no adverse reaction if incompatible blood is transfused.

After introduction of the indirect antiglobulin test (IAT) in 1945 *(2)*, it was possible to detect IgG antibodies, most of which react with protein antigens: These include antigens of the Rh, Kell, Duffy, Kidd, Lutheran, and Diego blood group systems. The antiglobulin test is also used as a "direct" test to demonstrate antibodies that have attached to RBCs in vivo, e.g., in the investigation of transfusion reactions, hemolytic disease of the newborn (HDN), and autoimmune hemolytic anemia (AIHA).

Table 1
Blood Group Systems and Collections with Associated Antigens
as Assigned by the ISBT and Listed in Alphabetical Order *(1)*

System name	Symbol	Associated antigens
Blood group systems		
ABO	ABO	A, B, A,B, A_1
Chido/Rodgers	CH/RG	CH1, CH2, CH3, CH4, CH5, CH6, WH, RG1, RG2
Colton	CO	Co^a, Co^b, Co3
Cromer	CROM	Cr^a, Tc^a, Tc^b, Tc^c, Dr^a, Es^a, IFC, WES^a, WES^b, UMC
Diego	DI	Di^a, Di^b, Wr^a, Wr^b
Dombrock	DO	Do^a, Do^b, Gy^a, Hy, Jo^a
Duffy	FY	Fy^a, Fy^b, Fy3, Fy4, Fy5, Fy6
Gerbich	GE	Ge2, Ge3, Ge4, Wb, Ls^a, An^a, Dh^a
Hh	H	H
Indian	IN	In^a, In^b
Kell	KEL	K, k, Kp^a, Kp^b, Kp^c, Ku, Js^a, Js^b, Ul^a, K11, K12, K13, + 9 others
Kidd	JK	Jk^a, Jk^b, Jk3
Knops	KN	Kn^a, Kn^b, McC^a, Sl^a, Yk^a
Landsteiner-Weiner	LW	LW^a, LW^{ab}, LW^b
Lewis	LE	Le^a, Le^b, Le^{ab}
Lutheran	LU	Lu^a, Lu^b, Lu3, Lu4, Lu5, Lu6, Lu7, Lu8, Lu9, Lu11, Lu12, + 7 others
MNS	MNS	M, N, S, s, U, He, Vw, Hut, Hil, M^g, Mur, St^a, Dantu, + 25 others
P	P1	P_1
Rh	RH	D, C, E, c, e, f, Ce, C^W, C^X, V, G, hr^B, hr^S, VS, CE, cE, + 28 others
Scianna	SC	Sc1, Sc2, Sc3
Yt	YT	Yt^a, Yt^b
Xy	XG	Xg^a
Kx	XK	Kx
Blood group collections		
Cost	COST	Cs^a, Cs^b
Er	ER	Er^a, Er^b
Globoside	GLOB	P, P^k, LKE
Ii	I	I, i
Unnamed		Le^c, Le^d
Low series		By, Sw^a, Bi, Bx^a, Tr^a, Bp^a, Wu, Jn^a, Rd, To^a, Pt^a, Mo^a + 25 others
High series		Vel, Lan, At^a, Jr^a, Ok^a, JMH, Emm, AnWj, MER2, Sd^a, Duclos, PEL

Antibodies recognizing antigens in the ABO blood group system are by far the most clinically significant. Other antibodies generally considered to be potentially clinically significant occur in the following order of frequency: anti-D, anti-K, anti-E, anti-C, anti-Fy^a, anti-c, anti-Jk^a, anti-S, anti-Jk^b *(3–5)*. In the United States, other clinically significant antibodies are found with an incidence of < 1% *(3–5)*. For a

Table 2
The Clinical Significance of Selected Alloantibodies to Blood Group Antigens *(43)*

Usually clinically significant	Sometimes clinically significant	Clinically insignificant if not reactive at 37°C	Clinically insignificant
ABO	Colton	A_1	Bg
Diego	Cromer	H	Chido/Rodgers
Duffy	Dombrock	I	Cost
Kell	Gerbich	Le^a	JMH
Kidd	Indian	Lutheran	Knops
P	Lan	M,N	Le^b
Rh	Landsteiner-Weiner	P1	Xg^a
Vel	S,s,U	Sd^a	
	Scianna		
	Yt		

summary of the clinical significance of some alloantibodies, *see* Table 2. Interested readers are referred to references *(3,4,6–8)*. Exceptions can always occur and it is important to evaluate each patient individually.

If an antibody to a low-incidence antigen is detected during crossmatching, it need not be identified in order to locate antigen-negative blood; another unit of donor blood from the stock supply is unlikely to be positive for the same uncommon antigen and will, therefore, be compatible with the patient's serum. In contrast, if an antibody to an uncommon antigen is detected during prenatal testing, its identification can be useful in predicting the likelihood and severity of HDN. Blood for exchange transfusion will not be hard to find. On the other hand, if a patient's serum contains an antibody to a high-incidence antigen, irrespective of whether the investigation is for transfusion purposes or prediction of HDN, it should be identified. This will aid both in the assessment of its clinical significance and in the location of appropriate blood for transfusion.

3.1.1. Approach to Antibody Identification

After an antibody has been detected by pretransfusion testing, we advise that its specificity be identified in order to assess its potential clinical significance. Tables 3–5 highlight some factors that influence the approach and extent of a serological workup. Table 6 summarizes the value of treating reagent RBCs with enzymes or dithiothreitol (DTT) in antibody identification. Figure 2 outlines the routine approach for antibody identification used in the Immunohematology Reference Laboratory of the New York Blood Center (NYBC).

3.1.2. Assessment of Clinical Significance of Antibody

Many alloantibodies detected in vitro do not induce in vivo destruction of incompatible RBCs. Even today, there is no technical procedure that reliably differentiates between clinically significant and insignificant antibodies. However, the following in vitro features can be used to predict the potential clinical importance of a particular antibody:

Table 3
Influencing Factors for Immunohematological Workup

Factor	Aspect
Clinical Situation	Life-threatening
	Urgent
	Elective
Primary purpose	Patient care
	Education
	Publication
Laboratory Level	Transfusion service
	Teaching facility
	Reference facility
	Research facility
Reason for transfusion	Acute
	Chronic
Resources	Reagents
	Equipment
	Techniques
	Staff available
	Experience
Economy	Direct and indirect costs
	Third-party payer versus direct patient billing

Table 4
Informative Predictors for Approaching Immunohematology Workups

Predictor	Considerations
Patient demographics	Clinical diagnosis, age, sex, ethnicity, history of transfusion and pregnancy, drugs, IV fluids (Ringer's lactate, IV-IgG, ALG, ATG), infections, malignancies, hemoglobinopathies, bone marrow transplantation
Initial serological results	ABO, Rh, DAT, phenotype, antibody detection (screen) results, autogeneic control, crossmatch results
Hematology/chemistry values	Hemoglobin, hematocrit, bilirubin, LDH, reticulocyte count, haptoglobin, hemoglobinuria, albumin:globulin ratio, RBC morphology
Sample characteristics	Site and technique of collection, age of sample, anticoagulant, visual hemolysis, lipemic
Other	Check records in current and previous institutions for identified antibody(ies) and history of transfusion reactions or HDN
Follow-up serological testing (antibody identification)	Phase of reactivity, reaction temperature, thermal amplitude, potentiator (saline, albumin, LISS, PEG), reaction strength, effect of chemicals on antigen (proteases, thio reagents), pattern of reactivity (single antibody or mixture of antibodies), characteristics of reactivity (mixed field, rouleaux), hemolysis, preservatives/antibiotics in reagents. See flow chart Fig. 2.

Table 5
Time Schedule for Testing and Selection of RBC Products
for Transfusion to Patients with Alloantibodies

Type of order	Time schedule for testing	Selection of RBC products*
Life-threatening	< 1 h	O D−, O D+, type-specific
Urgent	Within hours	Type-specific, XM compatible, antigen-negative if time allows
Elective	Within days	Type-specific, XM compatible, antigen-negative

*XM, crossmatch.

Table 6
Patterns of Reactivity After Treatment of RBCs with Ficin,
Papain, or DTT and Possible Antibody Specificity

Ficin/papain	DTT (200 mM)	Possible specificity
Nonreactive	Reactive	M,N,S,s*; Ge2,Ge4; Xg^a; Fy^a,Fy^b; Ch/Rg
Nonreactive	Nonreactive	Indian; JMH
Reactive	Weakly reactive	Cromer; Knops (weak in ficin); Lutheran; Dombrock; AnWj
Variable	Nonreactive	Yt^a
Reactive	Nonreactive	Kell; LW; Scianna
Reactive	Reactive	A,B; H; P1; Rh; Lewis; Kidd; Fy3; Diego; Co; Ge3; I,i; P, At^a; Cs^a; Er^a; Jr^a; Lan; Ok^a; Vel; Sd^a; PEL
Reactive	Reactive (Enhanced)	Kx

*s is variable with ficin/papain.

1. Reports of transfusion reactions caused by the same antibody specificity in other patients.
2. IgG antibodies are more likely to be harmful than IgM antibodies (main exception: antibodies in the ABO system). IgG subclasses are generally not predictive.
3. IAT-reacting antibodies are more likely to be significant than direct agglutinins.
4. High-titer antibodies are more likely to be pathogenic than low-titer antibodies.
5. Antibodies causing in vitro hemolysis are likely to be clinically significant.
6. The higher the thermal amplitude of an IgM antibody in vitro, the more likely it is to be clinically significant. If an antibody is active at room temperature or below, there is no need to identify it or to transfuse antigen-negative blood. A useful and simple test to predict the clinical significance of autoantibodies is to test, in a prewarm system, a patient's serum with antigen-positive RBCs in albumin at 30°C *(9)*.
7. Specialized tests such as the monocyte monolayer assay (MMA), antibody-dependent cellular cytotoxicity (ADCC) assay, and chemiluminescence test (CLT) may indicate the clinical significance of an antibody. However, such tests are technically demanding and should be performed only in a laboratory with adequate experience in performing them. The MMA measures phagocytosis and rosetting of sensitized RBCs, the ADCC assay measures lysis of sensitized RBCs, and the CLT measures the metabolic response of monocytes during erythrophagocytosis *(10)*.

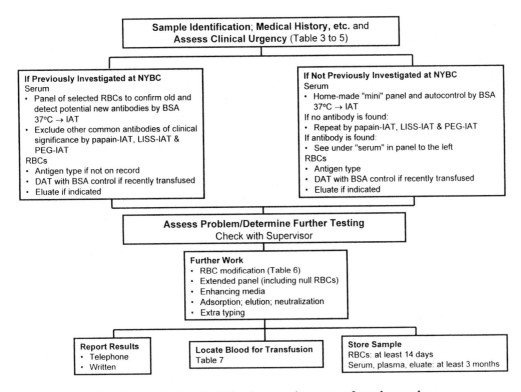

Fig. 2. Antibody identification workup on referred samples.

3.1.3. Factors that Influence the Extent of an Immunohematology Workup

The extent of an immunohematological workup is influenced by a variety of factors and the decision of which tests should be performed has to be individualized. Tables 3 and 5 summarize some relevant considerations and resulting consequences for the workup. Clearly, clinical aspects are most important as illustrated by the fact that in cases with acute transfusion needs it is not necessary to undertake sophisticated compatibility tests to obtain maximal RBC in vivo survival. However, in cases with chronic transfusion needs, the opposite is true: In order to reduce costs and risks for the patient, it is important to perform testing that allows selection of RBC units that have an optimal in vivo survival.

3.1.4. RBC Transfusion in the Presence of RBC Autoantibodies

Serum from some patients contains autoantibodies that recognize antigenic determinants on the patient's own RBCs and on RBCs from the majority of donors. Instances in which this may arise include AIHA, cold hemagglutinin disease, and paroxysmal cold hemoglobinuria. Autoantibodies may make it impossible to locate compatible blood and the patient's physicians may be asked by the transfusion service staff to sign for release of the incompatible blood. Transfusion of such blood (if clinically indicated) should not worsen the autoimmune process but may have a shortened in vivo RBC survival as is the case for the patient's own RBCs. The presence of autoantibodies complicates the detection and identification of underlying alloantibodies.

Table 7
Strategies for Localization of RBC Products for Transfusion

Antigen-negative RBC requirements of recipient	Source of RBC product
Not needed	Hospital transfusion service stocks Donor center stocks
Needed	
Antigen-negative incidence of > 1 in 200 (single or multiple antibodies	Screen hospital transfusion service stocks Screen donor center stocks
Antigen-negative incidence of < 1 in 200 (single or multiple antibodies)	Screen donor center stocks Use frozen blood from donor center Call in known antigen-negative donors by donor center Patient's siblings (and family) Rare donor registry Autogeneic

3.2. Locating RBC Products for Transfusion

Once a potentially clinically significant antibody has been identified, the patient must be transfused with antigen-negative RBCs for life. Neonates with passively acquired maternal antibodies are not actively immunized and, thus need to be transfused with antigen-negative RBCs only while the mother's antibody is still present in their serum (3–6 mo).

Selection of blood for transfusion to patients with blood group alloantibodies is the joint responsibility of the hospital transfusion service and the donor blood center (Table 7). If antigen-negative blood is indicated for transfusion, available donor units in the transfusion service should be tested first. If no antigen-negative units are found or the antibody(ies) present are such that it will be difficult to locate units, blood can be ordered from the donor center where usually a larger pool of donor blood is available for screening. It is important that the transfusion service staff communicate with the patient's physician to determine the predicted needs of the patient and with the donor center staff to insure that the needed blood is available for the patient. On the rare occasions when antigen-negative blood is not available locally, national and international rare donor registries can be accessed through the donor center.

If a patient has multiple alloantibodies, the number of units to be tested to locate one unit of compatible blood can be calculated by multiplying the incidence of antigen-negative donors for each antibody. For example, a patient has anti-S and anti-Jk^a. Compatible donors must be negative for S and Jk^a antigens. The incidence of S– and Jk(a–) donors in the general donor pool is, respectively, approx 0.45 and 0.25. If type-specific RBCs are selected, the incidence of compatible donors is $(0.45)(0.25) = 0.11$ or 1 in 9 *(6)*.

It has been suggested that patients who are expected to receive chronic transfusion therapy (sickle cell disease; thalassemia) should receive antigen-matched blood to prevent immunization. This practice should be a joint decision among the clinician, transfusion service physician, and donor center physician. Although transfusion of antigen-negative RBCs will prevent immunization, the community blood supply may not be sufficient to support this practice. We recommend strongly that RBCs from such a patient be phenotyped before transfusion or when the patient is transfusion free, i.e., at least 3 mo since the last transfusion.

3.3. What if Compatible RBCs Cannot be Found?

In emergency and catastrophic situations in which either immediate RBC transfusion therapy is crucial or unexpectedly large quantities of RBCs are required, a sophisticated immunohematological workup is often not possible. Experiences from World War II showed the importance of fluid resuscitation (not necessarily transfusion of RBCs) in patients with hypovolemic shock in preventing acute tubular necrosis *(11)*. If RBC support is considered necessary, the following rules are applicable: D-negative units should be used in women of childbearing age whenever possible to minimize the risk of Rh sensitization. Based on the clinical decision of the responsible physician, a patient with life-threatening bleeding may have to be transfused with incompatible RBCs. In such patients, large volumes should be transfused quickly and antigen-negative units reserved until the bleeding is controlled. Sensitized individuals with antibodies against high-incidence RBC antigens or multiple antibodies can be encouraged to deposit autogeneic RBCs for long-term storage and family members should be recruited as potential directed blood donors.

To prevent an acute hemolytic transfusion reaction, it is pivotal to observe the compatibility rules defined by the ABO system. Irregular antibodies in the serum of a patient that may be unknown at the time of RBC transfusion may reduce the survival of the transfused RBCs, however, serious clinical complications caused by such antibodies are unusual *(7,8)*. If immediate transfusion is indicated, use of RBCs should not be postponed because of minor immunohematological problems, that can be elucidated later and may then result in change of the transfusion therapy for the patient.

4. BLOOD GROUPS AND DISEASE ASSOCIATIONS

Blood group antigen profiles have been used to predict inheritance of diseases encoded by a gene in close proximity to the gene encoding the blood group antigen. The presence or absence of certain blood group antigens has been implicated in susceptibility or resistance to certain diseases.

4.1. Antigens and RBC Morphology

Null phenotypes that are associated with altered RBC morphology or other clinical manifestations are summarized in Table 8. Patients whose RBCs lack a protein carrying blood group antigens can make antibodies to that protein and, thereby create major problems should they require transfusion *(12)*. In special situations, specific blood-group antigen expression, paired with characteristic red cell morphology can be useful in clinical differential diagnosis. As an illustration, weakened expression of Kell antigens and absense of Kx antigen together with acanthocytosis are typical findings in McLeod Syndrome and separate this diagnosis from other causes of acanthocytosis *(13)*.

Table 8
Null Phenotypes Associated with Shape Change
of RBCs and Distinct Clinical Manifestations

RBC phenotype	RBC morphology	Clinical manifestation
Rh$_{null}$	Stomatocytes	Compensated hemolytic anemia
Ge$_{null}$ (Leach)	Elliptocytes	Compensated hemolytic anemia
		Reduced protein 4.1
McLeod	Acanthocytes	Compensated hemolytic anemia
		Muscular dystrophy
		Neuronal degeneration
		Weak Kell antigens
Lu(a–b–)	Acanthocytes	None
Jk(a–b–)	Discocytes	Unable to maximally concentrate urine.
		RBCs resist to lysis by urea

4.2. Other Associations Between Antigens and Diseases

There are three mechanisms by which blood group antigens have been associated with clinical entities.

1. Antigen-related susceptibility for certain infections, e.g., malaria, enteritis and bronchitis *(14–27)*.
2. Altered antigen expression of A, B, H, or D by gene rearrangement, e.g., CML, mye-lofbrosis; of T, Tn, or Tk by bacteremia or septicemia; and of A, B, H, or I by incomplete biosynthesis, e.g., myelodysplastic syndromes, stress hematopoiesis, thalassemia, sickle cell disease, Diamond Blackfan anemia, and hereditary erythoblastic multinuclearity with positive acidified serum test *(28–32)*.
3. Statistical associations *(29)*.

4.3. Antibodies Associated with Diseases

The occurrence of blood-group antibodies represents either the pathophysiological principle of a variety of clinically defined diseases and disorders or an epiphenomenon of a broad spectrum of diseases, disorders, and conditions (Table 9). For a transfusion reactions or HDN to occur, previous sensitization with the blood group antigen(s) is required. Blood group antibodies that occur as epiphenomena of other clinical conditions represent a common problem encountered in routine immunohematology. Although these antibodies are usually clinically "silent," occasionally, they can cause severe hemolysis (e.g., infection, lymphoproliferative disorders, autoimmune diseases). Some antibodies can be induced as a result of therapy, e.g., drugs, and use of formalin-sterilized filters in patients undergoing dialysis *(33,34)*. Therapeutic intervention should, therefore focus on treating the underlying disease or omitting iatrogeneic causes. In cases of transfusion needs, antigen-negative units are normally not indicated.

4.4. Serological Phenomena Associated with Clinical Conditions

Certain observations made during serological testing can be helpful in the overall judgment of the clinical picture. For example, rouleaux phenomenon of RBCs or precipitation of serum proteins on addition of polyethylene glycol indicate a high

Table 9
Blood Group Antibodies and Disease Associations *(28,44)*

Pathophysiology	Target antigens of induced antibodies
Antibody as cause of disease	
Transfusion reaction: intravascular hemolysis	ABO, Kidd, P, Vel, etc.
Transfusion reaction: extravascular hemolysis	Rh, Kell, Duffy, etc.
HDN	Rh, ABO, etc.
Warm autoimmune hemolytic anemia	Rh, Kell, MNS, Ge, etc.
Cold hemagglutination disease	I, rarely i
Paroxysmal cold hemoglobinuria	P (Donath-Landsteiner antibody), Pr
Antibody as epiphenomenon of disease	
Infectious mononucleosis (EBV)	i
Mycoplasma pneumonia	I
Viral infections	Rx, P, Pr, I
Parasitosis	P1, I
Neoplastic (e.g., Hodgkin's disease)	LW, I
Lymphoma	Pr
Spontaneous abortion	Anti-PP_1P^k
Dialysis	N_{form}
Drugs	En^a, e, Rhl7, Rh29, Ge3, Jk^b, Jk3, I, etc.

protein concentration with reversed albumin:globulin ratio that can be indicative of plasma cell dyscrasia or chronic active hepatitis. The identification of anti-Ch/Rg or anti-Kn^a may occur on reduced expression of, respectively, C4 or CR1 as is observed in systemic lupus erythematosis. Absent or weak anti-A/anti-B may suggest agammaglobulinemia or hypoglobulinemia. Polyagglutination (especially T) can be observed during sepsis or infection and such patients should not be transfused with plasma components containing anti-T *(35)*.

Unexpected hemagglutination should be questioned critically, because there are a number of iatrogenic causes: Mixed field agglutination, particularly in ABO typing, may be observed following transfusion of RBCs or bone marrow transplants. The ABO results may be other than expected in babies delivered to surrogate mothers after artificial insemination or in vitro fertilization. In these cases, it is helpful if the clinicians make such information available to the transfusion service staff.

5. MODERN MEDICAL PRACTICES AND FUTURE PERSPECTIVES

The revolutionary progress in molecular biology and biosciences have been major forces in developing new strategies and technologies in transfusion medicine. Since the introduction of polymerase chain reaction (PCR) *(36)* the technique has been widely applied in transfusion medicine. It allowed the elucidation of the genetic basis of polymorphisms in several blood group systems such as ABO, MNS, Kell, Duffy, LW, Gerbich, and Cromer *(37)*. Although PCR potentially provides an invaluable tool for prenatal evaluation of the presence of a blood-group antigen, more knowledge regarding the expression of a blood-group antigen is required before the test can be confidently used for clinical diagnosis. Further, the confounding variable of the persistence of fetal progenitor cells in maternal blood for decades *(38)* could lead to false typing when very sensitive PCR methods are applied.

To circumvent difficult antigen situations, future developments will supplement current therapies such as autogeneic predeposit and use of eryropoietin for treatment of chronic anemia in patients with kidney insufficiency or malignant diseases *(39)*. These developments include in vitro conversion of group A or group B RBC to group O *(40)* and systems for *ex vivo* expansion and differentiation of hematopoietic progenitors *(41,42)*.

ACKNOWLEDGMENTS

B. M. Frey was supported by a grant of the Fondazione San Salvatore, Lugano, Switzerland and the Dr. Arnold U. and Susanne Huggenberger-Bischoff Stiftung zur Krebsforschung, Zürich, Switzerland.

REFERENCES

1. Daniels GL, Anstee DJ, Cartron J-P, et al. Blood group terminology 1995. From the ISBT working party on terminology for red cell surface antigens. *Vox Sanguinis* 1995; 69:265–279.
2. Coombs RRA, Mourant AK, Race RR. A new test for detection of weak and "incomplete" agglutinins. *Br J Exp Path* 1945;26:255–259.
3. Giblett ER. A critique of the theoretical hazard of inter- vs. intraracial transfusion. *Transfusion* 1961;1:233–238.
4. Giblett ER. Blood group alloantibodies: an assessment of some laboratory practices. *Transfusion* 1977;4:299–308.
5. Hoeltge GA, Domen RE, Rybicki LA, Schaffer PA. Multiple red cell transfusions and alloimmunization: experience with 6996 antibodies detected in a total of 159,262 patients from 1985 to 1993. *Arch Pathol Lab Med* 1995;119:42–45.
6. Walker RH. *Technical Manual,* 11th ed., Bethesda, MD: American Association of Blood Banks, 1993.
7. Mollison PL, Engelfriet CP, Contreras M. *Blood Transfusion in Clinical Medicine,* 9th ed., Oxford, England: Blackwell, 1993.
8. Marsh WL, Reid ME, Kuriyan M, Marsh NJ. *A Handbook of Clinical and Laboratory Practices in the Transfusion of Red Blood Cells.* Moneta, VA: Moneta Medical Press, 1993.
9. Garratty G. Petz LD, Hoops JK. The correlation of cold agglutinin titrations in saline and albumin with haemolytic anaemia. *Br J Haematol* 1977;35:587–595.
10. Zupanska B. Cellular immunoassays and their use for predicting the clinical significance of antibodies. In: Garratty G. ed. *Immunobiology of Transfusion Medicine.* New York: Marcel Dekker, 1994, pp. 465–491.
11. Committee on Trauma—American College of Surgeons. *Early Care of the Injured Patient,* 3rd ed., Philadelphia: Sanders, 1982.
12. Issitt PD. Null red blood cell phenotypes: associated biological changes. *Transfusion Med Rev* 1993;7:139–155.
13. Marsh WL, Redman CM. The Kell blood group system: a review. *Transfusion* 1990; 30:158–167.
14. Lublin DM. Functional roles of blood group antigens. In: Silberstein LE, ed. *Molecular and Functional Aspects of Blood Group Antigens.* Bethesda, MD: American Association of Blood Banks, 1995.

15. Hadley TJ, Miller LH, Haynes JD. Recognition of red cells by malaria parasites: the role of erythrocyte-binding proteins. *Transfusion Med Rev* 1991;5:108–113.
16. Chaudhuri A, Polyakova J. Zbrzezna V, Williams K, Gulati S. Pogo AO. Cloning of glycoprotein D cDNA, which encodes the major subunit of the Duffy blood group system and the receptor for the Plasmodium vivax malaria parasite. *Proc Natl Acad Sci USA* 1993;90:10,793–10,797.
17. Dahr W. Immunochemistry of sialoglycoproteins in human red blood cell membranes. In: Vengelen-Tyler V, Judd WJ, eds. *Recent Advances in Blood Group Biochemistry.* Arlington, VA: American Association of Blood Banks, 1986, pp. 23–65.
18. Leffler H. Svanborg-Eden C. Chemical identification of a glycophingolipid receptor for *Escherichia coli* attaching to human urinary tract epithelial cells and agglutinating human erythrocytes. *FEMS Microbiol Lett* 1980;8:127–134.
19. Lomberg H. Cedergren B. Leffler H. Nilsson B. Carlstrom AS, Svanborg-Eden C. Influence of blood group on the availability of receptors for attachment of uropathogenic *Escherichia coli. Infect Immun* 1986;51:919–926.
20. Brown KE, Anderson SM, Young NS. Erythrocyte P antigen: cellular receptor for B19 parvovirus. *Science* 1993;262:114–117.
21. Boren T. Falk P. Roth KA, Larson G. Normark S. Attachment of *Helicobacter pyiori* to human gastric epithelium mediated by blood group antigens. *Science* 1993; 262:1892–1895.
22. Nowicki B. Hart A, Coyne KE, Lublin DM, Nowicki S. Short consensus repeat-3 domain of recombinant decay-accelerating factor is recognized by *Escherichia coli* recombinant Dr. adhesin in a model of a cell-cell interaction. *J Exp Med* 1993;178: 2115–2121.
23. Bergelson JM, Mohanty JG, Crowell RL, St. John NF, Lublin DM, Finberg RW. Coxsackievirus B3 adapted to growth in RD cells binds to decay-accelerating factor (CD55). *J Virol* 1995;69:1903–1906.
24. Ward T. Pipkin PA, Clarkson NA, Stone DM, Minor PD, Almond JW. Decay-accelerating factor CD55 is identified as the receptor for echovirus 7 using CELICS, a rapid immunofocal cloning method. *EMBO J* 1994;13:5070–5074.
25. Bergelson JM, Chan M, Solomon KR, St. John NF, Lin H. Finberg RW. Decay-accelerating factor (CD55), a glycosylphosphatidylinositol-anchored complement regulatory protein, is a receptor for several echoviruses. *Proc Natl Acad Sci USA* 1994;91:6245–6249.
26. van Alphen L, Poole J. Overbeeke M. The Anton blood group antigen is the erythrocyte receptor for *Haemophilis influenzoe. FEMS Microbiol Lett* 1986;37:69–71.
27. Moulds JM, Nowicki S. Moulds JJ, Nowicki BJ. Human blood groups: incidental receptors for viruses and bacteria. *Transfusion* 1996;36:362–374.
28. Reid ME, Bird GW. Associations between human red cell blood group antigens and disease. *Transfusion Med Rev* 1990;4:47–55.
29. Garratty G. Do blood groups have a biological role? In: Garratty G. ed. *Immunobiology of Transfusion Medicine.* New York: Marcel Dekker, 1994, pp. 201–255.
30. Reid ME. Associations of red blood cell membrane abnormalities with blood group phenotype. In: Garratty G. ed. *Immunobiology of Transfusion Medicine.* New York: Marcel Dekker, 1994, pp. 256–271.
31. Moulds JM. Association of blood group antigens with immunologically important proteins. In: Garratty G. ed. *Immunobiology of Transfusion Medicine.* New York: Marcel Dekker, 1994, pp. 273–297.
32. Grant SG and Jensen RH. Use of hematopoietic cells and markers for the detection and quantitation of human *in vivo* somatic mutation. In: Garratty G. ed. *Immunobiology of Transfusion Medicine.* New York: Marcel Dekker, 1994, pp. 299–323.
33. Ng YY, Chow MP, Wu SC, Lyou JY, Harris DCH, Huang TP. Anti-N_{form} antibody in hemodialysis patients. *Am J Nephrol* 1995;15:374–378.

34. Dahr W. Moulds J. An immunochemical study on anti-N antibodies from dialysis patients. *Immunol Commun* 1981;10:173–183.
35. Judd WJ. Review: polyagglutination. *Immunohematology* 1992;8:58–69.
36. Mullis KB. The unusual origin of the polymerase chain reaction. *Sci Am* 1990;262:56–65.
37. Reid ME. Molecular basis for blood groups and function of carrier proteins. In: Silberstein LE, ed. *Molecular and Functional Aspects of Blood Group Antigens.* Arlington, VA: American Association of Blood Banks, 1995, pp. 75–125.
38. Bianchi DW, Zickwolf GK, Well GJ, Sylvester S. DeMaria MA. Male fetal progenitor cells persist in maternal blood for as long as 27 years postpartum. *Proc Natl Acad Sci USA* 1996;93:705–708.
39. Whitsett CF. The role of hematopoietic growth factors in transfusion medicine. *Hem Onc Clinics North Am* 1995;9:23–68.
40. Goldstein J. Siviglia G. Hurst R. Lenny L, Reich L. Group B erythrocytes enzymatically converted to group O survive normally in A, B, and O individuals. *Science* 1982;215:168–170.
41. Palsson BO, Pack SH, Schwartz RM, et al. Expansion of human bone marrow progenitor cells in a high cell density continuous perfusion system. *Bio/Technology* 1993;11:368–372.
42. Koller MR, Emerson SG, Palsson BO. Large-scale expansion of human stem and progenitor cells from bone marrow mononuclear cells in continuous perfusion cultures. *Blood* 1993;82:378–384.
43. Shulman IA, Petz LD. Red cell compatibility testing: clinical significance and laboratory methods. In: Petz LD, Swisher SN, eds. *Clinical Practice of Transfusion Medicine.* New York: Churchill Livingstone, 1996, pp. 199–244.
44. Garratty G. Target antigens for red-cell-bound autoantibodies. In: Nance SJ, ed. *Clinical and Basic Science Aspects of Immunohematology.* Arlington, VA: American Association of Blood Banks, 1991, pp. 33–71.

Index